ANIMAL MODELS IN CARDIOVASCULAR RESEARCH

Developments in Cardiovascular Medicine

VOLUME 153

The titles published in this series are listed at the end of this volume.

Animal models in cardiovascular research

Second revised edition

by

DAVID R. GROSS, DVM, PhD
Professor & Director, Cardiovascular and Thoracic
Surgery Research Labs,
University of Kentucky,
Lexington, Kentucky, U.S.A.

Kluwer Academic Publishers
Dordrecht / Boston / London

Library of Congress Cataloging-in-Publication Data

```
Gross, David R., (David Ross)
    Animal models in cardiovascular research / by David R. Gross.
        p.   cm. -- (Developments in cardiovascular medicine ; v. 153)
    Includes bibliographical references and index.
    ISBN 0-7923-2712-8 (HB : alk. paper)
    1. Cardiovascular system--Diseases--Animal models.
  2. Cardiovascular system--Research--Methodology.   I. Title.
  II. Series.
    [DNLM: 1. Cardiovascular Diseases.  2. Animals, Laboratory.
  3. Cardiovascular System--drug effects.  4. Research.   W1 DE997VME
  v. 153 1994 / WG 20 G878a 1994]
  RC669.G76   1994
  616.1'027--dc20
  DNLM/DLC
  for Library of Congress                                 93-50932
```

ISBN 0-7923-2712-8

Published by Kluwer Academic Publishers,
P.O. Box 17, 3300 AA Dordrecht, The Netherlands.

Kluwer Academic Publishers incorporates
the publishing programmes of
D. Reidel, Martinus Nijhoff, Dr. W. Junk and MTP Press

Sold and distributed in the U.S.A. and Canada
by Kluwer Academic Publishers,
101 Philip Drive, Norwell, MA 02061, U.S.A.

In all other countries, sold and distributed
by Kluwer Academic Publishers Group,
P.O. Box 322, 3300 AH Dordrecht, The Netherlands.

Printed on acid-free paper

Cover illustration by:
Richard Gersony, MFA

To Ben Gross, my father,
my friend,
I still miss him.

Table of contents

Acknowledgements

Many have provided encouragement for this task. First and foremost my wife Rosalie who now has well over 30 years experience in bolstering my ego and pumping up my resolve. She is the primary reason this revision was finished. My sons Ted and Jeff have made their father very proud by finishing their training and embarking on their own scientific careers. They provided me with the security of their unquestioned support and encouragement. My good friend Professor Ned H.C. Hwang actually seems to believe I can do anything I say I can. He never doubted this revision would be completed. Finally Dr. Robert K. Salley, Chief, Division of Cardiovascular and Thoracic Surgery, Department of Surgery, College of Medicine, University of Kentucky provided both encouragement and practical support.

Preface

Proponents of animal rights claim that we have no right to use animals in ways that they define as objectionable. The most ethical of these proponents logically extend their ideas to prohibit the use of animal derived substances for food or clothing. However vegetarianism is not a central concept to the Judeo-Christian tradition.[1] The relationship between man and animals is well defined and central to that tradition. The tradition teaches that humans are the centerpiece of creation and that animals were created for our use.[2] These tenets are reinforced in the Talmud, the Midrash, and in the writings of rabbis, priests and ministers, both ancient and modern. The same tradition also clearly defines our responsibility for animals.[3] The concept is that we play a partnership role with God in responsibility for the welfare of the rest of God's creations. If you accept the premise that humans are the central figure, then it follows that everything else exists for our welfare. The concept of our preeminence is based upon our ability to reason, to understand the abstract difference between good and evil, and to have compassion and concern for all living entities.[3]

Somehow the animal rights advocates have been allowed to claim the moral high ground in this debate. They assume their position is more "correct" than the average person in society and certainly more ethical, moral and righteous than any scientist that does not agree with their position. This approach has been successful because many of us have a tendency to ascribe human-like emotions, reason and even the capability of communicating abstract thought to animals. The "Wild Kingdom" is, in fact, a very cruel, very inhumane place. Death infrequently comes swiftly. Many animals are injured or become ill and then die, sometimes in agony, much later. Animals in the wild frequently die of exposure, parasitism, or starvation. The Rabbis of old were well aware of this, as is evident from the large body of work dealing with the *Laws of Terefot* (ritual slaughter).

The *Laws of Terefot* appear to precede the Torah. Their existence is implied in Deuteronomy 12:21, the verse which instructs that slaughter of cattle or sheep should be conducted as per previous instructions. The laws appear to be so ancient that the talmudic sages could not agree on the meaning of several of the basic concepts. The original and most prevalent meaning of *terefah* was an animal mauled by wild beasts, though not killed outright. This was interpreted as encompassing all animals so seriously diseased or injured that they were unable to recover. The Rabbinic commentary on the subject discusses specific cases in great detail and lays down several important rules for defining categories of *terefah*. Basically the scholars decided that any animal with similar injuries or disease that cannot survive is classified as *terefah*. This obliged them to clarify numerous aspects of the anatomy and physiology of animals in order to determine which conditions rendered the animal *terefah*. Several scholars describe experiments designed to test if a condition or conditions actually meet these requirements.[4]

There are also very clear biblical injunctions against maltreating animals. The concept derives from a number of Old Testament passages.[5-9] While tradition clearly considers it improper to inflict pain or suffering upon animals there is no doubt that it is considered to be quite proper to sacrifice an animal for our benefit. Modern rabbis have even decided that, for the purpose of saving a life, no part of a nonkosher animal is considered taboo. For example, pig heart valves have been approved for use in the production of prosthetic heart valves. Although there is no question that we have an important moral and ethical responsibility to treat animals in a humane manner, it has never been suggested that animals have any responsibility, or indeed any capacity, to treat us or each other with similar concern.

There is no question that animal experimentation has played an essential role in the development of effective preventions for polio, measles, smallpox, and a host of other infectious diseases. Almost all of our modern surgical techniques, including coronary bypass and open heart surgery have been made possible only after being developed using animal models. Despite this, the activists clearly intend to do everything possible to block the use of animals in efforts to find new techniques of prevention, treatment and/or management for the illnesses that afflict both humans and animals.

The activists claim we can use computer models or cell or tissue cultures instead of animals for research. Computer models are only as good as the data used to calculate the parameters that comprise them. They are, without exception, very simplified when compared to mammalian systems. A basic tenet of the scientific method says that a hypothesis is of no real value unless it can be tested. A computer model is just another form of a hypothesis, without value unless verified and validated experimentally. Information obtained from cell or tissue cultures must, inevitably, be proven in the whole animal. Cells and/or tissues grown or maintained outside the body are frequently different in shape, size and/or morphology and sometimes different in function, compared to the same cells in the original animal.

If animal rights activists are willing to forgo a cure for cancer or heart disease, endure outbreaks of infectious diseases, and risk protein deficiency for themselves, their children and their grandchildren, that can be considered to be their choice. A moral and legal question can be raised about their right to decide the fate of their own children or grandchildren and this is an important moral and legal issue that will undoubtably be tested in our legal systems at some point. However, by what authority do they threaten my family or yours? Many of the most active of these groups have announced not only their intent to stop all use of animals in research but to stop all slaughter of animals, all use of products of animal origin. Their perceived Utopia is one in which all animals run free. Some groups have taken pride in unlawfully breaking into laboratories to release animals. The result of this criminal activity has been that multiple species have been "freed" to be injured or killed by each other or by environmental dangers - Utopia or Bedlam?!

Good researchers believe that animal subjects must be treated with care and compassion. Good researchers believe that we have a moral and an ethical obligation to insure the welfare of all animals. Law requires that all federally funded research done on animals be conducted under stringent guidelines which dictate a high level of care and concern for the animals used. All USA institutions in which federally funded animal research is conducted must have an Institutional Animal Care and Use Committee that oversees the total animal care program at that institution. National and International scientific organizations have instituted strong ethical codes and standards for the use of animals in research. Nongovernment agencies that award funds for research using animals uniformly insist that federal standards be followed. We cannot allow a small minority of dedicated activists with loud voices and deep pockets to convince the majority that research using animal models should be halted. They will not go away, this is a long term fight that will require perseverance, sound logic and continuous debate.

References

1. Exodus, 16:8; Deuteronomy 12:21, The Torah, The Five Books of Moses; A new translation of the Holy Scriptures according to the Masoretic Text, The Jewish Publication Society of America, First Edition, Philadelphia, 1962.
2. Genesis 1:26,29 and 9:3, The Torah, *Ibid.*
3. Kolatch, A.J.; The second Jewish book of Why, Jonathan David Publishers, Inc., Middle Village, NY, 1985.
4. Steinsaltz, A.; The essential Talmud, Basic Books Inc., Translated from the Hebrew by C. Calai, Basic Books, Inc. and Bantam Books, Inc., NY, 1976.
5. Deuteronomy 22:4, The Torah, *Ibid.*
6. Deuteronomy 22:10, The Torah, *Ibid.*
7. Exodus 23:5, The Torah, *Ibid.*
8. Exodus 23:12, The Torah, *Ibid.*
9. Exodus 23:23, The Torah, *Ibid.*

1. General principles of animal selection, preoperative care, preanesthesia, chemical restraint and analgesia

Animals used for meaningful experiments must be held long enough in approved facilities to insure that they are not incubating infectious diseases. They should be vaccinated against the diseases most likely to cause a problem in that species, and they should be verified free of internal and external parasites prior to use. These precautions can be expensive but are minuscule compared to the overall cost of conducting experiments where the results are suspect because of the physical condition and general health of the subject.

Physical examination

Prior to use, the animal should be given a thorough physical examination. One of the most neglected aspects of this examination is some history, easily supplied by observant animal care personnel, of the appetite displayed by the animal, and the character of the urine and feces. It is the responsibility of the investigator to ascertain that the animal care personnel are, in fact, observant and have been properly trained to record their observations appropriately for each animal. It is a rare animal that eats normally when it is ill. The physical examination should include an assessment of the rectal temperature, feasible in most species commonly used. A list of normal rectal temperatures is provided as Table 1.1.

The physical examination should also include an evaluation of the mucous membranes, with particular attention to abnormal discharges from the eyes, nose, and other orifices. Animals with inflamed mucous membranes should not be used. Judicious use of the stethoscope can rule out the possibility of using an animal for cardiovascular studies with a congenital or acquired heart murmur, unless that model is of particular interest. Animals which originate from areas where heartworms or parasitic blood diseases are a problem must be shown to be free of these afflictions. For cardiovascular studies, it is probably a good idea to take an electrocardiogram, especially if one of the giant breeds, or giant breed-crosses, is being used. Although congenital and acquired arrhythmias are relatively rare in dogs, they do occur.

It may not be necessary to do a complete hematological evaluation on every animal, but in studies where extensive surgical preparation is necessary and when considerable time and money are to be invested in the model, such an evaluation could be essential. Tables 1.2-1.8 provide normal hematological data for most of the species now in common use. It should be emphasized that these normal values may vary with geographical location (i.e., sea level versus high altitude) and with prevalent breeds in the particular region, as well as with gender and age. The values provided have been compiled by combining data from the Texas Veterinary Diagnostic Laboratory, the Clinical Pathology Laboratory of the Texas A&M Veterinary Teaching Hospital, the Texas A&M Laboratory Animal Resources Facility, the University of Kentucky Division of Laboratory Animal Resources, the University of Kentucky Cardiovascular and Thoracic Surgery Research Laboratories and the references listed at the end of this chapter.

The state of hydration is an important consideration in cardiovascular studies. All animals should be well hydrated before they are used, and if the procedure or preparation of the model requires extensive surgery, or is of long duration, the state of hydration must be maintained during the course of the experimental procedure. Again, these considerations seem obvious and redundant but, unfortunately, they are often ignored or forgotten. The choice of hydrating fluid is dependent upon the experimental protocol, but care should be taken to avoid iatrogenic changes in acid-base balance. Under most circumstances, this will mean the use of a balanced crystalloid solution with appropriate buffers and either lactate or bicarbonate added to maintain a normal blood pH.

Procedures in most species do not require that the animal be without water prior to the anesthesia. Free choice of water to a healthy subject should insure normal hydration. As a matter of convenience, and to prevent inspiration of ingesta, it is advisable to withhold food overnight or for 12 hours prior to general anesthesia.

Knowledge and understanding of blood coagulation and coagulopathies have created interest in hematological parameters related to this system. Platelet counts have been done on most species and found to range from about 2-5 X 10^5/ml. Cats, sheep and calves range slightly higher, 3-8 X 10^5/ml. Other commonly conducted tests include; activated clotting time (ACT), activated prothrombin time (A-PTT), prothrombin time (PT), thrombin time, and fibrinogen levels. The use of the heat precipitation method for the latter may result in falsely low values. The capillary tube clotting time is insensitive and limited to detection of severe clotting defects. Normal values of these parameters will vary with; the volume of the sample used, the incubation time, the commercial reagent used (including freshness), the anticoagulant used for sample collection, and the concentration of calcium ion present. There also appear to be optimal conditions for the assays which vary for each species. Most knowledgeable researchers in this field seem to agree that, if these data are required, it is best to compare subjects with normal controls at the time and in the same lab where the evaluation will be made.

Table 1.1: Range of normal rectal temperatures for some commonly used animal species

Species	°C	°F
Dogs	37.9 - 39.9	100.1 - 102.8
Cats	38.1 - 39.2	100.5 - 102.5
Cattle	36.7 - 39.1	98.0 - 102.4
Sheep	38.3 - 39.9	100.9 - 103.8
Goats	38.5 - 39.7	101.3 - 103.5
Horses and Ponies	37.2 - 38.2	99.0 - 100.8
Swine	38.7 - 39.8	101.6 - 103.6
Rabbits	38.6 - 40.1	101.5 - 104.2
Monkey, Rhesus	38.4	101.1

Guinea Pigs	36.4	98 - 101
Rats	37.5	99.5
Mice	37.4	99.3

Table 1.2: Averages (single values) or ranges of normal blood count data

Species	WBC (x10³)	Neutro-philes (%)	Lympho-cytes (%)	Mono-cytes (%)	Eosino-philes (%)
Dogs	6 -17	60 - 77	12 - 30	3 - 10	2 - 10
Cats	5.5 - 19.5	35 - 75	20 -55	1 - 4	2 - 12
Rats	9.76	25.6	73.9	0.29	0.48
Mice	13.5	17.5	72.3	2.19	2.25
Rabbits	8.45	44.7	40.4	8.5	2.0
Hamsters	8.10	25.6	70.7	2.45	0.8
Guinea Pigs	11.2	36.5	56.2	3.05	3.75
Pigs	14.8	34.0	55.5	4.3	0.24
Sheep	4 - 12	31.8	59.4	3.25	5.2
Goats	4 - 13	30 - 48	50 - 70	0 - 4	1 - 8
Horses	5.4 - 14.3	22 - 72	16 - 68	0 - 14	0 - 10
Calves	4 - 12	15 - 45	45 - 75	2 - 7	2 - 20
Primates (Old World)	10.8	38.6	58.8	1.10	1.85
Primates (New World)	4.3 - 28.5	46 - 82	13 - 54	0 - 3	0 - 4

Table 1.3: Averages (single values) or ranges of normal red blood cell parameters

Species	Hematrocrit (%)	Hemoglobin (g/100 ml)	RBC (x10⁶/µl)	Mean Corpuscular Volume (µm)³	Mean Corpus-cular Hb conc. (g%)
Dogs	35 - 55	12 - 18	5.5 - 8.5	60 - 77	32 - 36
Cats	24 - 45	3 - 15	5 - 10	39 - 55	30 - 36
Rats	45.8	14.2	8.47	56	31.1
Mice	41.8	11.1	9.2	49.25	26.5
Rabbits	40.6	13.4	6.51	62.8	32.8

Hamsters	50.7	16.4	7.35	70.0	32.3
Guinea Pigs	43.7	14.3	5.18	84	32.8
Pigs	41.0	12.4	6.99	58.5	30.2
Sheep	27 - 45	9 - 15	9 - 15	28 - 40	31 - 34
Goats	19 - 38	8 - 14	8.18	15 - 30	35 - 42
Horses	32 - 53	11 - 19	6.8 - 12.9	37 - 58.5	31 - 38.6
Calves	24 - 46	9.5 - 12.5	5.2 - 6.8	49.7 - 64.3	30.2 - 35.8
Primates (Old World)	27 - 44	9.5 - 12.5	5.2 - 6.8	49.7 - 64.3	30.2 - 35.8
Primates (New World)	17 - 48	5 - 12.5	1.97 - 4.22	54.8 - 55.4	15.4 - 38.5

Table 1.4: Averages with standard deviations (single values) or ranges for arterial blood gases

Species	pH	pO_2 (mmHg)	pCO_2 (mmHg)	HCO_3^- (mEq/l)	Total CO_2 (mmHg)
Dogs	7.31 - 7.42	85 - 95	38 ± 5.5	14.6 - 29.4	38 - 54
Cats	7.31 - 7.42	80 - 100	40 ± 5.4	12.6 - 32	16.7 - 42.9
Rats	7.35 ± 0.06	90 - 100	40 ± 5.4	12.6 - 32	40 - 55
Mice	7.35 ± 0.09	80 - 100	42 ± 5.7	25.5	40 - 55
Rabbits	7.44 ± 0.03	84.2 - 1.4	33.3 ± 0.6	16.2 - 31.8	35 - 55
Hamsters	7.39 ± 0.08	80 - 100	59 ± 5.0	32.7 - 44.1	38 - 56
Guinea Pigs	7.4 ± 0.08	80 - 100	40 ± 9.8	12.8 - 30	40 - 55
Pigs	7.4 ± 0.08	80 - 95	43 ± 5.6	24.5 - 35	36 - 56
Sheep	7.45 ± 0.06	80 - 95	38 ± 8.5	21.1 - 32.1	35 - 55
Lambs (2-4 days old)	7.37 ± 0.03	73 ± 5	33 ± 1	na	na
Goats	7.41 ± 0.09	80 - 95	50 ± 9.4	19.6 - 31.1	35 - 55
Horses	7.32 - 7.44	85 - 95	47 ± 8.5	19.5 - 36.2	35 - 55
Calves	7.30 - 7.60	85 - 100	38 - 46	24 - 30	54 - 72
Primates (Old World)	7.46 ± 0.06	85 - 95	44 ± 4.8	21.5 - 38.6	30 - 50
Primates (New World)	7.46 ± 0.06	85 - 95	44 ± 4.8	22 - 39	30 - 50

na = not available

Table 1.5: Averages (single values) or ranges for normal plasma electrolytes

Species	Na⁺ (mEq/l)	K⁺ (mEq/l)	Cl⁻ (mEq/l)	Mg⁺⁺ (mg/dl)
Dogs	139 - 153	3.6 - 5.2	103 - 121	1.5 - 2.8
Cats	147 - 164	3.5 - 4.7	113 - 127	2 - 3
Rats	143 - 156	5.4 - 7.0	100 - 110	1.6 - 4.4
Mice	128 - 145	4.8 - 5.8	105 - 110	0.8 - 3.9
Rabbits	138 - 155	3.7 - 6.8	92 - 112	2.0 - 5.4
Hamsters	106 - 146	4.0 - 5.9	85.7 - 118	1.9 - 3.5
Guinea Pigs	120 - 146	3.8 - 8.0	90 - 115	1.8 - 3.0
Pigs	135 - 152	4.9 - 7.1	94 - 106	1.2 - 3.7
Sheep	140 - 164	4.2 - 6.7	113 - 121	1.8 - 2.4
Goats	136 - 155	3.1 - 6.7	98 - 111	2.8 - 3.6
Horses	126 - 158	2.6 - 6.2	95 - 119	1.3 - 3.5
Calves	132 - 152	3.9 - 5.8	97 - 111	2.5 - 3.1
Primates (Old World)	143 - 164	3.8 - 6.7	103 - 118	1.0 - 2.7
Primates (New World)	148	3.6	110	na*

*na = no data available

Table 1.6: Averages (single values) or ranges for normal serum proteins

Species	Total Protein (g/100 ml)	Albumin (g/100 ml)	α-globulin (g/100 ml)	β-globulin (g/100 ml)	γ-globulin (g/100 ml)
Dogs	4.9 - 9.6	2.1 - 4.0	0.6 - 1.2	1.25 - 2.3	0.35 - 0.95
Cats	4.3 - 7.5	2.2 - 3.2	0.7 - 2.3	0.4 - 1.8	0.46 - 1.0
Rats	4.7 - 8.2	2.7 - 5.1	0.6 - 3.7	0.4 - 2.0	0.6 - 1.6
Mice	4.0 - 8.6	2.5 - 4.8	0.9 - 2.1	0.4 - 1.6	0.4 - 0.9
Rabbits	6.0 - 8.3	2.4 - 4.0	0.25 - 1.7	0.5 - 2.1	1.0 - 2.1
Hamsters	4.3 - 7.7	2.1 - 3.9	0.2 - 0.6	0.4 - 1.5	0.7 - 2.1
Guinea Pigs	5.0 - 6.8	2.1 - 3.9	0.2 - 0.6	0.4 - 1.5	-.7 - 2.1
Pigs	4.8 - 10.3	1.8 - 5.6	1.2 - 2.6	1.25 - 2.3	0.35 - 1.9
Sheep	5.7 - 9.1	2.7 - 4.5	0.6 - 1.5	0.25 - 1.2	0.9 - 1.9
Goats	5.9 - 7.8	2.5 - 4.3	0.6 - 1.5	1 - 2	0.5 - 1.5

Horses	5.2 - 9.9	1.7 - 4.0	1.0 - 3.7	0.35 - 1.6	0.95 - 2.7
Calves	6 - 8	2.4 - 2.9	0.6 - 1.2	0.5 - 1.2	1.2 - 2.4
Primates (Old World)	5.9 - 8.7	1.8 - 4.6	0.6 - 1.35	0.8 - 2.0	1 - 1.8
Primates (New World)	7.2	3.2	1.96	0.82	1.87

Table 1.7: Averages (single values) or ranges for some biochemical parameters

Species	Total Cholesterol (mg/dl)	BUN (mg/dl)	Creatinine (mg/dl)	SGOT (mU/ml)	Blood Glucose (mg/dl)
Dogs	137 - 275	10 - 26	0.8 - 1.7	20 - 85	70 - 110
Cats	83 - 135	14 - 32	0.8 - 1.8	20 - 83	70 - 110
Rats	10 - 54	5 - 29	0.2 - 0.8	46 - 81	50 - 135
Mice	26 - 82	14 - 28	0.3 - 1.0	23 - 48	63 - 126
Rabbits	10 - 80	13 - 29	0.5 - 2.6	43 - 98	78 - 155
Hamsters	10 - 80	12.5 - 27	0.35 - 1.6	38 - 168	33 - 118
Guinea Pigs	16 - 43	9 - 31	0.6 - 2.2	16.5 - 67	82 - 107
Pigs	76 - 174	4 - 22	1.2 - 6	15 - 72	55 - 110
Sheep	50 - 140	15 - 36	0.7 - 3.0	40 - 123	55 - 131
Goats	55 - 210	10 - 27	0.2 - 2.2	43 - 131	50 - 75
Horses	50 - 130	13 - 29	1.6 - 3.3	46 - 125	75 - 115
Calves	78 - 142	6 - 26	1.0 - 2.0	26 - 58	35 - 55
Primates (Old World)	100 - 270	7 - 23	1 - 2	12.5 - 45	43 - 148
Primates (New World)	161	31	na*	na*	80

*na = no data available

Animal behavior considerations

Another aspect of animal model selection is based upon species behavior patterns. If the experimental design dictates that data be collected over a prolonged period of time, without the interference of chemicals, it is necessary to select a species capable of remaining quiet for prolonged periods with minimal physical restraint. Many of the ruminant species are well suited for this. With minimal training goats, cattle and sheep will stand or lie quietly for prolonged periods with only their heads minimally restrained.

Most dogs and pigs can be restrained in a harness or sling if some pre-experiment training is conducted. Dogs are frequently trained to lie quietly on a table. However, occasionally even well trained and conditioned animals will struggle and even rage against confinement.

Cats can usually be restrained if confined in a close space, especially if their heads are covered and external stimuli are kept at a minimum. Almost all minor procedures, such as parenteral injections, can be conducted with minimal physical restraint in cats by an experienced handler.

Trained horses will stand quietly in a stock, but most individuals will react with some degree of violence to sudden or loud noises, painful stimuli, or sudden, startling movement. This is usually not a severe problem with small ponies, but adult horses can cause considerable damage to themselves, handlers and equipment. Excitement is also accompanied by sympathetic discharge the intensity of which varies with the species, and this may obscure results.

Special requirement considerations

If the experimental design can best be served by a particular animal model it is possible to learn to handle that animal and use it. All too frequently the animal model is chosen because the investigator and/or others in the lab are most familiar with that species, the normal physiological parameters for the species are known, and previous experience has been good. These are all valid reasons but should not dictate the choice when other factors may be involved. For example, experiments where the thermoregulatory system is involved should be conducted in a species that has thermoregulatory responses most similar to that of the human species. Dogs have only a few sweat glands in their paws, and rely on panting for thermal regulation. Pigs have very poor thermoregulation with thick subcutaneous fat and poorly developed sweating capabilities. Malignant hyperthermia is a practical problem in this species. Although horses sweat easily, have thin skins, and thermoregulate in a fashion very similar to that of humans, the pattern of autonomic innervation to the sweat glands is different. Human sweat glands have cholinergic sympathetic innervation, whereas horses have α-adrenergic.

Most herbivores, canines, and felines do not develop atherosclerosis. Swine, however, develop this disease with age, under normal conditions, and the condition can easily be accelerated with a slightly high cholesterol, high fat diet. The coronary circulation of pigs is most similar to that of man. The size and shape of the pig cardiovascular system is very similar to that in humans, although the pathways of ventricular excitation and distribution of Purkinje fibers are different. Dogs are more similar to humans in this respect.

Sometimes the choice of animal model is dictated by size considerations alone. When measuring blood flow velocity profiles, for example, the finite size of the velocimeter transducer and/or sample volume dictates that measurements must be made in a large vessel. If the histochemistry of a particular portion of the cardiovascular system is to be investigated, it might be wise to use mice, where the structure to be serially sectioned is small, rather than an adult horse, wherein the same anatomical structure might take a lifetime to analyze. The essential point is that the animal model must be matched to the experimental design. Specific models lend themselves to specific studies. This should not be ignored just because the investigator has no first hand experience with that species.

The use of anticholinergic drugs for preanesthesia

In the veterinary literature, atropine sulfate has long been recommended as a routine adjunct to general anesthesia, particularly with the inhalant anesthetic agents. This is probably a holdover from the days when the inhalant anesthetics were used for induction as well as maintenance of anesthesia and were administered with a cone or mask. Because the earlier available inhalant anesthetic agents were irritating to the mucous membranes, atropine was useful in controlling both salivary and, particularly, respiratory tract secretions. Atropine was also frequently given to reduce the salivary secretions associated with the use of morphine as a preanesthetic agent. Atropine also blocks the so-called "laryngeal reflex", which is purported to result in cardiac arrest. Modern inhalant anesthetics produce minimal respiratory irritation, and bronchiolar secretions are also minimal.

Atropine, however, does have pronounced effects on the cardiovascular system. The usual preanesthetic doses used do not markedly affect blood pressure, but do result in some degree of tachycardia. Small doses may produce an initial bradycardia, but tachycardia follows. Individual animals show varying degrees of tachycardia, depending upon the degree of vagal tone present in that individual at the time the injection takes effect. Cardiac output tends to increase as a result of the tachycardia. Since atropine blocks the cardiac vagal efferents, it will interfere with the response to any perturbation which is vagally mediated. The pressor effects of catecholamines are accentuated in animals given atropine. Large doses of atropine can act as direct cardiac depressants.[3]

When used as a preanesthetic agent in animals being prepared for chronic studies atropine has other effects of concern and interest. It causes an inhibition of gastrointestinal smooth muscle activity and may result in postoperative GI stasis. Rumen motility is consistently inhibited by recommended doses of atropine.[4] This can result in gas accumulation and bloat, which can be life threatening in these species. Rumen stasis can also cause less immediate, but still serious, gastrointestinal disturbances associated with inappetence and depression which will slow the course of recovery. The use of atropine in horses can result in colic, as a result of the GI stasis.[5] Secretions of the GI tract are also blocked by atropine, and this may add to postoperative complications, particularly in ruminants where salivary bicarbonate is very important to normal rumen pH and function. Atropine decreases bronchial and tracheal secretions, dilates the bronchioles, and changes the character of the respiratory muco-ciliary blanket resulting in prolonged muco-ciliary clearance. These respiratory tract effects can lead to atelectasis and other respiratory problems. Atropine also tends to cause urine retention because of its effect on urinary tract smooth muscle. There is a definite anhydrotic effect in species which normally sweat, and this may result in hyperpyrexia.

Based on the above discussion there seems to be little justification for the use of atropine, or any other parasympatholytic agent, as a preanesthetic. There will, however, be those who will persist in the face of these arguments. Those steadfast individuals should be aware of published recommended dosages: Dogs and cats should receive 0.045 mg/kg subcutaneously (SC), pigs 0.07-0.09 mg/kg intramuscularly (IM), goats and sheep 0.2 mg/kg intravenously (IV) every 15 minutes. Horses are given 0.01 mg/kg (IV) to block the second-degree heart block sometimes induced by xylazine.[6]

Preanesthetic agents

Each of the pharmacological agents reviewed in this text is discussed from the standpoint of directly measured effects on some aspect of the cardiovascular system in a particular species. Many of the results reflect complex interactions between the agent of interest and other pharmacological agents, usually general anesthetics. It is very easy, under these circumstances, to miscalculate the total effect of these agents by not considering the integrative response of the animal. Major differences, often in completely opposite directions, have been found in the response of conscious versus anesthetized animals for; reflex control of the circulation, effects of hemorrhage and alterations in preload and afterload. Experiments are also frequently conducted with positive pressure ventilation, animals suffering from surgical shock, and animals treated with muscle paralyzing agents. All of these perturbations are known to have marked direct effects on the cardiovascular system themselves.

The purpose of this text is to present a review of what direct effects have been documented, and the conditions under which the results were obtained. Any interpretation of how these effects may influence a particular experimental design are left to the investigator.

The psychotropic agents have been widely used in veterinary medicine since the 1950's when reserpine and the phenothiazine derivatives were first introduced in the USA. They have proven to be particularly valuable in quieting and calming unfriendly and apprehensive animals and in preparing animals for surgery. As a class of drugs, they seem to share one common problem; they are most effective when used in animals that are reasonably calm when the agents are administered. If the animal becomes extremely agitated before the agent is given, it is sometimes advantageous to not continue, to abandon the effort and return when the animal has calmed down. In some cases it may be advantageous to administer the agent orally, in a small bit of food. With particularly fractious or aggressive individuals and with most primates, some form of physical restraint is usually required before the agent can be administered. Under these circumstances it is best to give the drug via the intramuscular or subcutaneous, rather than the intravenous route, and then to leave the room and allow the animal to calm down before the agent starts to have its effect.

The major advantage in using preanesthetic agents are to make anesthetic induction easier and smoother, and to reduce the dose of anesthetic agent required. Major disadvantages are that drug interactions may occur, and it becomes difficult to separate drug effects from physiological responses in animals that have been given combinations of drugs. Many of the tranquilizers are α-adrenergic blocking agents and thereby have a direct effect on blood pressure and, in some cases, on heart rate. Although the cardiovascular effects of many of these agents have been documented, it is rare to find good documentation for the effects of various combinations of these agents and the anesthetic agents with which they are commonly used.

Recognition of pain and the use of analgesics

With the advent of cardiovascular studies being conducted on previously instrumented, intact, awake animals, the postoperative selection and use of analgesic agents has assumed greater importance. In most instances, experiments will not and should not be conducted while these agents are still causing cardiovascular effects. This statement presupposes that we are familiar with the elimination half-lives of all the various analgesic agents used in all species. This, of course, is not true, so extra care must be taken to assure that the analgesic agent being used is not having any influence on the cardiovascular parameter(s) being measured. We do have moral, legal and scientific obligations, however, to insure that all unnecessary pain is treated with appropriate analgesic agents.

Recognition of pain in some animal species, and in certain individual animals, can be difficult for the untrained observer. Any person who works or lives with a variety of animals on a regular basis comes to realize that individual animals have very different and individual personalities. These differences extend to the demonstration and perception of pain. Some animals are very stoic, while others can be extremely vociferous. There are species differences in the general manner in which pain is demonstrated, but individual variations within species can be greater than between species differences.

Animals experiencing pain may demonstrate a reluctance to move or may favor the painful site. They tend to focus their attention on the painful area by excessive licking, biting, scratching, kicking, or merely looking at the region. Occasionally, the attention becomes an obsession and may result in self-mutilation. Inappetence and a depressed attitude are commonly associated with pain.

Dogs tend to be vocal, although the loudness of their whining or howling is not necessarily directly correlated with the amount of pain, especially during recovery from general anesthesia. They will generally whine or cry out when the painful area is touched and, depending upon the individual, may react by biting or snapping at the offending hand. Cats tend to be very stoic until they are handled. They will then often respond violently, and vocalize loudly.

Most swine are very reluctant to move when in pain. If forced to move, they will vocalize with even greater enthusiasm than they generally display. The latter is usually sufficient for most people, particularly in a confined indoor area. They limp, or refuse to use an injured limb and will usually either stand or lie still rather than move unless vigorously prodded. Inappetence is not as reliable a sign in these animals as it is in other species. Pigs are social creatures and do better when in a group. If they are instrumented, however, they are very clever at removing tubes and wires from each other and usually require individual housing.

Goats tend to indicate pain by bleating. They will show a reluctance to move and refuse to eat, depending upon the degree of pain. They will often look at or nuzzle the painful portion of their anatomy. Joint pain is often evidenced by a lifting of the leg and looking at or nuzzling the painful location. Sheep tend to be stoic to the point of immobility. They often just give up and refuse to move, be aroused, eat or drink. Lameness or stiffness and reluctance to move in a certain manner usually indicates minor pain in this species. Sheep are very much flock animals and tend to do poorly when maintained individually. Cattle are also stoic and rarely vocalize pain unless it is acute and accompanied by psychological stress. Horses tend to become very defensive and aggressive when in pain. They will stand and look at the painful portion of their anatomy, nuzzle it, stamp their hooves, kick at their belly with abdominal pain and, rarely, vocalize with low whinnies. They lose appetite and will sometimes bite or kick at a handler when approached. They also tend to become hypersensitive and more apprehensive about being handled. They tend to react more violently to any form of stimulus, painful or otherwise.

Non-human primates tend to demonstrate pain behavior very similar to that of humans. The obvious problem with primates is that administration of the analgesic agent may be more traumatic than letting them cope with moderate amounts of discomfort. If the analgesic can be administered in food or water, this may solve the problem, but primates usually lose appetite when they are in pain, as do most other species.

Small laboratory rodents and other laboratory species pose more difficult problems in the diagnosis of pain. Careful observation of alterations in behavior make it abundantly clear, however, that these species also perceive and demonstrate pain with behavior patterns similar to the other species previously discussed.

Regardless of the species under consideration researchers may assume, as a general rule, that an animal will experience pain as a result of any procedure or surgical technique which would presumably cause pain in a human. Potentially painful procedures should be accompanied by careful observation of the involved animals, and demonstration of any of the above-mentioned signs or conditions should be treated appropriately.[18]

Special considerations concerning ruminant acid-base balance

When Na^+ intake is limited ruminants are capable of excreting K^+ in the urine. Urine K^+ ion concentrations approaching 700 mEq/L have been observed in sheep on a Na^+ free diet. The ruminant kidney seems to be capable of remarkable concurrent Na^+ and K^+ conservation. However there is a very large daily turnover of K^+. Chloride and HCO_3^- are the important anions in ruminant urine which is usually alkaline (pH 7.5-8.5) with $[HCO_3^-]$ as high as 300 mEq/L. The ruminant kidney is also capable of excreting hydrogen ions while maintaining K^+ output at normal levels.

Saliva of sheep contains as much as 140 mEq/L of HCO_3^-. Adult goats and sheep produce 2-4 L of saliva/day and cattle produce gallons. This high bicarbonate turnover is important for normal rumen function (the rumen is alkaline) and accounts for the high HCO_3^- turnover in these species. These specialized functions must be taken into consideration when managing acid-base and electrolyte balance in ruminants during an acute procedure or post-operatively.[16, 17]

References

1.   American Association for Laboratory Animal Science. Manual for Laboratory Animal Technicians. Publication 67-3, Dec. 1, 1979, Section II: page 140.
2.   Anderson, B.D. Temperature Regulation and Environmental Physiology in Duke's Physiology of Domestic Animals. 9th ed., ed. by M.J. Swenson, Cornell Univ. Press, Ithaca, NY, p. 687, 1977.
3.   Adams, H.R. Cholinergic Pharmacology: Autonomic Drugs, in Veterinary Pharmacology and Therapeutics. 5th ed., ed. by N.H. Booth and L.E. McDonald, The Iowa State University Press, Ames, Iowa, 1982.
4.   Garner, H.E., Mather, E.C., Hoover, T.R., Brown, R.E., Halliwell, W. C. Anesthesia of bulls undergoing surgical manipulation of the vas deferentia. *Can J Comp Med*, 39:250-255, 1975.
5.   Klavano, P.A. Anesthesia - Some developments in equine practice. *Proc Am Assoc Equine Pract,* 21st:149-155, 1975.
6.   Booth, N.H. Introduction to Drugs Acting on the Central Nervous System. Section 4 in Veterinary Pharmacology and Therapeutics, 5th ed., ed. by N.H. Booth and L.E. McDonald, The Iowa State University Press, Ames, Iowa, 1982.
7.   Fink, B.R., Schoolman, A. Arterial blood acid-base balance in unrestrained waking cats, *Proc Soc Exp Biol Med*, 112:328-330, 1963.
8.   Lunn, D.P., McGairk, S.M., Smith, D. F., MacWilliams, P.S. Renal net acid and electrolyte excretion in an experimental model of hypochloremic metabolic alkalosis in sheep, *Am J Vet. Res*, 51(11), 1990.
9.   Schalm, Jain and Carroll, eds. Veterinary Hematology, Lea and Feibiger, 1975.
10.   Guss. Management and Diseases of Dairy Goats, Dairy Goat Journal Publishing Corp., 1977.
11.   Kaneko, ed. Clinical Biochemistry of Domestic Animals, Academic Press, 1980.
12.   Mitruka and Rawnsley, eds. Clinical Biochemical and Hematological Reference Values in Normal Experimental Animals, Masson Pub. Inc., 1977.
13.   Archer and Jeffcott, eds. Comparative Clinical Haematology, Blackwell Scientific Public., 1977.
14.   Ohsumi, H., Sakamoto, M., Yamazaki, T., Okumura, F. Effects of Fentanyl on carotid sinus baro reflex control of circulation in rabbits, *Am J Physiol*, 256 (3): R625-R631, 1989.
15.   Yaster, M., Koehler, R.C., Traystman, R.J. Interaction of fentanyl and pentobarbital on peripheral and cerebral hemodynamics in newborn lambs, *Anesthesiol*, 70 (3): 461-469, 1989.
16.   Weinberg and Sheffner. Buffers in Ruminant Physiology and Metabolism, Church and Dwight Co., 1976.
17.   Gans, J.H. "The Kidneys" in, Duke's Physiology of Domestic Animals, M.J. Swenson ed., 8th ed., Cornell Univ. Press, 1970.
18.   Beynen and Solleneld, eds. New Developments in Biosciences: Their Implications for Laboratory Animal Science, Martinus Nijhoff, 1988.
19.   Chew, D.J., Leonard, M., Muir, W.W. Effect of sodium bicarbonate infusion on serum osmolality, electrolyte concentrations, and blood gas tensions in cats", *Am J Vet Res*, 52 (1), 1991.

2. Cardiovascular effects of the opiods

The following compilation of opiods also includes some agents which are more correctly classified as narcotic antagonists. However, these agents usually compete for the same receptor sites and have some analgesic and/or sedative properties when used alone. The list is not exhaustive but represents agents commonly cited as being used for cardiovascular studies in the recent literature. The effectiveness of these agents for chemical restraint, sedation and analgesia seems to be a matter of individual preference more than objective evaluation, but also involves considerable species variability. Cardiovascular effects, dosage and appropriate comments are tabulated for each of the agents in each of the species reviewed. In general, the opiods are reported to decrease preload, contractility, afterload and heart rate.[1] As a result cardiac output must also decrease. Actual reported cardiovascular responses to the various opiods do not always follow this scheme, especially in cats and horses, where the narcotic analgesics have repeatedly been reported to cause a paradoxical excitement and stimulation, usually as a result of central stimulation arising from ataxia.

Table 2.1: Morphine sulfate

Conditions of the Experiment	Dose	Cardiovascular Effects	Reference
2.1:1 Dogs			
Used as a preanesthetic. Onset of action within a few minutes following injection.	0.1-2 mg/kg, SC	Very young, aged and debilitated dogs seem to be more sensitive to respiratory depression.	2
Conscious, previously instrumented, intact	2 mg/kg, IV	Initial transient decrease in coronary resistance, initial increase in heart rate and in left ventricular dP/dt and dP/dt/P, decrease in left ventricular end-diastolic diameter and left ventricular end-systolic size. These responses followed by an increase in coronary resistance lasting 5-30 min. The heart rate, aortic pressure and left ventricular end-diastolic diameter returned to baseline values but left ventricular dP/dt/P remained elevated. Ten min. after injection late diastolic coronary flow had fallen from 44±3 ml/min to 25±3 ml/min, coronary resistance increased. With the heart rate held constant by pacing there was substantial coronary vasoconstriction.	3,4

Conditions of the Experiment	Dose	Cardiovascular Effects	Reference
2.1:1 Dogs			
Intact, awake, previously instrumented	0.25 mg/kg, IV, repeated every 15 min. total dose = 0.75 mg/kg	Significant coronary vasoconstriction after 3 doses	3
Intact, awake, previously instrumented	0.25 mg/kg, IV	No change in blood pressure, heart rate decreased	5
Intact, awake, previously instrumented	1 mg/kg, IV	Thirty % decrease in mesenteric vascular resistance, 11% decrease in renal vascular resistance, no change in iliac vascular resistance	6
Same	3 mg/kg, IV	One hundred and twenty % increase in mesenteric vascular resistance, 12% decrease in renal vascular resistance, no change in cardiac output, aortic pressure, systemic resistance or heart rate	6
Decerebrated or narcotized with ether, urethane, phenobarbital or "barbital" or given a preliminary "small" dose of morphine subcutaneously	>0.5 mg/kg, IV	Profound hypotension	7
Same	1-2 mg/kg, IV up to 50 mg/kg	Precipitous hypotension, duration 10-15 minutes	7
Chloralose (60 mg/kg IV) positive pressure ventilation, open thorax, heparin (3 mg/kg), total cardiopulmonary bypass using a rotating disc oxygenator	1 mg/kg into oxygenato r, i.e. intra arterial	Total peripheral vascular resistance decreased 46±20%	8
Pentobarbital anesthetized (30 mg/kg, IV)	2 mg/kg, IV	Coronary vasodilation (opposite effect of that seen in intact awake dog)	4

Conditions of the Experiment	Dose	Cardiovascular Effects	Reference
2.1:1 Dogs			
Pentobarbital anesthetized (35 mg/kg, IV)	2 mg/kg, IV	Increase arterial pCO_2, increased arterial pH, decreased arterial pO_2, slight increase in heart rate, dramatic decrease in aortic pressure and increase in plasma histamine levels	9
Pentobarbital anesthetized (30 mg/kg, IV)	Intra arterial injection no dose given	No effect on femoral artery flow or pressure	10
Anesthetized with thiamylal (18 mg/kg) 70% nitrous oxide in oxygen and halothane removed before injection of morphine, open chest extracorporeal reservoir	4 mg/kg, IV	Decrease in mean aortic pressure and reservoir volume, increased central hematocrit and decreased plasma volume. Concluded that morphine induced a decrease in extra corporeal reservoir volume at constant flow. There was also a drop in vena caval pressure caused by blood trapped in the liver, due to constriction of hepatic outflow, and plasma being filtered out at the liver sinusoids	11
Anesthetized with open chest, Thiamylal (18 mg/kg, IV) 70% nitrous oxide and 0.83% halothane. Right heart bypass preparation with separation of splanchnic and extra splanchnic venous returns	4 mg/kg, IV into pulmonary artery	No change in splanchnic compliance, peripheral compliance, or peripheral venous resistance. Increased splanchnic resistance, decreased % of cardiac output to the periphery. The aortic pressure, splanchnic arterial resistance, peripheral arterial resistance, systemic resistance and volume in the extracorporeal reservoir all decreased	12
Anesthetized with Pentobarbital (30 mg/kg, IV) and Atropine (3 mg total dose) Isoproterenol infusion of 0.1 g/kg/min	4 mg/kg, IV	Under these conditions, with the isoproterenol infusion, the heart rate, left ventricular dP/dt, cardiac index, stroke volume and aortic pressure all decreased. There was no change in systemic resistance or pulmonary arterial wedge pressure	13
Same as above with addition of 10 g/kg, IV propranolol	15 mg/kg, IV	Heart rate decreased but all other parameters did not change. Authors concluded that beta-blocking activity of propranolol is additive but not potentiated under these circumstances	13

Conditions of the Experiment	Dose	Cardiovascular Effects	Reference
2.1:1 Dogs			
Induction with thiopentone (10 mg/kg, IV), 70% nitrous oxide, 30% oxygen	4 mg/kg, IV	Severe and rapid fall in peripheral perfusion as measured by skeletal muscle surface pH. The calculated blood volume decreased by 20%	14
Anesthetized with pentobarbital (30 mg/kg, IV), 3 mg Atropine (total dose)	15 mg/kg, IV	Cardiac index and aortic pressure decreased, but no change in heart rate, left ventricular dP/dt, stroke volume, systemic resistance or pulmonary artery wedge pressure	13
Anesthetized with pentobarbital (30 mg/kg, IV), thorax open, positive pressure ventilation	Total dose 8 mg/kg given at 10 minute intervals of 0.25, 0.25, 0.5, 1.0, 2.0 and 4.0 mg/kg	Decreased aortic pressure, cardiac output, left ventricular dP/dt max, systemic resistance and heart rate, i.e. severe cardiac depression	15
Anesthetized with pentobarbital (25 mg/kg, IV), gallamine triethiodide (2 mg/kg, IV< repeated as necessary), beta-blockade with toliprolol (2.5 mg/kg IV and 2.5 mg/kg, S. C.	0.5 mg/kg intracister nal injection	Decreased heart rate, no change in aortic blood pressure, no increase in reflex bradycardia after angiotensin II injection	16
Same	0.5 mg/kg, IV	Decrease in heart rate but less than same dose given intracisternal injection. Aortic pressure and reflex bradycardia not affected	16
Anesthetized with pentobarbital (30 mg/kg, IV)	0.5 mg/kg, IV	Transient drop in arterial pressure with concomitant increase in heart rate	17
Anesthetized with halothane (0.75%) supplemented by succinylcholine (IV) and controlled ventilation	0.5 mg/kg, IV	Decreased cardiac output, heart rate and mean aortic pressure. Stroke volume and pulse pressure increased.	18

Conditions of the Experiment	Dose	Cardiovascular Effects	Reference
2.1:1 Dogs			
Anesthetized with alpha -chloralose (100 mg/kg) with additional doses of (50 mg/kg) to effect	0.125, 0.25 or 0.5 mg/kg, IV	Results indicate that central vagal activation by morphine may be protective against ventricular fibrillation	6
Anesthetized with alpha - chloralose (100 mg/kg, IV) open chest, heparin (3 mg/kg)	2 mg/kg, IV every 30 min.	Cardiac output decreased from 103±11 ml/kg/min to 43±6, mean aortic pressure decreased from 121±7 to 76±10 mmHg, left ventricular dP/dt decreased from 3134±439 to 1548±305 mmHg/sec. Myocardial blood flow decreased from 63±5 to 47±4 ml/min/100g and coronary resistance decreased from 1.66±0.14 to 0.74±0.17 mmHg/ml/100g. Myocardial lactate increased and myocardial lactate extraction decreased	19
Anesthetized with pentobarbital (30 mg/kg, IV) or phencyclidine (2 mg/kg, IM) plus alpha - chloralose (30 mg/kg IV)	2-3 mg/kg in increments	Failed to block serotonin induced cardiovascular reflex	20
Isolated pulmonary arteries and veins	not given	Failed to antagonize serotonin effects, induced contractile responses	21
Helical vascular smooth muscle strips from cutaneous hind limb arteries, experiments done at 20, 40 and 60% increased over initial length	10^{-2} mg/ml	No effect on norepinephrine dose-response curves for developed tension	22
Dogs anesthetized with pentobarbital (30 mg/kg, IV) helical strips of isolated lateral saphenous veins	5×10^{-5}M and 2×10^{-4}M	Measured evoked tension, dose-dependent depression of contractile response to transmural electrical stimulation. Contractile response to norepinephrine not affected. Decreased release of norepinephrine	23

Conditions of the Experiment	Dose	Cardiovascular Effects	Reference
2.1:1 Dogs			
Anesthetized with morphine sulfate (2 mg/kg, IM) and alpha - chloralose (100 mg/kg IV), sinus node artery perfused with blood from a femoral artery, morphine infused into sinus node artery, also isolated SA nodal preps	300 micro- g-1 mg	Concentrations equivalent to those which produce peripheral vasodilation when given IV had no effect on the SA pacemaker activity in <u>situ</u> or in the isolated prep. Decreased chronotropic response not prevented by atropine. Occas. 1 mg dose induced an increased chronotropic response followed by a decrease. Did not prevent effects of vagal stimulation or of ACH injected into the SA nodal artery	**86**
Anesthetized with Chloralose (60 mg/kg, IV), Heparin (3 mg/kg, IV), on a cardiopulmonary by pass system with systemic flow held constant	1 mg/kg, IV	13 normal dogs, decreased aortic blood pressure, transient decrease in peripheral resistance, blood volume increased 11±6 ml/kg	**100**
Same as above	0.5 mg/kg, IV	Venous tone decreased from 6.8±1.3 to 3.5±1.1 cm H_2O	**100**
Anesthetized with pentobarbital (30 mg/kg, IV), additional dose of 1-2 mg/kg after instrumentation	0.25, 0.5, 1.0, 2.0, and 4.0 mg/kg, IV	Decreased aortic blood pressure, left ventricular dP/dt max, cardiac output and heart rate, with same dose dependence. No change in peripheral resistance, stroke volume or pulmonary arterial pressure	**101**
Mongrels, n=25, anesthetized with pentothal (5-10 mg/kg, IV) and isoflurane to effect	1 mg/kg, IV	5 min. post injection had a decrease in heart rate, cardiac output, stroke volume and increases in peripheral resistance and pulmonary vascular resistance. There was no change in aortic blood pressure.	**102**
Chloralose anesthetized (80 mg/kg, IV)	2 mg/kg, IV	Decreased aortic pressure, effect not blocked by haloperidol but was blocked by naloxone	**103**
10-15 mm Segment of a cutaneous artery from dog hind limb	10^{-1} to 10^{-3} mg/ml of both	No contraction or relaxation over a variety of muscle lengths with or without norepinephrine	**125**
Excised saphenous vein rings	5×10^{-5} to 2×10^{-4} M	A dose-dependent decrease in contractile response to electrical stimulation, no effect at concentrations $< 5 \times 10^{-5}$ M	**126**

Conditions of the Experiment	Dose	Cardiovascular Effects	Reference
2.1:2 Cats			
Anesthetized with pentobarbital (42 mg/kg/IP), supplemented by 4.2 mg/kg every 1-2 hrs. Paralyzed with gallamine triethiodide (3 mg/kg, IV) positive pressure ventilation provided. Measured electrical activity of chemoreceptor units	0.1, 1, 10, 100 and 1000 micro-g intracarotid	Variable response that tended to be biphasic but generally causd inhibition of spontaneous chemoreceptor discharge from the carotid sinus nerve	**24**
Either decerebrated or narcotized with ether, urethane, phenobarbital or "barbital"	≥ 0.5mg/kg, IV	Profound hypotension	**7**
Anesthetized with chloralose	400 µg into lateral ventricle of brain	Increased heart rate, increase then decrease in mean aortic blood pressure	**126**
Same	0.5 mg/kg, sub-cutaneous	Decreased heart rate, decreased blood pressure	**126**
Same	400 µg intracistern al	Decreased heart rate and blood pressure	**126**
Anesthetized with chloralose (60mg/kg, IV), Thiopental (2.5 mg/kg, IV, as needed) gallamine triethiodide (2 mg/kg, IV), positive pressure ventilation, "debuffered", 1.3. the common carotid arteries were ligated and cut, vagus and depressor nerves cut bilaterally in the neck	500 micro g/kg into cisterna cerebellum	6 cats treated, 1 showed no changes, 5 had an initial increase in aortic blood pressure followed by a decrease. There was no change in heart rate or splanchnic nerve activity	**16**

Conditions of the Experiment	Dose	Cardiovascular Effects	Reference
2.1:2 Cats			
Same as above but not "debuffered"	Same	4 cats, 3 showed no changes in heart rate, aortic blood pressure or splanchnic nerve activity, the other cat showed a marked decrease in blood pressure and splanchnic nerve activity	16
Recommended analgesic dose - cats are not able to eliminate morphine by glyceronindation, this can result in increased sensitivity and toxicity	0.1 mg/kg, SC	No data provided	2
Anesthetized with chloralose, positive pressure ventilation provided	400 µg into lateral ventricle of the brain	Marked increase in heart rate, transient increase in aortic blood pressure with a subsequent decrease to below preinjection levels	25
Same	400 µg into the cisterna magna	Long lasting decrease in blood pressure with a mild decrease in heart rate	25
Isolated papillary muscle	1-10 g/ml up to 2,000 g/ml	No significant changes at low doses but then a dose dependent decrease in extent of shortening, velocity of shortening, rate of tension development, "cardiac work" and "cardiac power", 50% inhibition at high dose	26
Isolated, dissected pieces of pial arteries, approximately 5 mm long	perfusion, various concentrations	Dose dependent dilation, effect blocked by naloxone. Suggests presence of opiate receptors in the vessel walls	27
Isolated right ventricular papillary muscle	$10^{-5}M$ to $10^{-4}M$ concentrations	No change in maximum developed isometric tension or dT/dt at low dose but decreased both at higher dose	27
Acute preparation, open chest, anesthetized with thiopental, succinylcholine (1mg/kg/hr), positive pressure ventilation intermittent occlusion of the LAD coronary artery	1 mg/kg	When injected before coronary occlusion produced a significant increase in ST-segment elevation. There was no significant change in animals receiving saline or N_2O. Large doses of morphine may increase myocardial ischemia in this model	96

Conditions of the Experiment	Dose	Cardiovascular Effects	References
2.1:3 Rats and Mice			
Unanesthetized, intact awake rats	0.5 mg/kg	No effect on blood pressure	7
Intact, awake, previously instrumented rats	3 mg/kg, SC	Blood pressure decreased for 30 minutes along with decreased heart rate for 30 minutes	28
Anesthetized with pentobarbital, coronary artery ligation	3 mg/kg, SC 10 min. prior to anesthesia	Dose was injected approximately 30 min. prior to coronary artery ligation resulted in increased infarct size compared to identically handled control group, without morphine pretreatment	28
Midcollicular decerebrate, spontaneously breathing	2 mg/kg, right atrial injection	Dramatic decrease in heart rate with a slight and transient biphasic response in blood pressure. Bradycardia returned to baseline within 8-10 minutes	29
Conscious, previously instrumented drug naive (n=7)	7.5 mg/kg, IV, infusion over 15 min.	Transient but precipitous decrease in aortic pressure and heart rate with an increase in pulse pressure. Responses blocked by atropine.	104
Chronically injected i.e. daily doses prior to 15 min. infusion (n=6)	Same	Transient increase in aortic blood pressure with tachycardia seen during the later stages of the 15 min. morphine infusion	104
Conscious, instrumented 48 hours prior to recordings	7.5 mg/kg, IV	Decrease in heart rate and mean aortic pressure as a result of increased parasympathetic activity	105
Decapitated, isolated left atrium preparation. Electrically stimulated.	Dose response curves	Decreased contractility	106
300 g males killed by a blow to the head and atria excised, electrically stimulated	37-375 µM	Delayed decrease in atrial tension	107
Same as above but spontaneously beating	37-375 µM	Dose related decrease in heart rate and increase in atrial tension	107
Conscious, previously instrumented	4 mg/kg, IV, every 2 hrs. for 24 hrs.	Heart rate and blood pressure unchanged from baseline following all injections.	127
Anesthetized with ether, ligation of left coronary artery 2-3 mm from origin	3 mg/kg, Sub Q 10 min. prior to anesthesia	Developed significantly larger infarctions with the morphine than with sham injections	128

Conditions of the Experiment	Dose	Cardiovascular Effects	References
2.1:3 Rats and Mice			
Previously instrumented, intact awake	3 mg/kg, Sub Q	30 min. following injection decrease in heart rate and blood pressure	**128**
Decerebrate, previously instrumented, no anesthesia at time of study	2 mg/kg into right atrium	Decreased heart rate but no change in blood pressure	**129**
Aortic strips from decapitated rats	25 mg/kg, IP pretreated 30 min. prior to decapitation	Increased contractile sensitivity 130 to epinephrine and high concentrations of K^+. Decreased contractile sensitivity to Angiotensin II and low concentrations of K^+.	**130**
Decapitated 30 min. after morphine dose. Aortic strips and portal vein segments measured for isometric contractile tension, dose response curves to epinephrine, angiotensin II and potassium chloride	25 mg/kg, IP	Aortic strips showed increased sensitivity to high concentrations of K^+ and to epinephrine and decreased sensitivity to low concentrations of K^+ and to angiotensin II. The portal vein preparations did not show any effect on spontaneous mechanical activity or drug-induced activity as a result of morphine pretreatment	**30**
Response to sublethal doses of Doxapam	20 mg/kg	Sub-lethal doses of Doxapam appear to cause conduction defects in rat hearts, the toxic response is increased by morphine pretreatment	**31**
Isolated pulmonary artery strips	?	Fails to alter response to contraction inducing doses of serotonin or epinephrine	**21,32**
Recommended analgesic and sedative dose	2-5 mg/kg, SC or IM	Effects within 15 min. of SC injection. No data on cardiovascular effects	**2**
Anesthetized with urethane (1.2 g/kg, IP) acute instrumentation	0.01-0.75 mg/kg IV (Apo-morphine)	Dose-dependent decrease in aortic pressure, at higher doses a marked decrease in heart rate. Effects shown to be central in origin and mainly due to stimulation of a Dopamine receptor, some peripheral effects also probable.	**88**

Conditions of the Experiment	Dose	Cardiovascular Effects	References
2.1:4 Rabbits			
Unanesthetized, instrumented	≥0.5 mg/kg	No effect on blood pressure	7
Isolated spirally cut aortic strips, in an organ bath under 2g passive tension and equilibrated for 2 hrs.	5 x 10^{-6}g/ml	Potentiated responses to norepinephrine, no significant effect on responses to substance-P	33
Anesthetized with urethane (1g/kg, IV), Three different groups studied, one at each different morphine dose level	0, 3, 1.0 and 9 mg/kg, IV	Only high (9 mg/kg) dose resulted in significant changes. Heart rate and aortic pressures, systolic, diastolic and mean, all decreased, peak effect after 1 hour. Inhibited noradrenalin induced increase in blood pressure and reflex bradycardia, partially antagonized isoprenaline-induced decrease in blood pressure with no effect on tachycardia, norepinephrine release was enhanced. Resulted in an initial decrease then increase in tritiated norepinephrine uptake	34
Recommended dose	8 mg/kg, IM	No cardiovascular data provided, but results in profound CNS depression	2
Freshly stunned, excised papillary muscle preparation	Dose response, 1-10 μmol/l	No effect on action potential parameters or force of contraction, suggests morphine actions seen in intact preparations are mediated presynaptically.	108
Conscious, previously instrumented, (n=6)	4 mg/kg, IV, infusion in a volume of 400 μL/kg in 1 min.	Increased mean aortic pressure, decreased heart rate, hyperglycemia, increased plasma epinephrine and norepinephrine.	109
Conscious rabbits, previously instrumented	3 mg/kg, IV	Increased mean aortic blood pressure, decreased heart rate, increased plasma epinephrine and plasma glucose. Reactions were enhanced by antihistamine pretreatment.	110

Conditions of the Experiment	Dose	Cardiovascular Effects	References
2.1:4 Rabbits			
Anesthetized with urethane (1g/kg, IV) plus 30 min. of equilibration after instrumentation	9 mg/kg, IV	Decreased heart rate and blood pressure. Inhibited noradrenaline-induced increases in blood pressure and reflex bradycardia, partially antagonized isoprenaline-induced decrease in blood pressure with no effect on tachycardia, decreased then increased uptake of tritiated noradrenaline.	**131**

Conditions of the Experiment	Dose	Cardiovascular Effects	References
2.1:5 Hamsters			
Anesthetized with pentobarbital (no dose given), exposed *in vivo* cheek pouch preparation, superfused with Krebs solution	Dose - response	Dose-dependent dilation of arterioles	**35**
Same as above	10^{-8} to 10^{-9}M superfusate	Caused vasodilation but beta-endorphin 55 x more potent net - enkephalin 24x, leu enkephalin 20 x	**133**
Analgesia and sedation	2-5 mg/kg, SC	Effects within 15 min. of SC injection. No cardiovascular data provided.	**2**
Cheek-pouch preparation, anesthesia not described. Pre-treatment with increasing doses of morphine for 2 wks., sham treated control group	?	Relative potencies of the *in vivo* vasodilating effect after topical application decreases significantly, i.e. morphine tolerance develops	**36**
Cheek-pouch preparation, no anesthesia described	Topical application	Dilates arterioles, decreased potency and increases tolerance when chronically pretreated.	**111**

Conditions of the Experiment	Dose	Cardiovascular Effects	References
2.1:6 Guinea Pigs			
Unanesthetized	≥0.5 mg/kg	No effect on blood pressure	7
Isolated atrial preparation, no information on anesthesia	0.25 g/ml, 1 g/ml and 100 g/ml	85% decrease in heart rate at lowest dose, 79% decrease at 1 g/ml and only 63% decrease at 100 g/ml	37
Isolated papillary muscle preparation, from freshly stunned animals	Dose response from 1-10 μ Mol/l	No effect on action potential parameters or force of contraction. Results suggest presynaptic release of vasoactive substances as mediators of changes seen in intact animals	108
Spontaneously beating, excised atrial myocardial preparations	0.25 μg and 100 μg/ml of both	Lower dose had an enhanced effect on lowering heart rate	132

Conditions of the Experiment	Dose	Cardiovascular Effects	References
2.1:7 Pigs			
Halothane anesthesia, open chest, total and right heart by-pass preparations	10 mg/kg, IV	No change in stroke volume, during normoxia no change in myocardial oxygen consumption but during hypoxia myocardial oxygen consumption decreased. Coronary blood flow, myocardial lactate extraction and myocardia pO_2 and pCO_2 all decreased	38
Recommended analgesic dose, seems to have more CNS stimulation than depression	0.2-0.9 mg/kg IM	No data provided	4
Intact, awake, previously instrumented	1.0 mg/kg, IV	Induced an immediate but small increase in cardiac output, substantial increases in heart rate, mean systemic and pulmonary arterial pressures, left and right ventricular work, hematocrit and hemoglobin concentrations; no change in stroke volume or systemic vascular resistance	163

Conditions of the Experiment	Dose	Cardiovascular Effects	References
2.1:7 Pigs			
Intact, awake, previously instrumented	1.0 mg/kg, IV	Immediate increases in O_2 consumption, CO_2 production; hypermetabolic state persisted for approx. 1 hr, cause seemed to be an increase in skeletal muscle activity	**164**

Conditions of the Experiment	Dose	Cardiovascular Effects	References
2.1:8 Sheep			
Intact awake, pregnant ewes, previously instrumented	5 mg epidural	No change in maternal or fetal aortic blood pressure or acid-base status. No change in maternal central venous pressure, systemic resistance, pulmonary artery pressure, cardiac output or intrauterine pressure. Small but significant decrease in maternal heart rate and uterine blood flow at 120 min. post injection	**39**
Fetal lambs, chronically instrumented, n=28	Dose response, 0.075 to 40 mg/M, IV into fetus	Doses < 0.15 mg/hr had no effect on fetal heart rate or aortic blood pressure. Higher doses increased fetal heart rate, no change in aortic pressure, peak response at 2.5 mg/hr.	**112**
Intact, awake, previously instrumented pregnant ewes	0.6 mg/kg, SC	No change in umbilical blood flow or fetal O_2 consumption during 120 min. observation period. Transient maternal hyperglycemia. Umbilical vein glucose levels were significantly decreased and fetal glucose uptake was markedly decreased. No change in fetal uptake of lactate or pyruvate.	**40**

Conditions of the Experiment	Dose	Cardiovascular Effects	References
2.1:9 Horses			
Recommended dosage for pain	0.2-0.4 mg/kg, IM	No data provided	**2,41**

Conditions of the Experiment	Dose	Cardiovascular Effects	References
2.1:9 Horses			
Intact, awake, instrumented, adult, pain free	0.12 mg/kg, IV	Heart rate increased at 5 and 15 min., no change at 30 and 60 min. Respiratory rate increased at 5 min, no change at 15, 30 and 60 min. Cardiac output increased at 5 min, no change at 15, 30 and 60 min. No changes seen in pulmonary artery pressure, right atrial pressure, arterial pO_2 or pH. Arterial pO_2 decreased at 5 and 15 minutes	**42**
Recommended dosage for preanesthesia	0.12 mg/kg, IV	No data provided	**43**

Conditions of the Experiment	Dose	Cardiovascular Effects	References
2.1:10 Primates			
Recommended dose for chemical restraint and sedation of chimpanzees	1-3 mg/kg, SC or IM	No data provided	**44**
Recommended dose for adequate sedation and safe management for most primates	0.1-2 mg/kg,	No data provided	**2**

Table 2.2:   Meperidine

Conditions of the Experiment	Dose	Cardiovascular Effects	References
2.2:1 Dogs			
Intact, awake, previously instrumented	2 mg/kg, IV	Cardiac output decreased 30%, decreased stroke volume and heart rate, increased pulmonary arterial and systemic resistance. No change in arterial pH, pCO_2, or pO_2.	**45**

Conditions of the Experiment	Dose	Cardiovascular Effects	References
2.2:1 Dogs			
Intact, awake, previously instrumented	2 mg/kg, IV	Decreased cardiac output, decreased mean aortic pressure, mild renal vascular dilation characterized by a 10% decrease in renal vascular resistance and a 5% increase in renal blood flow. There was also a significant increase in systemic resistance.	**46**
Same	6 mg/kg, IV	Large renal vascular dilation characterized by a 22% decrease in resistance and an 18% increase in flow. There was an increase in heart rate, a decrease in mean aortic pressure, an increase in cardiac output initially and then a significant decrease. Systemic resistance decreased. The iliac vasculature showed a 39% decrease in resistance with a 40% increase in flow while the mesenteric vasculature had a 40% decrease in flow and an 89% increase in resistance.	**46**
Anesthetized with pentobarbital (30 mg/kg, IV), acute, open chest preparation	2.5 mg/kg, IV	Decreased left ventricular pressure, decreased mean aortic pressure, decreased left ventricular dP/dt max, decreased coronary sinus blood flow, decreased myocardial oxygen consumption and an increase in heart rate (possibly a baroreceptor response)	**47**
No specific data	10 mg/kg, IM	Decreased heart rate and a moderate decrease in aortic pressure 10-20 min. after IM injection. A return to baseline values occurs within 30 minutes.	**2**

Conditions of the Experiment	Dose	Cardiovascular Effects	References
2.2:2 Cats			
Analgesic dose	11 MG/KG, im	Half life of 0.7 hr at dose of 22 mg/kg, IV, no cardiovascular effects reported	**2**

Conditions of the Experiment	Dose	Cardiovascular Effects	References
2.2:2 Cats			
Isolated papillary muscle preparation. No information about euthanasia technique used.	Range of doses in perfusate.	Dose dependent decrease in inotropy.	**26**

Conditions of the Experiment	Dose	Cardiovascular Effects	References
2.2:3 Rats and Mice			
Analgesic dose	40-50 mg/kg, IP	No data	**2**
Pentobarbital anesthesia, 50 mg/kg, IP, isolated atria preparation	5×10^{-5}M	Increased developed force and dP/dt. The response not attenuated by naloxone, phentolamine, propranolol, polaramine, ranitidine, verapamil nor lidocaine.	**113**

Conditions of the Experiment	Dose	Cardiovascular Effects	References
2.2:5 Hamsters/Guinea Pigs			
Preanesthetic dose	2 mg/kg, IM	No data	**2**

Conditions of the Experiment	Dose	Cardiovascular Effects	References
2.2:6 Cattle			
Analgesic dose	1.1 mg/kg, IM	No data	**2**

Conditions of the Experiment	Dose	Cardiovascular Effects	References
2.2:7 Horses			
Pain free, adult, previously instrumented, awake	1.1 mg/kg, IV	Increased heart rate at 5 min. post injection but back to baseline at 15, 30 and 60 min. post injected. Cardiac output increased at 5 and 15 min. but same as baseline at 30 and 60 min. No change in pulmonary artery blood gases. No change in respiratory rate.	42
Analgesic dose	1.1 mg/kg, IV	No data - May require 4 mg/kg for visceral pain	2
Analgesic dose	2.2-3.0 mg/kg, IM	No cardiovascular data, onset of effect within 10 min.	41

Conditions of the Experiment	Dose	Cardiovascular Effects	References
2.2:8 Primates			
Rhesus monkeys, for analgesia	1.3-3.3 mg/kg	No cardiovascular data - some monkeys may require as much as 11 mg/kg. The Rhesus seems to be twice as sensitive as squirrel monkeys, on a body weight basis	2
Analgesic dose	1.1 mg/kg, IV	No data - May require 4 mg/kg for visceral pain	2

Table 2.3: Methadone

Conditions of the Experiment	Dose	Cardiovascular Effects	References
2.3:1 Dogs			
Preanesthetic dose	1.1 mg/kg, SC	Slight alterations in cardiovascular dynamics which can be blocked by prior administration of atropine. Reduces required dose of barbiturate anesthesia by 1/2.	2
Anesthetized with pentobarbital (15 mg/kg, IV) succinylcholine (2 mg/kg, IV)	0.5 mg/kg, IV	Modest decrease in heart rate, cardiac output, and aortic pressure	134

Conditions of the Experiment	Dose	Cardiovascular Effects	References
2.3:1 Dogs			
Anesthetized with pentobarbital (15 mg/kg, IV), succinylcholine (2 mg/kg, IV)	1.0, 1.5 and 2.0 mg/kg, IV	Decreases in all of above, dose response, with large decrease in heart rate	**134**
Anesthetized with pentobarbital (15 mg/kg, IV), succinylcholine (2 mg/kg, IV)	1.5 and 2.0 mg/kg, IV	Increased peripheral resistance. All of above responses blocked by atropine, 1.5 mg IM	**134**
Anesthetized with pentobarbital (15mg/kg, IV) succinylcholine (2 mg/kg, IV) positive pressure ventilation with 100% oxygen, plus atropine (1.5mg total dose)	0.3 mg/kg, IV	No change in heart rate, stroke volume, cardiac output, mean aortic pressure, mean pulmonary artery pressure, pulmonary arterial wedge pressure, mean right atrial pressure, systemic or pulmonary arterial resistance, i.e. responses blocked by atropine.	**48**
Same	0.8 mg/kg, IV cumulative dose using the above dose	No change in any of the above parameters	**48**
Same	1.8mg/kg, IV cumulative with above	Decrease in mean aortic pressure, all other parameters unchanged	**48**
Same	3.3mg/kg, IV cumulative with above	Decrease in mean aortic pressure only, other parameters unchanged	**48**
Same	5.3mg/kg, IV cumulative dose	Decreased mean aortic pressure, other parameters not affected	**48**
Anesthetized with pentobarbital (15mg/kg, IV), succinylcholine (2mg/kg, IV) positive pressure ventilation with 100% oxygen - no atropine	0.3 mg/kg, IV	No changes in heart rate, stroke volume, cardiac output, mean aortic pressures, mean pulmonary artery pressures, pulmonary artery wedge pressures, mean right atrial pressures, systemic resistance or pulmonary arterial resistance.	**48**

Conditions of the Experiment	Dose	Cardiovascular Effects	References
2.3:1 Dogs			
Same	0.8mg/kg, IV cumulative with previous dose	Decreased heart rate, cardiac output and mean aortic pressure with an increase in systemic resistance. All other parameters remained unchanged.	**48**
Same	1.8mg/kg, IV	Decreased heart rate and cardiac output with increase in resistance. All other parameters not affected.	**48**
Same	3.3mg/kg, IV	Decrease in heart rate, cardiac output, mean aortic pressure and increases in systemic resistance and pulmonary arterial resistance	**48**
Same	5.3mg/kg, IV	Decreased heart rate, cardiac output, mean aortic pressure and increases in systemic and pulmonary vascular resistance.	**48**
Pregnant bitches	?	Delays in normal maturational design of the brain and heart ornithine decarboxylase activity from puppies of treated mothers	**49**

Table 2.4: Pentazocine

Conditions of the Experiment	Dose	Cardiovascular Effects	References
2.4:1 Dogs			
No data given concerning conditions	5 mg/kg	Transient 18% decrease in aortic pressure with return to baseline within 1 minute	2
Same	3 mg/kg IM	Half life of 22.1 minute	2
Anesthetized with pentobarbital (35/kg IV)	8 mg/kg IV	Slight decrease in heart rate and mean aortic pressure, increase in arterial pCO_2 and a decrease in arterial pH and pO_2	9

Conditions of the Experiment	Dose	Cardiovascular Effects	References
2.4:2 Cats			
Analgesic dose	8 mg/kg IM	t 1/2 of 83.6 minutes	2

Conditions of the Experiment	Dose	Cardiovascular Effects	References
2.4:3 Guinea Pigs			
Isolated, spontaneously beating and electrically driven atria	1 x 10-6g/ml in bath	Rate reduced, decreased contractile amplitude. In the electrically driven atria there was an initial positive inotropic response which preceded the negative inotropic reaction. When the calcium ion concentration of the preparation was increased the Pentazocine induced decrease in contractility was antagonized. Pentazocine also antagonized the negative inotropic and chronotropic effects of adenosine and acetylcholine.	53

Conditions of the Experiment	Dose	Cardiovascular Effects	References
2.4:4 Horses			
Preanesthetic dose	0.9 mg/kg IV	No data	2
Determination of half life	3 mg/kg IM	Half life of 97.1 min	2
Analgesic dose	0.8 mg/kg IV repeated in 5-15 minutes	Onset in about 10 min. with duration of about 1 hour. Large volumes may lead to excitement in some individuals	41
Painfree, adult, intact, awake, previously instrumented	0.9 mg/kg IV	Heart rate increased at 5 and 15 min, no change at 30 and 60 min. Cardiac output increased at 5 and 15 min, no change at 30 and 60 min. No change in pulmonary, aortic or right atrial pressures. No change in blood gases or respiratory rate.	42

Conditions of the Experiment	Dose	Cardiovascular Effects	References
2.4:5 Pigs			
Analgesic dose	3 mg/kg IM	Half life = 48.6 min.	2

Conditions of the Experiment	Dose	Cardiovascular Effects	References
2.4:6 Goats			
Analgesic dose	3 mg/kg IM	Half life = 51.0 min.	2

Table 2.5 Fentanyl

Conditions of the Experiment	Dose	Cardiovascular Effects	References
2.5:1 Dogs			
Conscious, intact	50 µg/kg IV	Heart rate decreased from 111±11 to 42±3 beats/min, respiratory rate went from 38±5 to 9±2	54
Anesthetized with ether then an electrolytic decerebration. The ether was then removed for more than 2 1/2 hrs. to allow for equilibration	50 µg/kg IV	Mean aortic pressure decreased from 113±8 to 72±10 mmHg and heart rate decreased from 155±14 to 114±15 beats/min	54
Conscious, previously instrumented. Drug applied to 4th cerebral ventricle.	Not given	Pronounced bradycardia, blood pressure and the blood pressure response to baroreflex activation not affected by this perturbation	55
Anesthetized with pentobarbital (30mg/kg, IV) acute, open chest preparation	0.0025-0.03 mg/kg	Dose dependent increase in left ventricular dP/dt max and decrease in myocardial oxygen consumption, decreased pressure time index, decreased coronary sinus blood flow and heart rate	47
Same	0.03-0.16 mg/kg	No change in left ventricular dP/dt max, left ventricular pressure, left ventricular end diastolic pressure or mean aortic pressure. There was some evidence for tachyphylaxis.	47

Conditions of the Experiment	Dose	Cardiovascular Effects	References
2.5:1 Dogs			
Dogs anesthetized with 50mg/kg pentobarbital, IV. Left and right coronary arteries dissected free, helical strips mounted in superfusion chamber and electrical stimulation.	2×10^{-6} and 8×10^{-6} M added to superfusate	No dose effect seen. Caused significant increase in both stimulated and unstimulated preparations of norepinephrine and metabolites of norepinephrine, particularly 3, 4 dihydroxyphenylgycol a metabolite from intraneuronal metabolism of norepinephrine. However, this metabolite has no agonist activity and so fentanyl had minimal effects on adrenergic transformation in this preparation	56
Anesthetized with pentobarbital (30mg/kg, IV), autoperfused hindlimb preparation, positive pressure ventilation. Measurements made of pressures from the pre- and postcapillary small (resistance) vessels and the saphenous vein (capacitance). Constant flow with variable pressure	2.5 µg/kg intra-arterial (femoral)	First a decrease then, after 7 min, an increase in precapillary pressure. The initial drop could be antagonized by diphenhydramine (1.8mg/kg), atropine (1mg/kg), could not block the effect with propranolol (0.5mg/kg) or atropine (0.06mg/kg). There was also a moderate increase in saphenous vein pressure.	57
Anesthetized with chloralose (90mg/kg, IV), positive pressure ventilation	5 and 20 µg/kg, IV	Hypotensive, bradycardic and sympathoinhibitory response, not mediated by dopamine or serotonin	58
Same	5 µg/kg, IV	Augmented bradycardia produced by electrical stimulation of the carotid sinus nerves. Did not change the bradycardic response to stimulation of the nucleus of the solitary tract	58
Same	20 µg/kg, IV	Produced marked hypotension and bradycardia offsetting a fulminating hypertension and tachycardia produced by bilateral destruction of the nucleus of the solitary tract or by cutting the baroreceptor afferent fibers	58

Conditions of the Experiment	Dose	Cardiovascular Effects	References
2.5:1 Dogs			
Nitrous oxide analgesia	0.04 to 0.08 mg total dose	No effect on baroreceptor response	59
Preanesthetized with fluanisone (10 mg) & fentanyl (200 g/kg), Pentobarbital anesthesia (10mg/kg, IV) & maintained on 60% nitrous oxide. Open chest, acute. Left anterior descending coronary artery ligated, occluded once and then again	25 µg/kg, IV given before second LAD occlusion in treatment group	Compared to the control group at time of the second LAD occlusion the heart rate decreased 57%, left ventricular dP/dt max decreased 25%, aortic systolic pressure decreased 15% and diastolic pressure 33% while the mean aortic pressure decreased 26%. Mean coronary artery pressure decreased 30% and coronary artery flow decreased 47%.	60
Preanesthetized with haloanisone and fentanyl (1 ml/kg, IM, "Hypnorm"). Anesthetized with pentobarbital (10mg/kg, IV) and maintained with nitrous oxide and oxygen, open chest, positive pressure ventilation	25 µg/kg, IV given 5 min prior to 1st coronary artery stenosis	Decreased heart rate during second stenosis but not first, decreased left ventricular dP/dt max during second stenosis, no change in systolic aortic pressure but diastolic aortic pressure decreased during the second stenosis. Pressure in the coronary vasculature decreased during both stenoses. Decreased myocardial oxygen demand.	61
Anesthetized with methohexital (6mg/kg IV), positive pressure ventilation with 0.6-1.5% halothane in 70% nitrous oxide and 30% oxygen. Approximately 2 hrs of surgical preparation. No halothane for 1 hour prior to recordings. Pancuronium (0.1 mg/kg, IV plus 0.05 mg/kg, IV as needed) for immobilization	0.01 mg/kg, IV	Activated type A vagal efferents (cardioinhibitory), no effect on type B & C efferents. Effects antagonized by naloxone.	62
	0.0025 to 0.16 mg/kg, IV cumulative doses	With cumulative doses there was a progressive increase in the discharge rate of the type A efferents but with maximum effect at 0.04 mg/kg total dose	62

Conditions of the Experiment	Dose	Cardiovascular Effects	References
2.5:1 Dogs			
Preanesthetized with haloanisone and fentanyl (1ml/kg, IM), anesthetized with pentobarbital (10mg/kg, IV) and nitrous oxide. Open chest-positive pressure ventilation	?	Suggest that fentanyl prevents excessive breakdown of energy-rich phosphates and high anaerobic production rate of lactate by decreasing the energy demand of the ischemic myocardium	63
Anesthetized with chloralose (100mg/kg, IV)	20 µg/kg, IV	Decreased the spontaneous firing rate of the type A neurons found in the nucleus tractus solitarii (blood pressure dependent neurons) (NTS). There was a marked increase in one group of type A neurons in the nucleus ambiguus but decreased firing rates in another group of type A neurons in the same nucleus. Decreased firing rate of type B neurons in both the nucleus tractus solitarii and the nucleus ambiguus. Induced biphasic changes in firing rate of baroreceptor neurons in the NTS	64
Anesthetized with methohexital (6mg/kg, IV), intubation, positive pressure ventilation, halothane (0.6-1.5%) 70% N_2O, during a 2hr surgical preparation. Discontinued halothane 1 hr prior to experiment, Pancuronium (0.1 mg/kg,IV + 0.05 mg/kg, IV, as needed)	0.01 mg/kg, IV 0.0025-0.16 mg/kg, IV	Activated type A efferents (cardioinhibitory), no effect on type B and C efferents Progressive increase in discharge rate of type A afferents with decreased heart rate, effects maximized at 0.04 mg/kg	89 89
Anesthetized with ether, electrolytic decerebration, acute instrumentation, approx. 2.5 hr wait before experiment	50 µg/kg, IV	Decreased mean aortic pressure and heart rate	54

Conditions of the Experiment	Dose	Cardiovascular Effects	References
2.5:1 Dogs			
Anesthetized with methohexitone (13.6±0.9 mg/kg, IV), positive pressure ventilation, alpha - chloralose (33.9±0.1 mg/kg + 16.3±0.1 mg/kg/h, IV infusion), suxamethonium (2 mg/kg/h), acute instrumentation	100 µg/kg, IV	Decreased heart rate and mean aortic pressure, decreased somato-cardiovascular reflexes (stimulation of a cut cutaneous nerve), mean aortic pressure returned to baseline in approx. 70 min, back by 90 min as a result of changes induced by somato-cardiovascular stimulation	**90**
Premedicated with Hypnorm (1 ml/kg, IM) anesthetized with pentobarbital (10 mg/kg, IV), intubation, positive pressure, vent. with N_2O in O_2, open chest, acute instrumentation, 2 coronary occlusions (first as a control)	25 µg/kg, IV	When administered prior to the second occlusion decreased heart rate, mean aortic pressure and LVdP/dt max. Decreased release of lactate and inorganic phosphate during period of ischemia. Results suggest fentanyl prevents excessive breakdown of energy-rich phosphates and high anerobic production rate of lactate by decreasing the energy demand of the ischemic myocardium	**91**
Open chest, acute, intubated, positive pressure vent., acute mid left circumflex or LAD coronary occlusion	100 µg/kg loading + 27±4 µg/kg/h	Decreased regional blood flow within the infarct but not as bad as with halothane. Mean aortic pressure, cardiac index, LV minute work index and heart rate were all near the normal conscious animal values.	**93**
Intact, awake, previously instrumented	25 µg/kg and 50 µg/kg, IV over 10 min. period	Produced renal vascular constriction with renal blood flow maintained, i.e., increased renal vascular resistance (autoregulation), in anesthetized dogs renal vascular resistance decreased	**94**
Anesthetized with ketamine (7-9 mg/kg IM) and alpha chloralose (100 mg/kg + 50 mg/kg/hr)	60 µg/kg (2 doses of 30 µg/kg each	Progressive decrease in heart rate, decrease in mean aortic pressure, effects blocked by atropine. The second dose reduced the decline in ventricular fibrillation threshold caused by LAD occlusion.	**114**

Conditions of the Experiment	Dose	Cardiovascular Effects	References
2.5:1 Dogs			
Pentobarbital anesthetized (30 µg/kg IV) n=12	100 µg/kg	Increased R-R interval, atrial - HIS interval, paced atrial-HIS interval, AV nodal effective refractory period, AV nodel functional refractory period and retrograde ventricular effective refractory period. No change in HIS-ventricle interval.	**115**
Same	400 µg/kg	Same as above with larger increases in most cases	**115**
Isolated hindlimb preparation, halothane anesthesia n=5	5, 30 and 50 µg/kg of limb weight	Apparent dose-dependent decrease in resistance which was significant only at high doses in both innervated and dennervated limbs.	**116**
Anesthetized with 10 mg/kg thiopental IV, 20 mg Succinylcholine and 1.5% isoflurane in oxygen	30µg/kg IV	Decreased heart rate, mean aortic pressure, and plasma norepinephrine levels, no change in plasma epinephrine levels	**117**
Anesthetized with pentobarbital (30 mg/kg, IV) isolated Purkinje fiber preparation	94.6 n M, 0.19 µM, 0.95 µM - Dose response	Increased action potential duration at 50 and 90>o repolarization at all 3 doses	**118**
Anesthetized with pentobarbital (50mg/kg, IV), helical strips of anterior interventricular branches of left and right coronaries	2×10^{-6} and 8×10^{-6} M	Increased norepinephrine and the norepinephrine metabolite 3,4 dihydroxy-phenylglycol. Minimal effects on adrenergic neurotransmission in the coronary vascular bed	**119**
Chloralose anesthetized (100 mg/kg IV plus 50 mg/kg as needed) intact animal preparation	30 µg/kg, IV	Decreased heart rate, mean aortic blood pressure, increased ventricular fibrillation threshold (single stimulus technique). Direct sympatho-inhibitory effects, not vagally mediated. Some evidence that antifibrillatory effect is mediated through afferent component of the baroreflex.	**120**

Conditions of the Experiment	Dose	Cardiovascular Effects	References
2.5:1 Dogs			
Isolated coronary artery rings, with and without endothelium	100 ng/ml	With endothelium, no effect on serotonin induced contraction, without endothelium, minimal depressant effect on phenylephrine (10^{-5} M) induced contraction.	121
Constant volume perfused femoral artery preparation with pressures recorded from the femoral artery, small ventral foot artery, small metatarsal vein and the saphenous vein.	2.5 µg/kg intra-arterial	Initial decrease then, after 7 minutes, an increase in precapillary vascular smooth muscle tone. The initial decrease in resistance could be blocked by antihistamine or high doses of atropine, not blocked by propranolol or low doses of atropine.	123
Anesthetized with chloralose (90 mg/kg IV)	5 µg/kg, IV	Augmented bradycardia produced by electrical stimulation of carotid sinus nerves but no response to stimulation of the nucleus of the solitary tract (NTS)	124
Same	20 µg/kg, IV	After bilateral destruction of NTS and cutting of afferent baroreceptor fibers caused marked decrease in heart rate and blood pressure.	124
Conscious, previously instrumented dogs, Pancuronium added (0.1 mg/kg plus 0.02 mg/kg as needed)	500 µg/kg plus 1.5 µg/kg/min IV infusion	Increased mean aortic pressure and LV dP/dt, no change in heart rate, pulmonary vascular resistance, cardiac output, PR interval, carotid arterial flow, coronary arterial flow, renal flow or peripheral resistance.	136
Anesthetized with pentobarbital (30 mg/kg, IV)	100 µg/kg & 400 µg/kg, IV	Prolonged the RR interval 26 and 45% respectively, Prolonged AV node conduction by 28 & 25%, lengthened AV node conduction times during atrial pacing at fast enough rates to capture the atrial, lengthened AV node effective and functional refractory periods and ventricular refractory periods	162

Conditions of the Experiment	Dose	Cardiovascular Effects	References
2.5:1 Dogs			
Anesthetized with thiopental (20 mg/kg, IV), intubated and maintained with enflurane in O_2, vagotomy and spinal block for sympathetic	100 µg/kg, IV	No statistically significant changes in heart rate, mean aortic pressure, cardiac index, left ventricular end-diastolic pressure or systemic resistance	**165**
Effects of left circumflex ligation on regional myocardial function	Dose-response	With approx. 50% ligation there was an increase in fractional shortening and a tendency to shift the end-systolic pressure-length relationship to the left, i.e. no apparent deleterious effect of fentanyl on regional myocardial function	**166**

Conditions of the Experiment	Dose	Cardiovascular Effects	References
2.5:2 Cats			
Anesthetized with pentobarbital (25mg/kg, IV), gallamine triethiodide (2 mg/kg IV repeated as necessary), positive pressure ventilation adrenergic-blockade with toliprolal (2.5 mg/kg IV and 2.5 mg/kg SC	3 µg/kg intracisternal	Moderate decrease in aortic blood pressure, marked decrease in heart rate, no change in reflex bradycardia initiated by angiotensin II	**65**
Same	3 µg/kg, IV	No change in blood pressure, moderate decrease in heart rate, less than caused by intracisternal injection	**16**
Chloralose anesthesia (60 mg/kg, IV), Thiopental (2.5 mg/kg IV as necessary), gallamine (2mg/kg, IV), positive pressure ventilation	3 µg/kg, intracisternal	Decrease in blood pressure, heart rate and splanchnic nerve discharge rate	**16**
Same	30 µg/kg in both	Decreased blood pressure, heart rate and splanchnic nerve discharge rate	**16**

Conditions of the Experiment	Dose	Cardiovascular Effects	References
2.5:2 Cats			
Isolated papillary muscle	10 µg/kg in both	50% inhibition of inotropy	**26**
Halothane anesthesia with high conc. for induction, positive pressure ventilation, 0.7% halothane with 70% N₂O, selective perfusion of the 4th cerebral ventricle	5, 10, 20 & 50 µg/ml (0.15 ml/min)	Dose-dependent decrease in aortic pressure and heart rate, no cardiovascular effects with same infusions into the lateral ventricles or the 3rd ventricle. Effects were blocked with Naloxone.	**95**
Halothane (0.7%) plus nitrous oxide/oxygen (3:1) anesthesia, perfusion of the 4th cerebral ventricle	5, 10, 20 and 50 µg/ml at 0.15 ml/min infusion rate	Dose-dependent decrease in aortic blood pressure and heart rate	**122**

Conditions of the Experiment	Dose	Cardiovascular Effects	References
2.5:3 Rats			
Not given	Dose not given, administered either IV or inhaled as an aerosol	No effect on pulmonary vasoconstrictor response to alveolar hypoxia	**66**
Acute left anterior descending coronary artery ligation	0.2-1 µg/kg, IV	No overall beneficial effect on response to LAD coronary artery ligation. Arrhythmias, blood pressure changes, heart rate changes, ECG changes and mortality rates were all the same in control versus fentanyl treated groups	**67**
Anesthetized with diethyl ether, positive pressure ventilation, open chest, 100 IU heparin, isolated heart-lung prep	Plasma conc. same found in anesthetic practice given as nebulized form via the airways or in the perfusate	No effect on pulmonary vasoconstrictor response to hypoxia either if given as an aerosol or as an infusion	**92**

Conditions of the Experiment	Dose	Cardiovascular Effects	References
2.5:3 Rats			
Anesthetized with phenobarbital, ip, Isolated, perfused Langendorff preparation, 85 cm H$_2$O coronary perfusion pressure, paced at 250 beats/min.	100 ng/ml	No change in coronary blood flow, normal energy status	**121**

Conditions of the Experiment	Dose	Cardiovascular Effects	References
2.5:4 Rabbits			
Conscious, previously instrumented (n=9)	10 µg/kg, IV	No change in mean aortic pressure, decreased heart rate, no change in cardiac output or peripheral resistance. With bilateral carotid occlusion there was no change in mean aortic pressure response but fentanyl significantly attentuated the resistance response and augmented the heart rate response.	**135**
Same	15 µg/kg, IV	No change in cardiac output, mean aortic pressure, heart rate, cerebral blood flow, oxygen transport, oxygen consumption or GI blood flow. Decrease in renal blood flow (24>o)	**137**

Conditions of the Experiment	Dose	Cardiovascular Effects	References
2.5:5 Sheep			
Unanesthetized, previously instrumented lambs	3.0 mg/kg, IV	No change in cardiac output, mean aortic pressure, heart rate, cerebral blood flow, oxygen transport, oxygen consumption or GI blood flow. Decrease in renal blood flow (24>o)	**137**

Conditions of the Experiment	Dose	Cardiovascular Effects	References
2.5:5 Sheep			
Same	3.0 mg/kg, IV plus 20 min. then 4.0 mg/kg Pentobarbital	Significant decrease in cerebral blood flow, oxygen transport and consumption, renal blood flow and GI blood flow. When order of pentobarbital and fentanyl administration reversed magnitude of decrease was higher.	**137**

Conditions of the Experiment	Dose	Cardiovascular Effects	References
2.5:6 Horses			
Analgesia	2.2 µg/kg, IM or IV	Duration of approximately 1 hour	**2**

Conditions of the Experiment	Dose	Cardiovascular Effects	References
2.5:7 Pigs			
Anesthetized with halothane and nitrous oxide, open chest, acute preparation. Off halothane on 60-65% nitrous oxide for 60 min stabilization prior to dosing. Results compared to another group of pigs kept on halothane throughout the experiment.	50 µg/kg, IV plus 100 µg/kg/hr	Heart rate tended to increase but not significantly, two indices of contractility increased, left ventricular systolic pressure and the systolic pressure-time index both increased, but left ventricular end diastolic pressure tended to decrease. Coronary arterial oxygen content and blood flow both increased significantly.	**68**
Anesthetized with ketamine (1g/40kg), IM) plus 40-50 mg/kg IV infusion of ketamine with 80 mg thiopental and Heparin (125 IU/kg/hr).	50 and 250 µg/kg	No effect on coronary artery diameters	**121**

Conditions of the Experiment	Dose	Cardiovascular Effects	References
2.5:7 Pigs			
Sedated with 120 mg azaperitone, IM, anesthetized with 150 mg metomitate, IV intubated and anesthetized with N_2O and O_2 (2:1) plus 1% Halothane.	Dose penthothal and fentanyl not given.	No change in heart rate, cardiac output, LVdP/dt, mean aortic pressure, vascular resistance, left ventricular flow, oxygen delivery to the left ventricle or oxygen consumption of the left ventricle.	138
Anesthetized with Isoflurane or Desflurane 1.2 MAC	100 µg/kg, IV	Modest increase in peripheral resistance, no change in other parameters measured	167
Surgical preparation which enabled the investigators to induce a stepwise decrease in hepatic blood supply without induced hepatic hypoperfusion	100 µg/kg, IV + 50 µg/kg/hr	Higher values of hepatic O_2 delivery than in pigs anesthetized with halothane, enflurane or pentobarbital. Hepatic lactate uptake started to decrease at higher values of hepatic oxygen delivery than in pigs anes. with pentobarbital, halothane, isoflurane or enflurane	168

Conditions of the Experiment	Dose	Cardiovascular Effects	References
2.5:8 Primates			
Instrumented under isoflurane, allowed to awaken for 4 hours, measurements made while conscious (n=6).	2, 4, 16, 64 and 128 µg/kg (cumulative dose = 214 µg/kg) each dose administered over 1 min. with 10 min. between doses.	Stroke volume decreased for 10 min. after final dose, cardiac output and mean aortic pressure decreased for 175 min, peripheral resistance decreased for 125 min, central venous pressure, and pulmonary arterial wedge pressure all not changed.	139

Table 2.6 Alfentanil

Conditions of the Experiment	Dose	Cardiovascular Effects	References
2.6:1 Dogs			
Anesthetized with methohexitone (13.6±0.9 mg/kg, IV), positive pressure ventilation, alpha - chloralose (33.9±0.1 mg/kg/h, IV infusion) suxamethonium (2 mg/kg/h) acute instrumentation.	500 µg/kg	Decreased heart rate and mean aortic pressure, decreased somato-cardiovascular reflexes (less effect than fentanyl). Dissociation between the maximum effect of alfentanil on the resting circulation and on the evoked cardiovascular reflexes.	90
Isolated hindlimb preparation, anesthetized with halothane (n=5).	50, 300 and 500 µg/kg of limb weight	Apparent dose-dependent decrease in resistance, significant only at high dose (48% decrease) in both innervated and denervated limb.	116

Conditions of the Experiment	Dose	Cardiovascular Effects	References
2.6:2 Rats			
Previously instrumented, conscious	50, 130, 260 and 500 µg/kg repeated after 1 hr, IV	Decreased heart rate and mean aortic blood pressure, second injection caused less response, i.e., tachyphylaxis	140

Conditions of the Experiment	Dose	Cardiovascular Effects	References
2.6:3 Rabbits			
Isolated cardiac tissues from animals killed by captive bolt.	Cumulative dose - response 0.001-0.5 mM	Atrial preps; no change in frequency of contraction, developed force, peak in developed force, max. rate of rise of developed force, time-to-peak developed force, max. rate of fall of developed force. Papillary muscle: no change in peak developed force, peak developed tension, dT/dt max, time-to-peak developed force, - dT/dt max, t50% relaxation.	141

Table 2.7 Sufentanil

Conditions of the Experiment	Dose	Cardiovascular Effects	References
2.7:1 Dogs			
Intact, awake previously instrumented, autonomic nervous system blocked with atropine (2 mg/kg) and hexamethonium (20mg/kg).	100-150 µg/kg over 15 min as loading dose then 150 µg/kg/hr IV infusion	No change in heart rate, left ventricular end-diastolic pressure, cardiac output, stroke volume, pH, arterial pCO_2, regional preload recruitable mark, (PRSW) length intercept, slope of PRSW/EDL, dP/dt, dP/dt 50, segmental shortening, increased mean aortic pressure, left ventricular systolic pressure, peripheral resistance and arterial pO_2	**142**
Isolated canine cardiac Purkinje fibers, dogs were anesthetized with pentobarbital (30 mg/kg, IV)	86-4 nM, 0.17 µM and 0.26 µM	Increased action potential duration at 50 and 90% repolarization at all three dose levels with dose response reaction. There was no change at 8.6 nM concentration.	**118**
Isoflurane anesthesia at IMAC.	12.7 ± 6.5 µg/kg plus 0.01 ± 0.00^2 µg/kg/min, titrated to maintain PET CO_2 at 50 mm/kg.	Reduction in the contribution of the central chemoreflexes to ventilatory drive and, consequently, a relative increase in the contribution from the peripheral chemoreflexes, decreased heart rate, mean arterial pressure, peripheral resistance; no change in cardiac output. Pulmonary arterial pressure, peripheral vascular resistance, wedge pressure, or central venous pressure; increase in stroke volume and pulmonary vascular resistance.	**143**
Isolated hind limb preparation, halothane anesthesia.	0.6, 3.6 and 6 µg/kg of limb weight.	Apparent dose-dependent decrease in resistance but only statistically significant at the high dose in both innervated and dennervated limbs.	**116**

Conditions of the Experiment	Dose	Cardiovascular Effects	References
2.7:1 Dogs			
Intact, awake, chronically instrumented	25 and 50 µg/kg, IV	Rate pressure product decreased at high dosage. No changes seen in left ventricular systolic pressure, or end diastolic pressure. dP/dt of the left ventricle, coronary blood flow diastolic velocity, segmental shortening, mean coronary blood flow velocity, diastolic coronary vascular resistance, mean coronary vascular resistance.	**144**
Intact, awake, previously instrumented	25 & 50 µg/kg, IV	Significant sinus or junctional brady-arrhythmia, no change in systemic or coronary hemodynamics	**169**

Table 2.8: Oxymorphone

Conditions of the Experiment	Dose	Cardiovascular Effects	References
2.8:1 Dogs			
Analgesic, chemical restraint dose-mixed in same syringe with triflurpromazine (1.1 mg/kg)	0.165 mg/kg SC, IM or IV	No data	**2**
Intact, awake, previously instrumented	0.4 mg/kg loading, plus 0.2 mg/kg x 3 total dose 1 mg/kg, IV	Decreased tidal volume, alveolar total volume, arterial pO_2, heart rate and a transient decrease in cardiac output. Increased breathing rate, arterial pCO_2, physiological dead space, base deficit, hemoglobin concentration, mean arterial pressure, transient increase in peripheral resistance, central venous pressure, mean pulmonary arterial pressure and pulmonary wedge pressures.	**145**

Conditions of the Experiment	Dose	Cardiovascular Effects	References
2.8:2 Cats			
Analgesic, chemical restraint dose-mixed in same syringe with triflurpromazine (1.1 mg/kg)	0.167 mg/kg SC, IM or IV	No data	2

Conditions of the Experiment	Dose	Cardiovascular Effects	References
2.8:3 Horses			
Analgesic dose	22-30 micro-g/kg	No data	2
Pain-free, adult, previously instrumented, awake	0.03 mg/kg, IV	Heart rate increased at 5 and 15 min post injection, back to baseline levels at 30 & 60 min. Cardiac output increased at 5 & 15 min. Back to baseline at 30 & 60 min. No change in pulmonary artery, right atrial or aortic pressures & no change in blood gases or respiratory rate.	42

Table 2.9: Naloxone

Conditions of the Experiment	Dose	Cardiovascular Effects	References
2.9:1 Dogs			
Anesthetized with piritamide (Dipitor, Janssen-2 mg/kg, IV), plus 0.5% halothane with nitrous oxide and oxygen, positive pressure ventilation, morphine (2.0 mg/kg) stabilized for 45 min then given naloxone dose.	15 mg/kg, IV bolus	Heart rate increased 73%, cardiac output increased 20%, mean aortic pressure increased 20%, no change in systemic resistance, left ventricular dP/dt max increased 25%, left ventricular dP/dt max IP increased 14%, however when preload and heart rate changes are taken into consideration probably no change in contractility. There was a 60% increase in myocardial oxygen demand and a 59% increase in coronary blood flow.	69

Conditions of the Experiment	Dose	Cardiovascular Effects	References
2.9:1 Dogs			
Anesthetized with pentobarbital (30 mg/kg, IV) acute open chest preparation	Increasing doses up to 5 mg/kg	No change in cardiovascular parameters being monitored	47
Anesthetized with pentobarbital (30 mg/kg, IV) additional pentobarb (1-2 mg/kg) as needed, acute preparation. Hemorrhagic shock to 45-58 mmHG for 60 mnin, then given dose of naloxone.	2 mg/kg, IV	Increased mean aortic pressure, cardiac output and left ventricular dP/dt max, also increased systemic resistance.	70
Anesthetized with pentobarbital (30 mg/kg, IV) endotoxic shock.	1 mg/kg, IV plus 1 mg/kg/hr and 2 mg/kg, IV plus 2 mg/kg, hr	Showed a dose dependent reversal of hypotension along with a dose dependent increase in left ventricular dP/dt and cardiac output.	71
Anesthetized with pentobarbital (30 mg/kg, IV)	2 mg/kg, IV	Slight increase in mean aortic pressure, no effect on other cardiovascular parameters measured.	72
Same as above plus *E. coli* endotoxin induced shock.	2 mg/kg, IV	Counteracted depressant effects of endotoxin on mean aortic pressure, cardiac output, and left ventricular dP/dt, 5 of 6 dogs survived.	72
Same	1 mg/kg, IV	Same as above but less effective and no effect on survival.	72
Anesthetized with ether, electrolytic decerebration, ether removed for more than 2½ hrs to allow for equilibration	1 mg/kg, IV	Pulse pressure increased from 88±13 to 96±15 mmHg, mean aortic pressure increased from 128±12 to 139±10 mmHg, heart rate increased from 138±24 to 157±22 beats/min and respiratory rate increased from 23±3 to 34±4 breaths/min.	54

Conditions of the Experiment	Dose	Cardiovascular Effects	References
2.9:1 Dogs			
Anesthetized with thiopental (12.5 mg/kg, IV0, gallamine (2 mg/kg, IV), repeated doses of thiopental (1 mg/kg, IV0 every 30 min.	0.1 mg/kg, IV	No change in blood pressure or heart rate prior to sino-aortic dennervation. After sino-aortic dennervation blood pressure and heart rate increased, this change not affected by Naloxone.	146
Anesthetized with piritamide (2.0 mg/kg) and halothane (0.5%) with nitrous oxide.	15 µg/kg, IV	Increased heart rate, cardiac output, mean aortic pressure, dP/dt max, dP/dt max/IP, coronary blood flow, coronary A-V O_2, and left ventricular O_2 consumption. Decreased stroke volume, central venous pressure, ejection fraction and coronary resistance. No change in peripheral resistance or left ventricular end diastolic pressure.	147
Anesthetized with pentobarbital (30 mg/kg, IV)	40 µg/kg	Significantly blunted baroreflex function, i.e., decreased by 55%.	148
Intact, awake, chronically instrumented, response to clonidine (10 µg/kg, IV)	1-10 µg/kg, IV	Clonidine decreased heart rate and mean arterial pressure and increased ventricular refractoriness. Naloxone blocked clonidine effects in a dose dependent fashion.	149
Intact, awake, previously instrumented, exercising.	1 mg/kg + 20 µk/kg/min	Increased plasma beta-endorphin and adrenocorticotropic hormone at rest, no effect on heart rate, mean aortic pressure, cardiac output, left ventricular dP/dt, dP/dt at 50 mmHg, dP/dt/P or plasma catecholamines. With exercise plasma beta-endorphin and adrenocorticotropic hormone increased. Normal exercise induced increases in the cardiovascular parameters were not blocked by Naloxone.	150

Conditions of the Experiment	Dose	Cardiovascular Effects	References
2.9:2 Cats			
Anesthetized with pentobarbital (42mg/kg, IP) supplemented with pentobarbital (4.2 mg/kg every 1-2 hr, IV), paralyzed with gallamine triethiodide (3 mg/kg, IV) positive pressure ventilation. measured electrical activity of chemoreceptor units.	0.2 g intra-carotid	Slight increase of spontaneous chemoreceptor discharge rate from carotid sinus nerve, greatly reduced chemoinhibition caused by morphine and caused a substantial reduction of the rapid, powerful inhibition of the chemoreceptor discharge caused by Methionine-enkephalin. Did not block the excitatory action of adenosine but did antagonize the depressant effect of intracarotid morphine.	**73-74**
Chloralose anesthesia (no dose given), artificial ventilation.	200 μg, IV, intra-ventricular brain or intracisternal	No effect on heart rate or blood pressure.	**151**

Conditions of the Experiment	Dose	Cardiovascular Effects	References
2.9:3 Rats			
Conscious, previously instrumented spontaneously hypertensive rats.	10 mg/kg, IV followed by 20-25 mg/kg/hr.	Blocked the long-lasting depressor response induced by a prolonged low frequency stimulation of the sciatic nerve.	**75**
Unanesthetized, previously instrumented.	0.1 mg/kg, IV	Reversed hypotensive effects of endotoxic, hypovolemic and spinal transection shock.	**71**
Isolated atria, spontaneously beating. Methionine-enkephalin antagonist action on positive chronotropic action of norepinephrine	10^{-7}M in bath.	Completely blocked the methionine-enkephalin blockade of the norepinephrine response.	**76**

Conditions of the Experiment	Dose	Cardiovascular Effects	References
2.9:3 Rats			
Anesthetized with urethane (1.4 g/kg, IP) acute occipital craniotomy, injection directly into the nucleus tractus solitarii (NTS)	10 ng	Depressor and bradycardia response to endorphin reduced by pretreatment into the NTS.	**77**
Anesthetized with thiopental (50 mg/kg, IP) and urethane (375 mg/kg, IV) for 5 min. + heparin 150 IU/kg, IV	2.5-10 mg/kg, IV	Potentiated pressor responses to epinephrine (2 µg/kg). At 5 mg/kg dose potentiated pressor responses to norepinephrine (1-4 µg/kg) and phenylephrine (10-50 µg/kg) and reflex pressor responses to 60 sec carotid occlusion. Naloxone had no effect on pressor responses to methoxamine (100 µg/kg), Angiotensin (0.5-2 µg/kg) or isoproterenol (1 µg/kg).	**152**
Pithed	2.5-10 mg/kg, IV	No effect on Naloxone induced potentiation of norepinephrine (0.25-0.5 µg/kg) pressor response.	**152**
Acute adrenalectomy	2.5-10 mg/kg, IV	Same as above.	**152**
Chemical sympathectomy, (6-hydroxydopamine)	Same.	Abolished the Naloxone response.	**152**
Isolated atrial preparation, following decapitation.	$1.4\text{-}2.8 \times 10^{-5}$ M	Potentiated chronotropic response to norepinephrine.	**152**
Conscious, previously instrumented.	0.03-3 mg/kg, IV increasing bolus doses over 3-4 min.	No change in mean aortic pressure or heart rate in either WKY or SHR rats.	**153**
Isolated atrial preparation, rats killed by a blow to the head.	51-340 µM	Electrically stimulated: there was a delayed dose-related decrease in atrial tension. Spontaneously beating: the same doses resulted in decrease heart rate and increased atrial tension.	**107**

Conditions of the Experiment	Dose	Cardiovascular Effects	References
2.9:4 Guinea Pigs			
Isolated atrial preparation, spontaneously beating.	0.25 g/ml 1 g/ml 100 g/ml	84% decrease in rate. 69% decrease in rate. 72% decrease in rate.	**37**
Excised atrial preparation, spontaneously beating.	0.25, 1 and 100μg/ml of both.	Decreased heart rate with lower dose having an enhanced effect.	**132**

Conditions of the Experiment	Dose	Cardiovascular Effects	References
2.9:5 Rabbits			
Intact, awake, previously instrumented.	4 mg/kg + 0.1 mg/kg/min.	Transient decrease in heart rate, no change in blood pressure or cardiac output.	**154**
Anesthetized with pentothal (15 mg/kg, IV), endotracheal tube then halothane. After instrumentation removed from halothane and given alpha-chloralose (45 mg/kg, IV) then pancuronium 0.8 mg, IV plus 0.2 mg each 30-40 min.	20 n mol in a 100 nl bilateral injection into the rostral ventrolateral medulla pressor region.	An initial decrease then an increase in mean aortic pressure and a decrease in heart rate.	**155**

Conditions of the Experiment	Dose	Cardiovascular Effects	References
2.9:6 Sheep			
Fetal sheep (120-130 days gestation) acute preparation	1 mg/kg into fetus	No change in fetal arterial blood gases or pH, heart rate tended to decrease but not significantly and a non-significant increase in aortic pressure, i.e. no significant changes seen.	**78**
Isolated Purkinje fiber preparation, slaughter house hearts.	10^{-4} to 10^{-7} M.	A direct electrophysiological effect on cardiac cells, probably explains its antiarrhythmic action.	**156**

Conditions of the Experiment	Dose	Cardiovascular Effects	References
2.9:6 Sheep			
Chronically catheterized fetal lambs, in utero.	2 mg/kg, IV infusion.	Augmentation of catecholamine response to hypoxia. No change in pH, pO_2, norepinephrine levels, heart rate or mean aortic pressures in the fetuses.	157

Conditions of the Experiment	Dose	Cardiovascular Effects	References
2.9:7 Primates			
Cynomolgus monkeys, conscious, previously instrumented.	10 mg/kg	Decreased mean aortic pressure response to Angiotensin II.	158
Same.	3 mg/kg.	Decreased heart rate response to Angiotensin II.	158

Table 2.10 Butorphanol

Conditions of the Experiment	Dose	Cardiovascular Effects	References
2.10:1 Dogs			
Halothane anesthetized.	No dose given.	No change in aortic systolic pressure, cardiac output, stroke volume, peripheral resistance, pH, $PaCO_2$, PO_2, bicarbonate, pulmonary arterial pressure and pulmonary arterial wedge pressure. Significant decreases in diastolic and mean aortic pressures.	160
Excised saphenous vein rings.	5×10^{-6}	Decreased contractile response to electrical stimulation, apparent presynaptic action, significant decrease in endogenous norepinephrine release.	162

Conditions of the Experiment	Dose	Cardiovascular Effects	References
2.10:2 Guinea Pigs			
Excised atrial preparation, spontaneously beating.	0.25, 1 and 100 µg/ml of both.	Potent decrease in heart rate.	**132**

Table 2.11 Buprenorphine

Conditions of the Experiment	Dose	Cardiovascular Effects	References
2.11:1 Dogs			
Ketamine (7-9 mg/kg/M) alpha-chloralose (100 mg/kg)	0.3 mg/kg, IV	Decreased heart rate and mean aortic pressure. Second dose had less effect on heart rate, further depressed blood pressure.	**114**

Table 2.12: Etorphine

Conditions of the Experiment	Dose	Cardiovascular Effects	References
2.12:1 Dogs			
Anesthetized with pentobarbital (36mg/kg, IV)	1 mg/kg, IV	Heart rate decreased with marked sinus arrhythmia, mean aortic pressure decreased about 33 mmHg. Effects developed in 1-10 min. with a >60 min duration.	**79**

Conditions of the Experiment	Dose	Cardiovascular Effects	References
2.12:2 Cats			
Anesthetized with ether and maintained with chloralose (50 mg/kg, IV)	0.1-5 µg/kg, IV	Heart rate decreased about 50%, mean aortic pressure decreased about 48 mmHg, onset 5-10 min, duration >60 min.	**79**

Conditions of the Experiment	Dose	Cardiovascular Effects	References
2.12:3 Rats			
Awake, instrumented	6, 12 and 24 μg/kg, SC	Heart rate decreased, mean aortic pressure decreased, respiratory rate decreased. Maximum effect 20 min. following injection, duration of 30-60 min.	**79**
Pentobarbital (50 mg/kg, IP), ventilated with room air.	0.1 μg/kg, IV	Decreased heart rate and mean aortic pressure.	**159**

Conditions of the Experiment	Dose	Cardiovascular Effects	References
2.12:4 Guinea Pigs			
Isolated atrial prep.	1-4 M	Dose dependent reduction in sympathetic response induced by trains of field pulses in atria stimulated at 4 Hz. Effect was antagonized by 10 M naloxone. Did not modify dose dependent inotropic effect curve of exogenous norepinephrine in same preparation, therefore depressant effect may be due to stimulation of presynaptic inhibitory opiate receptors on adrenergic nerve terminals in the heart.	**80**

Conditions of the Experiment	Dose	Cardiovascular Effects	References
2.12:5 Rhesus Monkeys			
Anesthetized with pentobarbital (30 mg/kg, IP)	1 μg/kg, IV	Decreased heart rate and blood pressure. Respiration usually completely arrested for 1-2 min. but recovered spontaneously.	**79**

Conditions of the Experiment	Dose	Cardiovascular Effects	References
2.12:6 Horses			
Awake	22 µg/kg, IV	Increased heart rate and blood pressure, remained elevated until deprenorphine (antagonist) given. Plasma noradrenaline levels increased from 0.73 p mole/ml to 4.04 p mole/ml.	**81**

Table 2.13: Etomidate

Conditions of the Experiment	Dose	Cardiovascular Effects	References
2.13:1 Dogs			
Nitrous oxide analgesia, stimulation of the carotid baroreceptors using a neck pressure device.	0.3-1.2 mg total dose.	No impairment of baroreceptor response.	**59**
Intact, awake, previously instrumented.	4 mg/kg, IV	No change in heart rate, decreased aortic pressure and LV dP/dt max. Cardiac output decreased while the dogs were anesthetized.	**96**

Conditions of the Experiment	Dose	Cardiovascular Effects	References
2.13:2 Pigs			
Premedicated with Azaperone (120 mg IM), 30 min later sedated with metomidate (150 mg, IV), Pancuronium (2 mg/kg/h), positive press. vent. with N_2O in O_2 (2:1), open chest, acute instrumentation.	30 min infusions of 0.03, 0.06, 0.12 and 0.24 mg/kg/min.	Moderate but dose-dependent decrease in cardiac output, aortic pressure and LV dP/dt max. Decreased myocardial wall thickening, no change in heart rate, myocardial blood flow distribution, myocardial metabolism of lactate, glucose or free fatty acids. Decreased cerebral blood flow substantially, slight decrease in renal blood flow but ony after the first dose.	**97**

Conditions of the Experiment	Dose	Cardiovascular Effects	References
2.13:3 Rabbits			
Decerebrated or pithed, anesthetized with 3% halothane in O_2, after surgery completed were allowed to recover, gallamine (1 mg/kg every 40 min), positive pressure vent. with 100% O_2	0.5-8 mg/kg	Decerebrate, dose-related (after ≥2 mg/kg) decrease in mean aortic pressure and preganglionic sympathetic nerve activity. No change in heart rate or baroreceptor reflex. Pithed-effects of shorter duration and less magnitude. Decerebrate results probably due to depression of central cardiovascular control. At anesthesia levels from 0.5-1 mg/kg no effects, larger doses marked decrease in central CV control, myocardium and peripheral vasculature.	**98**

Conditions of the Experiment	Dose	Cardiovascular Effects	References
2.13:4 Cats			
Isolated heart-lung preparations	0.5-8 mg/kg	Decerebrate, dose-related (after ≥2 mg/kg) decrease in mean aortic pressure and preganglionic sympathetic nerve activity. No change in heart rate or baroreceptor reflex. Pithed-effects of shorter duration and less magnitude. Decerebrate results probably due to depression of central cardiovascular control. At anesthesia levels from 0.5-1 mg/kg no effects, larger doses marked decrease in central CV control, myocardium and peripheral vasculature.	**98**

Table 2.14 Dynorphin A and Dynorphin A (1-13)

Conditions of the Experiment	Dose	Cardiovascular Effects	References
2.14:1 Rats			
Conscious, previously instrumented.	10-20 nmol, Intrathecal infusion into the lower thoracic spinal space.	Increased blood pressure and decreased heart rate, mediated by spinal cord mu-opiod receptors independent of arginine vasopressin receptors.	**161**

Table 2.15: Nalbuphine

Conditions of the Experiment	Dose	Cardiovascular Effects	References
2.15:1 Dogs			
Excised saphenous vein rings.	$< 5 \times 10^{-5}$ M	No effect on contractile response to electrical stimulation.	**162**

Conditions of the Experiment	Dose	Cardiovascular Effects	References
2.15:2 Guinea Pigs			
Excised atrial preparations, spontaneously beating.	0.25, 1 and 100 μg/ml of bath.	Lower dose had enhanced effect on lowering heart rate.	**132**

Table 2.17: d-Codeine

Conditions of the Experiment	Dose	Cardiovascular Effects	References
2.17:1 Cats			
Anesthetized with Pentobarbital (35mg/	1 mg/kg, IV	No change in mean aortic pressure or heart rate.	**83**
	2 mg/kg, IV	30% decrease in mean aortic pressure, 20% decrease in heart rate.	
	3 mg/kg, IV	64% decrease in mean aortic pressure, 20% decrease in heart rate.	
	4 mg/kg, IV	65% decrease in mean aortic pressure, 22% decrease in heart rate.	

Table 2.18: l-Codeine

Conditions of the Experiment	Dose	Cardiovascular Effects	References
2.18:1 Cats			
Same as above.	0.54 mg/kg,IV 2.5 mg/kg,IV	18% decrease in mean aortic pressure. 30% decrease in mean aortic pressure.	**83**

Table 2.19: Propoxyphene

Conditions of the Experiment	Dose	Cardiovascular Effects	References
2.19:1 Cats			
Isolated right ventricular papillary muscle.	10^{-5}M in bath.	Decrease maximum developed isometric tension and dT/dt. Not responsive to electrical stimulation at this concentration.	**84**

Table 2.20: Norpropoxyphene

Conditions of the Experiment	Dose	Cardiovascular Effects	References
2.20:1 Horses			
Awake, previously instrumented, pain-free, apparently causes dose-dependent excitatory effects similar to the narcotic analgesics.	0.5 and 1.0 mg/kg 2.2 mg/kg	No change in measured parameters. Increased heart rate and mean aortic pressure t 1/2 61-135 min, dose-dependent, rate-related decrease in P-R and Q-T intervals.	**82**

References

1.   Parker, J.L., Adams, H.R. The influence of chemical restraining agents on cardiovascular function: a review, Ketamine, *Lab Anim Sci*, 28 (5):575-583, 1978.

2.   Booth, N.H. Introduction to Drugs Acting on the Central Nervous System. Section 4 in *Veterinary Pharmacology and Therapeutics, 5th ed.*, ed. by N.H. Booth and L.E. McDonald, The Iowa State University Press, Ames, Iowa, 1982.

3.   Vatner, S.F., Marsh, J.D., Swain, J.A. Effects of morphine on coronary and left ventricular dynamics on conscious dogs, *J Clin Invest*, 55:207-217, 1975.

4.   Vater, S.F. Effects of anesthesia on cardiovascular control mechanisms, *Environ Health Perspect*, 26:193-206, 1978.

5.   DeSilva, R.A., Verrier, R.L., Loron, B. The effects of psychological stress and vagal stimulation with morphine on vulnerability to ventricular fibrillation in the conscious dog, *Am Heart J*, 95(2):197-203, 1978.

6.   Priano, L.L., Vatner, S.F. Morphine effects on cardiac output and regional blood flow distribution in conscious dogs, *Anesthesiology,* 55(3):236-243, 1981.

7.   Schmidt, C.F., Livington, A. The action of morphine in the mammalian circulation, *J Pharmacol Exp Ther*, 47:411-441, 1933.

8.   Henney, R.P., Vasko, J.S., Brawley, R.K., Oldham, H.N., Morrow, A.G. The effects of morphine on the resistance and capacitance vessels of the peripheral circulation, *Am Heart J*, 72:242-250, 1966.

9.   Lewis, A.J., Kirchner, T. A comparison of the cardiorespiratory effects of ciramadol, dezocine, morphine and pentazocine in the anesthetized dog. Morphine/Pharmacodynamics, *Arch Int Pharmacodyn Ther,* 250(1):73-83, 1981.

10.   Buylaert, W.A., Williems, J.L., Bogaert, M.G. Vasodilatation produced by apomorphine in the hindleg of the dog, *J Pharmacol Exp Ther*, 201(3):738-746, 1977.

11.   Green, J.F., Jackman, A.P., Krohn, K.A. Mechanism if morphine-induced shifts in blood volume between extracorporeal reservoir and the systemic circulation of the dog under conditions of constant blood flow and vena caval pressures, *Circ Res*, 42(4):479-486, 1978.

12.   Green, J.F., Jackman, A.P., Parsons, G. The effects of morphine on the mechanical properties of the systemic circulation in the dog, *Circ Res*, 42(4):474-478, 1978.

13.   Slogoff, S., Keats, A.S., Hibbs, C.W., Edmonds, C.H., Bragg, D.A. Failure of general anesthesia to potentiate propranolol activity, *Anesthesiology*, 47(6):504-508, 1977.

14.   Berthelsen, P., Erksen, J., Ahn, N.C., Rasmussen, J.P. Peripheral circulation during sufentanyl and morphine anesthesia, *Acta Anaesthesiol Scand*, 24(3):241-244, 1980.

15.   Lind, R.E., Reynolds, D.G., Ganes, E.M., Jenkins, J.T. Morphine effects on cardiovascular performance, *Am Surg*, 47(3):107-111, 1981.

16.   Kobinger, W., Pichler, L. Differentiation of drugs acting centrally upon the cardiovascular system by means of sympathetic and vagal responses, *Clin Exp Hypertens*, 1(2):229-249, 1978.

17.   DeSilva, R.A., Verrier, R.L., Loron, B. Protective effect of the vagotonic action of morphine sulphate on ventricular vulnerability, *Cardiovasc Res*, 12:167-172, 1978.

18.   Lee, D.C., Clifford, D.H., Lee, M.O., Nelson, L. Reversal by acupuncture of cardiovascular depression induced with morphine during halothane anaesthesia in dogs, *Can Anaesth Soc J*, 28(2):129-135, 1981.

19.   Schrank, K.P., Fewel, J.G., Arom, K.V., Trinkle, J.K., Webb, G.E., Grover, F.L. Effects of morphine anesthesia on myocardial contractility, blood flow and metabolism, *J Surg Res*, 28(4):319-327, 1980.

20.   Hageman, G.R., Urthaler, F., James, T.N. Cyproheptadine blockade of a cardiogenic hypertensive chemoreflex, *Proc Soc Exp Biol Med*, 154(4):578-581, 1977.

21.   Chand, N., Altura, B.M. Reactivity and contractility of rat main pulmonary artery to vasoactive agents, *J Appl Physiol*, 49(6):1016-1021, 1980.

22.   Flaim, S.F., Vismara, L.A., Zelis, R. The effects of morphine on isolated cutaneous canine vascular smooth muscle, *Res Commun Chem Path Pharmacol*, 16(1):191-194, 1977.

23.   Muldoon, S., Otto, J., Freas, W., Watson, R.L. The effects of morphine, nalbuphine and butorphanol on adrenergic function in canine saphenous vein, *Anesth Analg*, 62:21-28, 1983.

24.   McQueen, D.S., Ribeiro, J.A. Inhibitory actions of methionine-enkephalin and morphine on the cat carotid chemoreceptor, *Br J Pharmacol*, 71(1):297-305, 1980.

25.   Feldberg, W., Wei, E. The central origin and mechanism of cardiovascular effects of morphine as revealed by naloxone in cats, *J Physiol*, 272:99-100, 1977.

26.   Strauer, B.E. Contractile responses to morphine, piritramide, meperidine and fentanyl: A comparative study of effects on the isolated ventricular myocardium, *Anesthesiology*, 37:304-310, 1972.

27.   Hamko, J.H., Hardebo, J.E. Enkephalin-induced dilatation of pial arteries in vitro probably medicated by opiate receptors, *Eur J Pharmacol*, 51(3):295-297, 1978.

28.   Markiewicz, W., Finberg, J.P.M., Lichtig, C. Morphine increases myocardial infarction size in rats, *Anesth Analg,* 61:843-846, 1982.

29.   Willette, R.N., Sapree, H.N. Peripheral versus central cardiorespiratory effects of morphine, *Neuropharmacol*, 21:1019-1026, 1982.

30.   Weinberg, J., Altura, B.M. Morphine pretreatment influences reactivity of isolated rat arterial smooth muscle, *Substance Alcohol Actions/Misuse*, 1:71-81, 1980.

31.   Pleuvry, B.J. A study of enhanced toxicity of doxapram in rodents treated with narcotic analgesics, *Br J Anaesth*, 50(5):451-458, 1978.

32. Chand, N., Altura, B.M. Serotonin receptors subserve only contraction in canine and rat pulmonary arteries and veins, *Artery*, 7(3):232-245, 1980.

33. Moore, A.F. The interaction of enkephalins with substance P on vascular smooth muscle, *Res Commun Chem Pathol Pharmacol*, 23(2):233-242, 1979.

34. Bhargara, H.N., Kasabdji, D., Thompson, E.B. Subsensitivity to noradrenaline and isoprenaline in rabbits acutely pre-treated with morphine, *Gen Pharmac*, 8:257-261, 1977.

35. Raye, J.R., Dubin, J.W., Blechner, J.N. Alterations in fetal metabolism subsequent to maternal morphine administration, *Am J Obstet Gynecol*, 136(4):505-508, 1980.

36. Koo, A., Wong, T.M. Cross tolerance between morphine and alpha-endorphin in the in vivo vasodilating effect in the hamster cheek pouch, *Life Sci*, 32:475-477, 1983.

37. Gintautas, J., Kraynack, B.J., Cockings, E., Harasi, G. Depression of atrium function by narcotics, *Proc West Pharmacol Soc*, 25:55-56, 1982.

38. Moores, W.Y., Weiskopf, R.B., Dembitsky, W.P., Utley, J.R. Comparative effects of halothane and morphine anesthesia on myocardial function and metabolism during cyanosis in swine, *Surg Forum*, 30:221-223, 1979.

39. Craft, J.B. Jr, Bolan, J.C., Coaldrake, L.A., Mondino, M., Mazel, P., Gilman, R.M., Shokes, L.K., Woolf, W.A. The maternal and fetal cardiovascular effects of epidural morphine to sheep model, *Am J Obstet Gynecol*, 142(7):835-839, 1982.

40. Wong, T.M., Li, C.H. Alpha-endorphin, vasodilating effect on the microcirculatory system of hamster cheek pouch, *Inst J Peptide Protein Res*, 18:420-422, 1981.

41. Kohn, C.W. Preparative management of the equine patient with an abdominal crisis, *Vet Clin N Am (Lg Anim Proc)*, 1(2):289-311, 1979.

42. Muir, W.W., Sams, R.A., Huffman, R. Cardiopulmonary behavioral and pharmacokinetics effects of propoxyphene in horses, *Am J Vet Res*, 41(4):575-580, 1980.

43. Muir, W.W., Skarda, R.T., Sheehan, W. In Equine Pharmacology, ed. by J.D. Powers, Proceedings of the 2nd Equine Pharmacology Symposium, Golden, CO: *Am Assoc Eq Pract*, p.173, 1978.

44. Clifford, D. in Textbook of Veterinary Anesthesia, ed. by L.R. Soma, Williams & Wilkins, Baltimore. 385-393, 1971.

45. Goldberg, S.J., Linde, L.M., Wolfe, R.R., Griswold, W., Momma, K. The effects of meperidine, promethazine and chlorpromazine on pulmonary and systemic circulation, *Am Heart J*, 77:214-221, 1969.

46. Priano, L.L., Vatner, S.F. Generalized cardiovascular and regional hemodynamic effects of meperidine in conscious dogs, *Anesth Analg*, 60(9):649-654, 1981.

47. Freye, E. Cardiovascular effects of high dosages of fentanyl, meperidine and naloxone in dogs, *Anesth Analg*, 53:40-47, 1974.

48. Stanley, T.H., Liu, W.S., Webster, L.R. Haemodynamic effects of intravenous methadone anaesthesia in dogs, *Can Anaesth Soc J*, 27:52-56, 1980.

49. Slotkin, T.A., Seidler, F.J., Whitmore, W.L. Effects of maternal methadone administration on ornithine decarboxylase in brain and heart of the offspring: relationships of enzyme activity to dose and to growth impairment in the rat, *Life Sci*, 17:26(11):861-867, 1980.

50. Bareis, D.L., Slotkin, T.A. Responses of heart ornithine decarboxylase and adrenal catecholamines to methadone and sympathetic stimulants in developing and adult rats, *J Pharmacol Exp Ther*, 205(1):164-174, 1978.

51. Lee, C.H., Berkowitz, B.A. Calcium antagonist activity of methadone, I-acetylmethadol and I-pentazocine in the rat aortic strip, *J Pharmacol Exp Ther*, 202(3):646-653, 1977.

52. Bareis, D.L., Slotkin, T.A. Maturation of sympathetic neurotransmission in the rat heart. I. Ontogeny of the synaptic vesicle uptake mechanism and correlation with development of synaptic vesicles, *J Pharmacol Exp Ther*, 2012(1):120-125, 1980.

53. Kucukhusseyin, C. Some effects of pentazocine and cyclazocine on the isolated guinea-pig atria, *Arch Int Pharmacodyn Ther*, 225(1):114-123, 1977.

54. Wu, K.M., Martin, W.R. Effects of naloxone and fentanyl inacutely decerebrated dogs, *Life Sci*, 31(2):151-157, 1982.

55. Freye, E., Arndt, J.O. Perfusion of the fourth cerebral ventricle with fentanyl induces naloxone-reversible bradycardia, hypotension and EEG synchronization in conscious dog, *Naunyn-Schmiedeberg's Arch Pharmacol*, 307:123-128, 1979.

56. Henney, R.P., Vasko, J.S., Brawley, R.K., Oldham, H.N., Morrow, A.G. The effect of morphine on the resistance and capacitance vessels of the peripheral circulation, *Am Heart J*, 72(2):242-250, 1966.

57.   Freye, E. The effect of fentanyl on the resistance and capacitance vessels of the dog's hindlimb, *Arzneim-Forsch/Drug Res*, 27(5):1037-1039, 1977.

58.   Laubie, M., Schmitt, H., Drouillat, M. Central sites and mechanisms of the hypotensive and bradycardic effects of the narcotic analgesic agent fentanyl, *Naunyn-Schmiedeberg's Arch Pharmacol*, 296:255-261, 1977.

59.   Arndt, J.O., Mameghani, F. The effect of etomidate, fentanyl and dehydrobenzperidol on baroreflex function. A study on dog's carotid sinus reflex (author's transl.), *Anaesthesist*, (4):200-207, 1980.

60.   van der Vusse, G.J., Coumans, W.A., Kruger, R., Verlaan, C., Reneman, R.S. Effect of fentanyl ion myocardial fatty acid and carbohydrate metabolism and oxygen utilization during experimental ischemia, *Anesth Analg (Cleve)*, 59(9):644-654, 1980.

61.   Reneman, R.S., van der Vusse, G.T. Effect of fentanyl on myocardial metabolism during ischemia, *Angiology*, 33(1):51-63, 1982.

62.   Inoue, K., Samodelor, L.F., Arndt, J.O. Fentanyl activates a particular population of vagal efferentes which are cardioinhibitory, *Naunyn-Schmiedebergs Arch Pharmacol*, 312(1):57-61, 1980.

63.   van der Vusse, G.J., van Belle, H., van Gersen, W., Kruger, R., Reneman, R.S. Acute effect of fentanyl on haemodynamics and myocardial carbohydrate utilization and phosphate release during ischaemia, *Br J Anaesth*, 51(10):927-935, 1979.

64.   Laubie, M., Schmitt, H. Action of the morphinometric agent, fentanyl, on the nucleus tractus solitarii and the nucleus ambiguous cardiovascular neurons, *Eur J Pharmacol*, 67(4):403-412, 1980.

66.   Kedem, J., Zurouski, Y., Miller, H., Batter, A. Effect of reserpine upon the haemodynamic cause of recovery following experimental myocardial infarction, *Arch International e de Physiol et de Bioch*, 88:427-436, 180.

67.   MacLeod, B.A., Augereau, P., Walker, M.J. Effects of halothane anesthesia compared with fentanyl anesthesia and no anesthesia during coronary ligation in rats, *Anesthesiology*, 58(2):84-92, 1982.

68.   Merin, R.G., Verdouw, P.D., de Jong, J.W. Myocardial functional and metabolic responses to ischemia in swine during halothane and fentanyl anesthesia, *Anesthesiology*, 56(2):84-92, 1982.

69.   Patschke, D., Eberlein, H.J., Hess, W., Tarnow, J., Zimmerman, G. Antagonism of morphine with naloxone in dogs: Cardiovascular effects with special reference to the coronary circulation, *Br J Anaesth*, 49:525-533, 1977.

70.   Vargish, T., Reynolds, D.G., Gurll, N.J., Ganes, E.M., Lutz, S.A. The interaction of corticosteroids and naloxone in canine hemorrhagic shock, *J Surg Res*, 32(3):289-295, 1982.

71.   Faden, A.I., Holaday, J.W. Experimental endotoxin shock: the pathophysiologic function of endorphins and treatment with opiate antagonists, *J Infec Dis*, 142(2):229-238, 1980.

72.   Reynolds, D.G., Gurll, N.J., Vargish, T., Lechner, R.B., Faden, A.I., Holaday, J.W. Blockade of opiate receptors with naloxone improves survival and cardiac performance in canine endotoxic shock, *Circ Shock*, 7(1):39-48, 1980.

73.   McQueen, D.S., Ribeiro, J.A. Inhibitory actions of methionine-enkephalin and morphine on the cat carotid chemoreceptor, *Br J Pharmacol*, 74(1)297-305, 1980.

74.   McQueen, D.S., Ribeiro, J.A. Effects of adenosine on carotid chemoreceptor activity in the cat, *Br J Pharmacol*, 74(1):129-136, 1981.

75.   Yao, T., Anderson, S., Thoren, P. Long-lasting cardiovascular depressor response following sciatic stimulation in spontaneously hypertensive rats. Evidence for the involvement of central endorphin and serotonin systems, *Brain Res*, 244(2):295-303, 1982.

76.   Eiden, L.E., Ruth, J.A. Enkephalins modulate the responsiveness of rat atria in vitro to norepinephrine, *Peptides*, 3(3):475-478, 1982.

77.   Petty, M.A., de Jong, W., de Wild, D. An inhibitory role of beta-endorphin in central cardiovascular regulation, *Life Sci*, 30(21):1835-1840, 1982.

78.   La Gamma, E.F., Itskovitz, J., Rudolph, A.M. Effects of naloxone on fetal circulatory responses to hypoxemia, *Am J Obstet Gynecol*, 143(3):933-940, 1982.

79.   Blane, G.F., Boura, A.L.A., Fitzgerald, A.E., Lister, R.E. Actions of Etorphine HCI, (M99): A Potent Morphine-like Agent, *Br J Pharmacol Chemotherapy*, 30:11-22, 1967.

80.   Ledda, F., Mantelli, L. Possible presynaptic inhibitory effect of etorphine on sympathetic nerve terminals of guinea-pig heart, *Eur J Pharmacol*, 85(2):247-250, 1981.

81.   Bogan, J.A., MacKenzie, G., Snow, D.H. An evaluation of tranquilizers for use with etorphine as neuroleptanalgesic agents in the horse, *Vet Rec*, 103(21):471-472, 1978.

82. Muir, W.W., Skarda, R.T., Sheehan, W.C. Cardiopulmonary effects of narcotic agonists and a partial agonist in horses, *Am J Vet Res*, 39:1632-1635, 1978.

83. Chau, T.T., Harris, L.S. Comparative studies of the pharmacological effects of the d- and l-isomers of codeine, *Natl Inst Drug Abuse Res Monogr Series*, 34:58-63, 1981.

84. Amsterdam, E.A., Rendig, S.V., Henderson, G.L., Mason, D.T. Depression of myocardial contractile function by propoxyphene and norpropoxyphene, *J Cardiovasc Pharmacol*, 3(1):129-138, 1981.

85. Lees, P., Hillidge, C.J. Neuroleptanalgesia and cardiovascular function in the horse, *Equine Vet J*, 7(4):184-191, 1975.

86. Chiba, S. Effect of morphine on the S.A. node of the dog, *Arch Int Pharmacodyn*, 206:129-134, 1973.

87. Kisin, I., Markiewica, W., Birkhahn, J. Effect of large doses of morphine on experimental myocardial ischemia in cats, *Isr J Med Sci*, 15(7):588-591, 1979.

88. Ramirez, A.J., Enero, M.A. Blood pressure and heart rate response to apomorphine in urethane anesthetized rats, *Acta Physiol Lat Am*, 30(3):199-203, 1981.

89. Inoue, K., Samodelov, L.F., Arndt, J.O. Fentanyl activates a particular population of vagal efferents which are cardioinhibitory, *Naunyn-Schmiedebergs Arch Pharmacol*, 312(1):57-61, 1980.

90. skitopoulou, H., Whitwam, J.G., Sapsed, A., Chakrabarti, M.K. Dissociation between the effects of fentanyl and alfentanil on spontaneous and reflexly evoked cardiovascular responses in the dog, *Br J Anaesth*, 55(2):155-161, 1983.

91. van der Vusse, G.J., van Belle, H., van Gerven, W., Kruger, R., Reneman, R.S. Acute effect of fentanyl on haemodynamics and myocardial carbohydrate utilization and phosphate release during ischaemia, *Br J Anaesth*, 51(10):927:935, 1979.

92. Bjertnaes, L., Hauge, A., Kritz, M. Hypoxia-induced pulmonary vasoconstriction: effects of fentanyl following different routes of administration, *Acta Anaesthesiol Scand*, 24(1):53-7, 1980.

93. Mergner, G.W., Gilman, R.W., Woolf, W.A., Patch, J.H. Effect of halothane and fentanyl on myocardial infarct size and regional blood flow distribution, *Anesthesiol*, 57(3), A17, 1982.

94. Priano, L.L. Renal vasculature and high dose fentanyl, *Anesthesiol*, 57(3), A32, 1982.

95. Freye, E., Gupta, B.N. Cardiovascular effects on selective perfusion of the 4th cerebral ventricle in cats with fentanyl, naloxone and methohexital, *Indian J Exp Biol*, 18(1):29-31, 1980.

96. Twissell, D.J., Dodds, M.G. The systemic hemodynamic effects of minaxolone: A comparison with other anesthetics in the dog. Meeting of the Anaesthetic Research Society, Glasgow, Scotland, *Br J Anaesth*, 1979.

97. Prakash, O., Dhasmana, K.M., Verdouw, P.D., Saxena, P.R. Cardiovascular effects of etomidate with emphasis on regional myocardial blood flow and performance, *Br J Anaesth*, 53(6):591-600, 1981.

98. Hughes, R.L., MacKenzie, J.E. An investigation of the centrally and peripherally mediated cardiovascular effects of etomidate in the rabbit, *Br J Anaesth*, 50(2):101-108, 1978.

99. Fischer, K.J., Marquort, H. Experimental Investigations on the Direct Effect of Etomidote on Myocardial Contractility. Anesthesiology and Resuscitation, Vol. 106, ed. by A. Doenicke, Springer-Verlag: Berlin, West Germany. 95-112, 1977.

100. Lind, R.E., Reynolds, D.G., Ganes, E.M., Jenkins, J.T. Morphine effects on cardiovascular performance, *Am Surg*, 47:107-11, 1981.

101. Alcaraz, C., Barnsinath, M., Turndorf, H., Puig, M.M. Cardiovascular effects of morphine during hypothermia, *Arch Int Pharmacodyn Ther*, 29:133-147, 1989.

102. Agarwal, R.K., Pandey, U.S., Dixit, K.S., Shukla, N. Role of dopaminergic system in opioid-induced cardiovascular responses in dogs, *Indian J Med Sci*, 43(12):323-328, 1989.

103. Thornhill, J.A., Townsend, C., Gregor, L. Intravenous morphine infusion (IMF) to drug-naive, conscious rats evokes bradycardic, hypotensive effects, but pressor actions are elicited after IMF to rats previously given morphine, *Can J Phys Pharmacol*, 67(3):213-222, 1989.

104. May, C.N., Ham, I.W., Heslop, K.E., Stone, F.A., Mathias, C.J. Intravenous morphine causes hypertension, hyperglycemia and increases sympathoadrenal outflow in conscious rabbits, *Clin Sci*, 75(1):71-77, 1988.

105. Laorden, M.L., Hernandez, J., Carceles, M.D., Miralles, F.S., Puig,, M.M., Interaction between halothane and morphine on isolated heart muscle, *Eur J Pharmacol*, 175(3):285-290, 1990.

106.   Thornhill, J., St Onge, R., Gregor, L. Naloxone's effect on the inotropic and chronotropic responses of isolated, electrically stimulated or spontaneously beating rat atria, *Can J Physiol Pharmacol*, 68(3), 392-401, 1990.

107.   Nawrath, H., Rupp, J., Jakob, H., Sack, U., Mertzlufft, F., Dick, W. Failure of opioids to affect excitation and contraction in isolated ventricular heart muscle, *Experientia*, 45(4):337-339, 1989.

108.   May, C.N., Whitehead, C.J., Heslop, K.E., Mathias, C.J. Evidence that intravenous morphine stimulates central opiate receptors to increase sympathoadrenal outflow and cause hypertension in conscious rabbits, *Clin Sci*, 76(4):431-437, 1989.

109.   May, C.N., Ham, I.W., Heslop, K.E., Stone, F.A., Mathias, C.J. Intravenous morphine causes hypertension, Hyperglycemia, and increases sympathoadrenal outflow in conscious rabbits, *Clin Sci*, 75:71-77, 1988.

110.   Koo, A., Wong, T.M. Cross tolerance between morphine and B-endorphin in the in vivo vasodilating effect in the hamster cheek pouch, *Life Sci*, 32:475-477, 1983.

111.   Zhu, Y.S., Szeto, H.H. Morphine-induced tachycardia in fetal lambs: a bellshaped dose-response curve, *J Pharmacol Exp Ther*, 249(1):78-82, 1989.

112.   Helgesen, K.G., Ellingsen, O., llebekk, A. Inotropic effect of meperidine: influence of receptor and ion channel blockers in the rat atrium, *Anesth Analg*, 70(5):499-506, 1990.

113.   Saini, V., Carr, D.B., Verrier, R.L. Comparative effects of the opioids fentanyl and buprenorphine on ventricular vulnerability during acute coronary artery occlusion, *Cardiovasc Res*, 23(12):1001-1006, 1989.

114.   Royster, R.L., Keeler, D.K., Haisty, W.K., Johnson, W.E., Prough, D.S. Cardiac electrophysiologic effects of fentanyl and neuromuscular relaxants in pentobarbital-anesthetized dogs, *Anesth Analg*, 67(1):15-20, 1988.

115.   White, D.A., Reitan, J.A., Kien, N.D., Thorup, S.J. Decrease in vascular resistance in the isolated canine hindlimb after graded doses of alfentanil, fentanyl, and sufentanil, *Anesth Analg*, 71(1):29-34, 1990.

116.   Mills, C.A., Flacke, J.W., Miller, J.D., Davis, L.J., Bloor, B.C., Flacke, W.E. Cardiovascular effects of fentanyl reversal by naloxone at varying arterial carbon dioxide tensions in dogs, *Anesth Analg*, 67(8):730-736, 1988.

117.   Blair, J.R., Pruett, J.K., Introna, R.P., Adams, R.J., Balser, J.S. Cardiac electrophysiologic effects of fentanyl and sufentanil in canine cardiac Purkinje fibers, *Anesthes*, 71(4):565-570, 1989.

118.   Rorie, D.K., Muldoon, S.M., Tyce, G.M. Effects of fentanyl on adrenergic function in canine coronary arteries, *Anesth Analg (Cleve)*, 60(1):21-27, 1981.

119.   Saini, V., Carr, D.B., Hagestad, E.L., Lown, B., Verrier, R.L. Antifibrillatory action of the narcotic agonist fentanyl, *Am Heart J*, 115(3):598-605, 1988.

120.   Blaise, G.A., Witzeling, T.M., Sill, J.C., Vinay, P., Vanhoutte, P.M. Fentanyl is devoid of major effects on coronary vasoreactivity and myocardial metabolism in experimental animals, *Anesthes*, 72(3):535-541, 1990.

121.   Freye, E., Gupta, B.N. Cardiovascular effects on selective perfusion of the fourth cerebral ventricle in cats with fentanyl, naloxone and methohexital, *Ind J Exp Biol*, 18:29-31, 1980.

122.   Freye, E. The effect of Fentanyl on the resistance and capacitance vessels of the dog's hindlimb, *Arzneim Forsch Drug Res*, 27(5), 1977.

123.   Laubie, M., Schmitt, H., Drouillat, M. Central sites and mechanisms of the hypotensive and bradycardiac effects of the narcotic analgesic agent fentanyl, *Naunyn-Schmiedeberg Arch Pharmacol*, 296:255-261, 1977.

124.   Flaim, S.F., Vismara, L.A., Zelia, R. The effects of morphine on isolated cutaneous canine vascular smooth muscle, *Res Comm Chem Path Pharmacol*, 16(1):191-194, 1977.

125.   Feldberg, W., Wei, E. The central origin and mechanism of cardiovascular effects of morphine as revealed by naloxone in cats, *J Physiol*, 272(1):998-1008, 1977.

126.   Chang, P.-L., Dixon, W.R. Role of plasma catecholamines in eliciting cardiovascular changes seen during naloxone precipitated withdrawal in conscious, unrestrained morphine-dependent rats, *J Pharmacol Exp Ther*, 254(3):857-863, 1990.

127.   Markiewiez, W., Finberg, J.P.M., Lichtig, C. Morphine increases myocardial infarction size in rats, *Anesth Analg*, 61:843-846, 1982.

128.   Willette, R.N., Sepru, H.N. Peripheral versus central cardio respiratory effects of morphine, *Neuropharmacology*, 21:1019-1026, 1982.

129. Weinberg, J., Altura, B.H. Morphine pretreatment influences reactivity of isolated rat arterial smooth Muscle, *Substance Alcohol Actions/Misuse*, 1:71-81, 1980.

130. Bhargana, H.N., Kasabdj, D,. Thompson, E.B. Subsentivity to noradrenaline and isoprenaline in rabbits acutely pretreated with morphine, *Gen Pharmacol*, 8:257-261, 1977.

131. Gintautas, J., Kraynack, B.J., Cockings, E., Havosi, G. Depression of atrium function by narcotics, *Prac West Pharmacol Soc*, 25:55-56, 1982.

132. Wong, T.M., Koo, A., Li, C.H. β-Endorphin, vasodilating effect on the microcirculation of hamster cheek pouch, *Int J Peptide Protein Res*, 18:420-422, 1981.

133. Stanley, T.H., Lui, W.S., Webster, L.R., Johansen, R.K. Haemodynamic effects of intravenous methadone anesthesia in dogs, *Can Anaesth Soc J*, 27(1):52-56, 1980.

134. Ohsumi, H., Sakamoto, M., Yamazaki, T., Okumura, F. Effects of fentanyl on carotid sinus baroreflex control of circulation in rabbits, *Am J Physiol*, 256(3,Pt.2):625-631, 1989.

135. Hill, D.C., Chelly, J.E., Dlewati, A., Abernathy, D.R., Doursout, M.F., Merin, R.G. Cardiovascular effects of and interaction between calcium blocking drugs and anesthetics in chronically instrumented dogs, *Anesthesiol*, 68(6):874-879, 1988.

136. Yaster, M., Koehler, R.C., Traystman, R.J. Interaction of fentanyl and pentobarbital on peripheral and cerebral hemodynamics in newborn lambs, *Anesthesiol*, 70(3):461-469, 1989.

137. vanDaal, G.J., Lachmann, B., Schairer, W., Tenbrinck, R., vanWoerkens, L.J., Verdouw, P., Erdmann, W. The influence of different anesthetics on the oxygen delivery to and consumption of the heart, *Adv Exp Med Biol*, 248:527-532, 1989.

138. Nussmeier, N.A., Benthuysen, J.L., Steffey, E.P., Anderson, J.H., Carstens, E.E., Eisele, J.H., Stanley, T.H. Cardiovascular respiratory and analgesic effects of fentanyl in unanesthetized rhesus monkeys, *Anesth Analg*, 72:221-226, 1991.

139. Doorley, B.M., Knight, V.V., Spaulding, T.C. Development of acute tolerance to the cardio-respiratory effects of alfentanil after subsequent bolus injection in conscious rats, *Life Sci*, 43(4):365-372, 1988.

140. Zhang, C.C., Su, J.Y., Calkins, D. Effects of alfentanil on isolatec cardiac tissues of the rabbit, *Anesth Analg*, 71(3):268-274, 1990.

141. Pagel, P.S., Kampine, J.P., Schmeling, W.T., Warltier, D.C. Effects of nitrous oxide on myocardial contractility as evaluated by reload recruitable stroke work relationship in chronically instrumented dogs, *Anesthesiol*, 73(6):1148-1157, 1990.

142. Abdul-Rasool, I.H., Ward, D.S. Ventilatory and cardiovascular responses to sufentanil infusion in dogs anesthetized with isoflurane, *Anesth Analg*, 69(3):300-306, 1989.

143. Schmelling, W.T., Kampine, J.P., Warltier, D.C. Negative chronotropic actions of sufentanil and vecuronium in chronically instrumented dogs pretreated with propranolol and/or diltiazem, *Anesth Analg*, 69(1):4-14, 1989.

144. Copland, V.S., Haskins, S.C., Patz, J. Naloxone reversal of oxymorphone effects in dogs, *Am J Vet Res*, 50(11):1854-1858, 1989.

145. Montastruc, J.L., Montastruc, P. Naloxone and acute neurogenic hypertension in anaesthetized dogs, *Arch Farmacol Toxicol*, 8:45-48, 1982.

146. Patschke, D., Eberlein, H.J., Hess, W., Tarnow, I., Zimmerman, G. Antagonism of morphine with naloxone in dogs: cardiovascular effects with special reference to the coronary circulation, *Br J Anaesth*, 49:525-533, 1977.

147. Szilagyi, J.E. Opioid modulation of baroreceptor reflex sensitivity in dogs, *Am J Physiol*, 252, 21:H733-H737, 1987.

148. Pinto, J.M., Kirby, D.A., Verrier, R.L. Abolition of clonidine's effects on ventricular refractoriness by naloxone in the conscious dog, *Life Sci*, 45(5):413-420, 1989.

149. Imai, N., Stone, C.K., Woolf, P.D., Liang, C.S. Effects of naloxone on systemic and regional hemodynamics responses to exercise in dogs, *J Physiol*, 64(4):1493-1499, 1988.

150. Feldberg, W., Wei, E. The central origin and mechanism of cardiovascular effects of morphine as revealed by naloxone in cats, *J Physiol*, 272(1):998-1008, 1977.

151. Feria, M., Alvarez, C., Dominguez, J., Sanchez, A., Boada, J. Naloxone Potentiation of cardiovascular responses to sympathomimetic amines in the rat, *J Pharmacol Exp Thera*, 255(2):523-528, 1990.

152. Cader, S., Wright, J., Wong, S.M. The action of naloxone on the blood pressure and heart rate in conscious SHR and WKY rats, *Proc West Pharmacol Soc*, 32:299-301, 1989.

153. Ludbrook, J., Rutter, P.C. Effect of naloxone on haemodynamic responses to acute blood loss in unanesthetized rabbits, *J Physiol*, 400:1-14, 1988.

154. Morilak, D.A., Drolet, G., Chalmers, J. Cardiovascular effects of opioid antagonist naloxone in rostral ventrolateral medulla of rabbits, *Am J Physiol*, 258(2Pt 2):325-331, 1990.

155. Cerbai, E., DeBonfioli-Cavalcabo, P., Masini, I., Porciatti, F., Mugelli, A. Antiarrhythmic properties of naloxone: an electrophysiological study on sheep cardiac Purkinje fibers, *Eur J Pharmacol*, 162(3):491-500, 1989.

156. Martinez, A., Padbury, J., Shames, L., Evans, C., Humme, J. Naloxone potentiates epinephrine release during hypoxia in fetal sheep: dose response and cardiovascular effects, *Pediat Res*, 23(4):343-347, 1988.

157. Kirby, D.A., Spealman, R.D. Attenuation by naloxone of the pressor effects of angiotensin II in conscious cynomolgus monkeys, *Life Sci*, 43(5):453-458, 1988.

158. Roquebert, J., Delgoulet, C. Cardiovascular effects of etorphine in rats, *J Auton Pharmacol*, 8(1):39-43, 1988.

159. Greene, S.A., Hartsfield, S.M., Tyner, C.L. Cardiovascular effects of butorphanol in halothane-anesthetized dogs, *Am J Vet Res*, 51(8):1276-1279, 1990.

160. Thornhill, J.A., Pittman, Q.J. Hemodynamic responses of conscious rats following intrathecal injections of prodynorphin-derived opioids: independence of action of intrathecal arginine vasopressin, *Can J Physiol Pharmacol*, 68(2):174-182, 1990.

161. Muldoon, S., Otto, J., Freas, W., Watson, R.L. The effects of morphine, nalbuphine and butorphanol on adrenergic function in canine saphenous veins, *Anesth Analg*, 62:21-28, 1983.

162. Royster, R.L., Keeler, D.K., Haisty, W.K., Johnston, W.E., Prough, D.S. Cardiac electrophysiologic effects of fentanyl and combinations of fentanyl and neuromusclular relaxants in pentobarbital-anesthetized dogs, *Anesth Analg*, 67:15-20, 1988.

163. Hannon, J.P., Bossone, C.A. Cardiovascular and pulmonary effects of morphine in conscious pigs, *Am J Physiol*, 261:R1286-R1293, 1991.

164. Bossone, C.A., Hannon, J.P. Metabolic actions of morphine in conscious chronically instrumented pigs, *Am J Physiol*, 260:R1051-R1057, 1991.

165. Flacke, J.W., Davis, L.J., Flacke, W.E., Bloor, B.C., Van Etten, A.P. Effects of fentanyl and diazepam in dogs deprived of autonomic tone, *Anesth Analg*, 64:1053-1059, 1985.

166. Chinzei, M., Morita, S., Chinzei, T., Takahashi, H. *et al.* Effects of isoflurane and fentanyl on ischemic myocardium in dogs: assessment by end-systolic measurements, *J Cardiothorac Vasc Anesth*, 5:243-249, 1991.

167. Weiskopf, R.B., Eger, E.I., Holmes, M.A., Yasuda, N., Johnson, B.H., Targ, A.G., Rampil, I.J. Cardiovascular actions of common anesthetic adjuvants during desflurane (I-653) and isoflurane anesthesia in swine, *Anesth Analg*, 71(2):144-148, 1990.

168. Nagano, K., Gelman, S., Parks, D.A., Bradley, E.L. Jr. Hepatic oxygen-supply-uptake relationship and metabolism during anesthesia in minature pigs, *Anesthesiology*, 72:902-910, 1990.

169. Schmeling, W.T., Kampine, J.P., Warltier, D.C. Negative chronotropic actions of sufentanil and vecuronium in chronically instrumented dogs pretreated with propranolol and/or diltiazem, *Anesth Analg*, 69:4-14, 1989.

3. Cardiovascular effects of the tranquilizers

Most of these agents are more correctly classified as psychotropic or neuroleptic agents. This indicates a primary mode of action on certain functions of the central nervous system. Many of these agents have a profound effect on the cardiovascular system in addition to, or perhaps as a result of, their CNS activity. Much of the CNS activity seems to be linked to the blockade of dopamine within the basal ganglia complex. The stereochemical model of chlorpromazine (one of the phenothiazine derivatives) is similar to the structures of epinephrine, norepinephrine and dopamine, but two-dimensional models of these compounds do not usually make the similarities apparent. Many of these compounds are apparently dopamine antagonists which act on dopamine excitatory receptors.[1] The drugs are widely used for chemical restraint and preanesthetic agents when working with animals.

The phenothiazine tranquilizers are reported to decrease preload, contractility and afterload and to increase heart rate.[2] They have been reported to produce arrhythmias along with their paradoxical antiarrhythmic properties. They have been shown to: decrease the rate of rise of phase 0 of the myocardial action potential, decrease the duration and amplitude of phase 2, and prolong phase 3. Repolarization abnormalities induced by these agents seem to be dose related.[3] This class of agents not only have strong central α-adrenergic blocking actions, they also block peripheral α-adrenergic receptors. It may be that the major action of these agents is stimulation of peripheral β_2 receptors resulting in intense vasodilation. Whatever the mechanics of action, arterial hypotension is a result.[141] The Butyrophenones are a group of agents which were developed from efforts to increase the analgesic potency of a series of 4-phenylpiperidines related to meperidine. They are related to the antihistamines and spasmolytics. In veterinary practice they are most frequently used in combination with narcotic analgesics, which seems to potentiate the sedative action of both agents. They also act as dopamine antagonists on dopamine excitatory receptors.[141]

The Benzodiazepines induce taming effects in animals probably by affecting neurotransmitter systems, including acetylcholine, catecholamines, serotonin, GABA and glycine. A widespread distribution of benzodiazepine receptors in the grey matter of the CNS has been demonstrated in all species studied, as opposed to a lack of receptors in white matter.[1] These agents are frequently used for their calming or taming effects as preanesthetics, and also for their antiarrhythmic effects.

The Rauwolfia derivatives are known to result in depletion of catecholamine stores and, therefore, act by reducing the normal physiological response to stress. Reserpine is the major Rauwolfia derivative used, but its use has most recently been limited to studies which are designed to investigate the role of catecholamines in the cardiovascular response to a wide variety of perturbations. The recent literature using reserpine in this manner in rats, mice, rabbits, guinea pigs, and hamsters is overwhelming.

In veterinary medicine xylazine HCl, which is pharmacologically classified as an analgesic, sedative and skeletal muscle relaxant, has supplanted most psychotropic agents, particularly in larger species, because of its superior effects as a sedative without causing ataxia. When used as a preanesthetic agent in cardiovascular studies, it is extremely important to know that xylazine is a mixed α-adrenoceptor agonist. Its α1 to α2 selectivity ratio is believed to be near unity (1.28), indicating a near equal affinity for peripheral α1 and α2 adrenoceptors.[87] It has CNS effects which effectively reduce release of norepinephrine. It is reported to cause initial hypertension following IM or IV injection followed by prolonged hypotension, probably as a result of its central α_2-adrenergic receptor action.[86]

Xylazine provides excellent sedation and calming and is widely used for that purpose in horses and cattle. It also may potentiate second degree heart block in horses. It has severe hypotensive and bradycardic effects which have a duration of approximately 1 hour with normal doses. The effects are dose-dependent, and ruminants require only 1/10 of the dose used in horses. If the animal is ill lower doses may be required.[4] The drug is reported to cause decreases in preload, afterload, and heart rate with no change in contractility.[2] These effects all seem to be attributable to either direct or indirect effects on the autonomic nervous system. Initially, following an intravenous injection, there is a transitory hypertension, via vasoconstriction of the splanchnic and peripheral vasculature. These effects have been enhanced by beta-adrenergic-blockers and blocked by alpha-adrenergic-blockers in a variety of species so tested. Bradycardia and second degree A-V block are commonly seen, probably as a result of an increase in vagal tone resulting from the hypertension. Atropine has been shown to block this reaction.[80] Xylazine is sold under the trade name of Rompun[R] and Bay Va 1470.

Table 3.1 The Phenothiazine Derivative Tranquilizers; Chlorpromazine and Promazine

Conditions of the Experiment	Dose	Cardiovascular Effects	Reference
3.1:1 Dogs			
Intact, awake	4.4 mg/kg, IV (Promazine) 1.25 mg/kg, IV (Chlorpromazine)	Initial, short-lived, tachycardia followed by bradycardia	5
Intact, awake, previously instrumented, injection into pulmonary artery	1 mg/kg, IV (Chlorpromazine)	Approximate 20% increase in cardiac output, decrease in pulmonary artery resistance, significant decrease (approx. 15%) in aortic pressure, systemic resistance increased approximated 30%, no change in heart rate, stroke volume increased, peak stroke velocity decreased and no change in stroke acceleration	6

Conditions of the Experiment	Dose	Cardiovascular Effects	Reference
Intact, awake, previously instrumented, drug injected slowly over 30 sec	2.2 mg/kg, IV (Chlorpromazine)	Aortic pressure did not change at 5 min but decreased at 15 and 30 min, back to baseline levels at 60 min. No changes occurred in arterial pH or pCO_2	7
Anesthetized with Thiopental sodium (20 mg/kg, IV), alpha-Chloralose (60 mg/kg IV), positive pressure ventilation with room air, acute, open chest, dT/dt measured with Walton-Brodie strain gauge	1 mg/kg, IV (Chlorpromazine)	Decreased mean aortic pressure, left ventricular dT/dt decreased, increased conduction time and decreased conduction velocity in AV-nodal tissue, His-Purkinje tissue and ventricular tissue. Caused a biphasic response in A-V nodal tissue	8
Anesthetized with Pentobarbital (50 mg/kg, IP), positive pressure ventilation	1 mg/kg, IV (Chlorpromazine)	Decreased the ventricular multiple response threshold (the minimum current necessary to induce more than 3 serial ventricular extrasystoles), decreased mean aortic pressure. Caused mitochondrial dysfunction which derived from a disturbance in the first segment of the electron transport chain. Decreased calcium ion binding activity which is probably responsible for the antiarrhythmic effects	9
Isolated tissues. No indication of how animals were anesthetized for removal of hearts and preparation of cardiac sarcolemma	Chlorpromazine, a range of concentrations	Inhibition of the sodium-calcium ion exchange mechanism which was strongly dependent on the ratio between the chlorpromazine concentration and the concentration of the vesicles in the suspension	10
Isolated tissues, cardiac sarcolemma preparation	Chlorpromazine, range of concentrations	Inhibited the hydrolysis of lysosomal lipases	11

Conditions of the Experiment	Dose	Cardiovascular Effects	Reference
Intact, awake, n=4	4.4 mg/kg, IV (Promazine)	Transient tachycardia, decreased heart rate, in 1 dog a 9-sec. episode of sinus arrest.	86
Intact, awake, n=4	1.25 and 3.5 mg/kg, IV (Chlorpromazine)	Transient tachycardia then bradycardia	86
Intact, awake, previously instrumented	2.2 mg/kg, IV	Decreased mean aortic pressure, no change in arterial pH or $PaCO_2$	87

Conditions of the Experiment	Dose	Cardiovascular Effects	Reference
3.1:2 Cats			
Anesthetized with pentobarbital (36 mg/kg, IP), gallamine triethiodide (6 mg/kg IV), positive pressure ventilation, additional pentobarbital as needed (5 mg/kg, IV). Measured carotid body output activity	Chlorpromazine, 1 mg/kg, IV	Decreased spontaneous chemoreceptor activity, decreased responses to sodium cyanide and dopamine. Effects were much more brief and less marked than same effects caused by Properidol	12
Dial-urethane anesthetized, pretreatment with chlorpromazine	5, 10, 20, 30, 40, or 60 mg/kg, IV	No dose-response sensitivity to Ouabain-induced arrhythmia (2µg/kg/min, IV) Decreased aortic pressure without reflex tachycardia. Suggests agent may interfere with baroreflexes	88
Spinal cord transections at atlanto-occipital junction	1 mg/kg/min, IV	No protection against Ouabain-induced arrhythmia or death	89
Alpha-chloralose anesthetized	0.5 mg intracerebro-ventricular injection (Chlorpromazine)	Did not induce arrhythmias or death. Initial decrease in blood pressure. Conclude there is a direct myocardial effect, not central.	89

Conditions of the Experiment	Dose	Cardiovascular Effects	Reference
3.1:3 Rats			
Decapitated, isolated subcellular membranes	Chlorpromazine, a range of concentrations	Significantly decreased calcium ion binding, magnesium ATPase and sodium-potassium ATPase activities of the sarcolemmal fraction. Significantly decreased calcium ion binding and uptake abilities of the microsomal and mitochondrial fractions. Mitochondrial respiratory and oxidative phosphorylation activities were depressed at higher concentrations.	**13**
Stunned, decapitated, hindquarter perfusion with Krebs solution and glucose (95% oxygen, 5% CO_2), a flow through, non-recirculating, system	Chlorpromazine, intra-arterial injection at various concentrations	Showed competitive antagonist action towards 5-hydroxytryptamine	**14**
Ether anesthesia with ligation of left coronary artery, allowed to recover and then groups killed at various periods post ischemia	45 mg/kg, IP 1 hour prior to surgery and every 6 hours thereafter (chlorpromazine)	Treatment prevented appearance of ischemic cell death in the main portion of the free-wall myocardium for at least 24 hours without affecting the reaction of the subepicardial and subendocardial cells. Inhibited the second phase of calcium ion accumulation. Presented accelerated degradation and loss of phospholipid. Protected against loss of phospholipid, inhibition of calcium ion uptake and increased calcium ion permeability of the sarcoplasmic reticulum	**15**

Conditions of the Experiment	Dose	Cardiovascular Effects	Reference
Decapitation and heart removal, Langendorff preparation of spontaneously beating hearts	5 g/ml in perfusate (Chlorpromazine)	Decreased heart rate, transient but significant increase in coronary flow after 15 min. of perfusion with the drug but then decreased and at 60 min. was back to baseline, decreased isometric systolic tension, increased PR and Q-T intervals, decreased QRS amplitude, no change in phosphorylase activity	16
Decapitation, excised aortas, stripped of adventitial tissue, incubated in a bath	0.25 mM in incubation medium (Chlorpromazine)	Significantly decreased the incorporation of ^{14}C-acetate into free fatty acids and total phospholipids but not triglycerides. Altered the pattern of arterial phospholipids synthesized. Also is an inhibitor of sterol biosynthesis in these tissues.	17
Exsanguinated to kill, isolated right atrial preparations	0.01-10 g/ml (Chlorpromazine)	Failed to prevent arrhythmic contractions induced by electrical stimulation during rhythmic spontaneous contractions	18
Exsanguinated to kill, isolated atrial and papillary muscle preparations	1.0 g/ml (Chlorpromazine)	Increased the refractory period of papillary muscle, no effect on refractory period of left atrium. Decreased the maximum driving frequency of the left atrium by 33.3%	18
Same	0.01-1.0 g/ml (Chlorpromazine)	Had little effect on either the rate or force of spontaneous contraction of the right atrium. No change in contractile force of the left atrium driven by electrical stimulation but decreased force in the papillary muscle	18

Conditions of the Experiment	Dose	Cardiovascular Effects	Reference
Decapitated, isolated sarcolemmal, microsomal and mitochondrial fractions	25-120 µM (chlorpromazine)	Decreased; calcium ion binding, magnesium ATPase and sodium/potassium ATPase activities of sarcolemmal fraction. Decreased calcium ion binding and uptake of microsomal and mitochondrial fractions. Mitochondrial respiratory and oxidative phosphorylation activities were depressed at higher concentrations.	90
Isolated left atrium, right atrium and papillary muscle	0.01=10 µg/ml (chlorpromazine)	Did not prevent arrhythmic contraction by threshold electrical stimulation in rhythmic spontaneously contracting right atrium	91
Same	1.0 µg/ml (Chlorpromazine)	Increased refractory period of papillary muscle by 42.8% but no effect on left atrium	91
Same	1.0 µg/ml (Chlorpromazine)	Decreased maximum driving frequency by 33.0%, no effect on papillary muscle	91
Same	0.01-1.0µg/ml (Chlorpromazine)	No effect on rate or force of spontaneous right atrial contractions	91
Same	2.0 µg/ml (Chlorpromazine)	Decreased contractile force of electrically stimulated left atrium and papillary muscle	91
Same	0.01-1.0 µg/ml (Chlorpromazine)	No effect on contractile force of electrically driven left atrium but a dose-response decrease in contractile force of papillary muscle	91

Conditions of the Experiment	Dose	Cardiovascular Effects	Reference
In vitro rat aortas, incubated with radiolabeled acetate and mevalonate as lipid precursors	0.25 mM (Chlorpromazine)	Significant decrease in incorporation of labeled acetate into free fatty acids and total phospholipids but not triglycerides. Altered the pattern of arterial phospholipids synthesized from acetate and decreased acetate incorporation into the combined fractions of sterol esters, hydrocarbons, sterols and diglycerides. Mevalonate uptake studies indicated chlorpromazine is also an inhibitor of sterol biosynthesis	92
Isolated right ventricular strips	1-5 μM (Chlorpromazine) calcium ion repletion following calcium ion depletion	Inhibition of calmodulin	93
Newborn cat myocardial cells in culture	1.6×10^{-4} M (Chlorpromazine)	Caused severe damage to the cells, not related to calcium ion concentrations. Is a fairly specific inhibitor of calmodulin-calcium complex. Also capable of blocking net calcium ion influx and inhibition activation of phospholipases.	94
Anesthetized with ether, papillary muscle preparation, isotonic and isometric contractions	10^{-6}, 10^{-5}, 10^{-4} M (Chlorpromazine)	Slight positive inotropic effect at 10^{-6}M, slight negative effects at 10^{-5} and 10^{-4} M. Apparently modulates intrinsic energetics and mechanics by modifying sarcoplasmic reticulum, myofilament calcium ion sensitivity and cross-bridge kinetics. Is both load- and dose-dependent.	95

Conditions of the Experiment	Dose	Cardiovascular Effects	Reference
3.1:4 Guinea Pigs			
Isolated right ventricular papillary muscle preparation. Animals heparinized prior to killing	1×10^{-6} M (Chlorpromazine)	Decreased maximum upstroke velocity of the action potential, decreased contractile force and flattened the repolarization phase	19
Same	1×10^{-5} M (Chlorpromazine)	Decreased overshoot and decreased resting potential, a much larger decrease in the maximum upstroke velocity of the action potential	19
Cervical dislocation and removal of the heart, left atrial isolated preparation	Hydroxylated metabolites of Chlorpromazine, a range of concentrations	Release catecholamines from cardiac sympathetic nerve terminals and increase myocardial contractile force	20
Stunned and exsanguinated, Mesenteric artery dissection, parts in an isolated bath	5×10^{-7} M and greater (Chlorpromazine)	Depolarized the vessels' cellular membranes and reduced membrane resistance, as measured by the current-voltage relationship. Suppressed contractions evoked by excess potassium ions and by caffeine	21
Skinned muscle preparation	1×10^{-6} M and greater (Chlorpromazine) (Chlorpromazine)	Suppressed the calcium ion induced contraction in a dose dependent manner. This suggests that the drug acts on the surface membrane and suppresses calcium ion influx. This results in vascular relaxation (alpha-blocking effects?)	21
Isolated right ventricular papillary muscle, animal heparinized prior to euthanasia	10-6 M (Chlorpromazine)	Decreased maximum upstroke velocity of the action potential, flattening of repolarization phase	96
Same	10^{-5} M (Chlorpromazine) (Chlorpromazine)	Decreased overshoot and resting potential and a large decrease in maximum upstroke velocity of the action potential	96

Conditions of the Experiment	Dose	Cardiovascular Effects	Reference
Anesthetized with pentobarbital, 40 mg/kg, IP. Langendorff-Tyrodes' perfused hearts. Suction pipettes used to record from individual cells. Space-clamp control and patch-clamp techniques used	5 µM (Chlorpromazine)	Sodium ion current decreased 10% within 1 min., reached a steady state within 5 min. Profound use-dependent block. Blocked sodium ion-channels reversibly in a voltage-dependent manner	97

Conditions of the Experiment	Dose	Cardiovascular Effects	Reference
3.1:5 Rabbits			
Atherosclerotic diet fed, decapitated and exsanguinated under light Pentobarbital anesthesia, incubated aortas until cell fractions isolated	Chlorpromazine in a range of concentrations	Inhibited cholesterolacyltransferase in isolated arterial microsomes	22
Isolated SA node preparation. Both double sucrose gap and microelectrode techniques were used to study the electrophysiology	2.5×10^{-5} M (Chlorpromazine)	Arrested spontaneous activity which could then be restored with norepinephrine	23
Heparinized and anesthetized with Pentobarbital (50 mg/kg, IP). Isolated, perfused interventricular septal preparation.	Chlorpromazine in a range of concentrations	Inhibits calcium ion influx and phospholipase activation. Resulted in better functional recovery following ischemia of contractile parameters. Also protected against ischemia induced structural and membrane permeability alterations	24
Anesthetized, exsanguinated, helically cut aortic strips	1×10^{-6} M (Chlorpromazine)	Antagonized the norepinephrine, serotonin and histamine induced contractions but did not antagonize the PGF_2 and Angiotensin II induced contractions	25

Conditions of the Experiment	Dose	Cardiovascular Effects	Reference
Isolated pulmonary artery and aortic vascular preparations	10^{-8} to 10^{-5} M (Chlorpromazine)	Dose responses decreased pulmonary artery contractions evoked by electrical field stimulation. Inhibitory effect was not reversible.	98
Same	10^{-8} to 10^{-4} M (Chlorpromazine)	Decreased accumulation of tritiated-noradrenaline by the aorta	98
Same	10^{-8} to 10^{-6} M (Chlorpromazine) (Chlorpromazine)	Antagonized aortic contractions evoked by exogenous noradrenaline. Concluded that chlorpromazine is a potent inhibitor of postsynaptic alpha-1-adrenoceptors and also inhibits uptake.	98

Conditions of the Experiment	Dose	Cardiovascular Effects	Reference
3.1:6 Pigs			
Isolated carotid artery helical strips from slaughtered pigs	0.01 mM concentration (Chlorpromazine)	75% decrease in tension generated by norepinephrine induced contraction, also inhibited light chain phosphorylation	26

Conditions of the Experiment	Dose	Cardiovascular Effects	Reference
3.1:7 Chickens			
Isolated cardiac cells from 7-day old chicks, cell culture	10^{-5} M (Chlorpromazine)	Increased incorporation of choline into both phosphocholine and phospholipid. Presented anoxia-induced changes in phosphocholine.	99
Same	10^{-4} M (Chlorpromazine)	Damaged myocardial cells, i.e., decreased cellular protein and decreased choline incorporation.	99

Table 3.2: The Phenothiazine Tranquilizers (Acetylpromazine)

Conditions of the Experiment	Dose	Cardiovascular Effects	Reference
3.2:1 Dogs			
Preanesthetic dose	0.4 mg/kg, IV or IM	Prolonged hypotension and cardiac depressant activity with vasodilation	**4**
Twenty minutes following preanesthetic dose anesthetized with Thiamylal sodium and Halothane	0.4 mg/kg	Displayed protection against epinephrine-induced arrhythmias	**27**
Intact, awake, previously instrumented	0.11 mg/kg, IV over 30 sec.	Mean aortic pressure decreased at 5, 15, 30 and 60 min., arterial pH increased at 5 and 30 min., no change at 15 and 60 min., no change in arterial pCO_2	**7**
Intact, awake, previously instrumented	0.2 mg/kg, IV	Decreased mean aortic pressure, stroke volume, left ventricular work, respiratory rate, minute ventilation and oxygen consumption	**100**
Intact, awake, previously instrumented	0.11 mg/kg, IV	Decreased mean aortic pressure and pH. No change in $PaCO_2$.	**87**
Intact, awake, left lateral recumbency (n=13)	0.2 mg/kg, IV	No change in heart rate, mean pulmonary arterial pressure, central venous pressure, cardiac output and peripheral resistance. Decrease in mean aortic pressure, stroke volume, left ventricular work and left ventricular stroke work.	**101**

Conditions of the Experiment	Dose	Cardiovascular Effects	Reference
3.2:2 Cats			
Anesthetized with Chloralose (30 mg/kg, IV), positive pressure ventilation	1.5 mg/kg, IV	Increased toxicity to ouabain, decreased blood pressure and increased heart rate	**28**

Conditions of the Experiment	Dose	Cardiovascular Effects	Reference
Same	500 g intra-cerebro-ventricular	Decreased blood pressure, no change in heart rate	28
Intact, awake, previously instrumented	0.2 mg/kg, IM (Acepromazine) 4.0 mg/kg, IM (Meperidine) 0.05 mg/kg, IM (Atropine)	Measurements after 20 min. Decreased cardiac output. No change in stroke volume, heart rate, PaO_2, $PaCO_2$, pH or respiratory rate	102

Conditions of the Experiment	Dose	Cardiovascular Effects	Reference
3.2:3 Sheep			
Conducted in awake, anesthetized with Thiopental and anesthetized with a combination of Thiopental and Halothane	0.5 mg/kg, IV	Prevented epinephrine-induced arrhythmias in all 3 preparations	29

Conditions of the Experiment	Dose	Cardiovascular Effects	Reference
3.2:4 Horses			
Intact, awake	0.5 mg/kg, IM	Slight increase in heart rate, no change in packed cell volume, slight increase in serum cortisol levels	30
Intact, awake, previously instrumented	0.09 mg/kg, IV	No change in heart rate, cardiac output or mean pulmonary artery pressure, significant decreases in respiratory rate, central venous pressure and mean aortic pressure, no change in arterial pCO_2, pO_2 or pH	31
Intact, awake, instrumented	0.1 mg/kg, IV	Decreased mean aortic pressure and partially antagonized the pressor action of 1.5 micro-g/kg adrenaline IV challenge	32

Conditions of the Experiment	Dose	Cardiovascular Effects	Reference
Intact, awake	0.05 mg/kg, IV	20 minutes after acepromazine decreased mean aortic pressure and cardiac index, slight increase in heart rate	**103**
Intact, awake	0.01 mg/kg, IV	20 minutes post-injection, decreased systolic and diastolic aortic pressures, no change in heart rate	**104**

Table 3.3: The Phenothiazine Tranquilizers (Triflupromazine and Thioridazine)

Conditions of the Experiment	Dose	Cardiovascular Effects	Reference
3.3:1 Cats			
Dial-urethane, 0.6 ml/kg, IP, spinal cord transection	1 mg/kg/min, IV (Thioridazine)	Does not appear to produce arrhythmia or death via a central locus, i.e. direct myocardial arrhythmogenic effects	**89**

Conditions of the Experiment	Dose	Cardiovascular Effects	Reference
3.3:2 Rats			
Stunned and decapitated, hindquarter perfusion with Krebs and glucose, O_2 and CO_2 controlled, non-recirculating, flow-through system	Range of intra-arterial doses (Triflupromazine)	A very strong competitive antagonist for 5-hydroxytryptamine	**14**
Isolated right ventricular strips. Calcium repletion following calcium depletion.	1-5 μM (Trifluoperazine)	Significant improvement in recovery of contractility after calcium repletion, i.e., calmodulin inhibition	**93**

Conditions of the Experiment	Dose	Cardiovascular Effects	Reference
Isolated "working" hearts, globally ischemic, 40 minutes of normothermic arrest, rats anesthetized with 20-25 mg pentobarbital, IP	2.45 µM in perfusate added before ischemia or during reperfusion (Trifluoperazine)	Increased membrane stabilization, inhibits calmodulin and binds to other calcium-dependent protein-treated hearts recovered mechanically after 40 min. of normothermic ischemic arrest. Untreated hearts failed after 20 minutes of ischemia. No effect on tissue high energy phosphate levels or mitochondrial oxidative phosphorylation.	105

Conditions of the Experiment	Dose	Cardiovascular Effects	Reference
3.3:3 Pigs			
Helical strips from isolated carotid arteries of slaughtered pigs	0.1 mM (Triflupromazine)	75% decrease in tension generated by norepinephrine challenge	26
	0.5 mM (Triflupromazine)	Complete inhibition of tension generated by norepinephrine challenge and inhibition of light chain phosphorylation	26

Conditions of the Experiment	Dose	Cardiovascular Effects	Reference
3.3:4 Chickens			
Isolated cardiac cells from 7-day old chicks, cell culture	10^{-5} M (Trifluoperazine)	Increased incorporation of choline into both phosphocholine and phospholipids prevented anoxia-induced changes in phosphocholine	99
Same	10^{-4} M (Trifluoperazine)	Damaged myocardial cells, i.e. decreased cellular protein and decreased choline incorporation	99

Table 3.4: The Butyrophenones (Droperidol)

Conditions of the Experiment	Dose	Cardiovascular Effects	Reference
3.4:1 Dogs			
Nitrous oxide analgesia	0.5-1 mg/kg, IV	No effect on baroreceptor function	**33**
Pentobarbital anesthetized (30 mg/kg, IV), helical isolated strips of saphenous veins and pulmonary arteries and longitudinal strips of anterior mesenteric veins. Measured developed tension	Range of concentrations	Concluded that the vasodilator properties of smaller doses, in these vessels, are as a result of the ability to block alpha-adrenergic receptors	**34**
Anesthetized with Pentobarbital (30 mg/kg, IV), positive pressure ventilation, open chest, acute preparation, Heparin (3 mg/kg, IV), isolation of sinus node artery form the right coronary	500-1000 µg infused directly into the sinus node artery	Sino-arterial arrest followed by HIS bundle rhythm	**35**
Anesthetized with pentobarbital (50 mg/kg, IP), exsanguination. Helical strips of LAD coronary and interlobar renal arteries, isolated and perfused. Preparation treated for 60 min. with phenoxybenzamine, washed repeatedly and equilibrated for 40-50 min. in control media. Contracted with PGF^2.	3×10^{-5} and 3×10^{-4} M	Dose-related response relaxation caused by Dopamine (2×10^{-7} to 10^{-4} M) shifted to the right	**36**
Anesthetized with pentobarbital (30 mg/kg, IV)- helical strips of saphenous veins	3.9×10^{-6} 3.9×10^{-7} M	This concentration seems to act as an antagonist of the postsynaptic, but not the presynaptic, alpha-adrenoceptor. Promotes leakage of norepinephrine from intraneuronal storage vesicles	**37**

Conditions of the Experiment	Dose	Cardiovascular Effects	Reference
Anesthetized with pentobarbital (30 mg/kg, IV) open thorax, sinus node artery cannulation	500-1000 mcg into sinus node artery	Sinus arrest followed by HIS bundle rhythm	**106**
Helical strips of saphenous vein, pulmonary arteries and longitudinal strips of anterior mesenteric veins. Dogs were anesthetized with 30 mg/kg, IV, pentobarbital, electrically paced.	Dose-response 1.10×10^{-2} to 10^{-8}	Inhibited the spontaneous activity of portal and mesenteric veins. Inhibited the contractile response to nerve stimuli, no effect on the evoked release of tritiated norepinephrine. Demonstrates alpha-adrenergic receptor blockade.	**107**

Conditions of the Experiment	Dose	Cardiovascular Effects	Reference
3.4:2 Cats			
Isolated papillary muscle preparation	range of concentrations	Increased effective refractory period but no change in developed tension	2
Halothane anesthetized, intact, epinephrine-induced arrhythmias	250 micro-g/kg, IV	Blocked epinephrine-induced arrhythmias in 5 of 7 cats	2
Anesthetized with pentobarbital, coronary artery occlusion-induced arrhythmias	250 micro-g/kg, IV	Decreased arrhythmias	2
Anesthetized with pentobarbital (36 mg/kg, IP), gallamine triethiodide (6 mg/kg, IV) positive pressure ventilation, additional pentobarbital as needed (5 mg/kg, IV). Measured carotid body output activity.	range of doses	Low doses resulted in a transient increase in rate of chemoreceptor afferent activity. High doses caused a transient increase, then depression. High doses reduced or abolished the normal increase in afferent activity associated with stagnant asphyxia.	12

Conditions of the Experiment	Dose	Cardiovascular Effects	Reference
Isolated adrenal glands, perfused with Krebs-bicarbonate, release of catecholamine as a result of nicotine (5 µM) exposure.	Dose response 0.05-50 µM	Lower concentrations markedly increase the secretory response induced by nicotine. High concentrations decreased the secretory response.	**108**

Conditions of the Experiment	Dose	Cardiovascular Effects	Reference
3.4:3 Rats			
Isolated vas deferens preparation	range of doses	Dose-dependent inhibition of norepinephrine-induced contractions. Demonstrates alpha-adrenergic blocking activity.	**38**
Isolated helical strips of thoracic aorta	range of doses	Alpha-adrenoreceptor blocking activity, dose-related blocking of epinephrine-induced contractions	**38**

Conditions of the Experiment	Dose	Cardiovascular Effects	Reference
3.4:4 Rabbits			
Anesthetized, agent not described	250 micro-g/kg, IV	Reduced preload, afterload and contractility and increased heart rate. Alpha-adrenergic blockade which protected against catecholamine-induced ventricular tachycardia and arrhythmias	**2**

Conditions of the Experiment	Dose	Cardiovascular Effects	Reference
Killed by a blow to the head, isolated descending aortic and left atrial strips, maintained in a tissue chamber. Atrial preparations were electrically stimulated, dose response curve for phenylephrine induced contractions, isometric contracting tension measured (aortic strips). Potentiation by tyramine measured from atrial strips.	1×10^{-9}, 10^{-8}, and 10^{-7} M	Shifted phenylephrine dose-response curve to the right for aortic strips. The potentiation of contraction by dynamine in the electrically stimulated left atrial preparations was markedly depressed.	39
Isolated spleen preparation	range of doses	Dose related inhibition of norepinephrine induced contractions	38
Isolated central ear artery segments	range of doses	Alpha-adrenergic blocking activity, blocking to epinephrine induced contractions was dose related	38
Isolated perfused middle cerebral and central ear arteries, constant flow, measured change in pressure	?	Antagonized dopamine induced relaxation of these vessels	38
Stunned, hearts excised, isolated perfused Langendorff type preparations	?	Blocked recovery of excitability induced by isoproterenol after depolarization with KCl, same effect as Verapamil. Inference is that Droperidol hinders myocardial membrane permeability to calcium ions in a manner similar to that of Verapamil, however, calcium ion permeability was not directly measured	40

Conditions of the Experiment	Dose	Cardiovascular Effects	Reference
Stunned, excised hearts, isolated right atrial preparation, measured transmembrane action potentials from the SA nodal area	1 mg/l in bath	Prolonged the spontaneous rate by reducing the phase 4 slope of the action potential	41
	5 mg/l in bath	More pronounced effect than at lower dose and after 20 min. decreased the upstroke velocity and threshold potential. After 45 min. only subthreshold oscillations were recorded. At high concentrations seems to cause total blockade of Na^+-Ca^{++} slow channels	
Stunned and exsanguinated, isolated mesenteric artery helical strips	3×10^{-6} to 3×10^{-5} M	Blocked Dopamine induced relaxation after pre-treatment with phenoxybenzamine and contraction with PGF_2. Alpha-adrenoceptor blocker (Pindolol) did not block this effect. Considered to be a dopamine-receptor antagonist but at high concentrations (10^{-5} M) there are some beta-adrenolytic effects	42
Aortic strips, left atrial strips isolated from rabbits killed by a blow to the head	Dose response 10^{-9} to 10^{-5} M	Alters dose-response curves to phenylephrine, phentolamine, tyramine, all compared to reserpine effects. Evidence that Droperidol may block alpha-adrenergic receptors and also inhibit norepinephrine uptake at adrenergic terminals.	109

Conditions of the Experiment	Dose	Cardiovascular Effects	Reference
3.4:5 Guinea Pigs			
Isolated perfused hearts	250 micro-g/kg, IV	Delayed ventricular fibrillation induced by perfusion with substrate-free Tyrodes' solution	2

Conditions of the Experiment	Dose	Cardiovascular Effects	Reference
Stunned and exsanguinated, isolated papillary muscle preparation, measured transmembrane potential with sucrose gap	10^{-6} to 4×10^{-5} M	Slows ventricular pacemaker activity, reversible with epinephrine. The maximum upstroke velocity of the action potential (V_{max}) was decreased. Time constant for V_{max} was prolonged during reduced membrane potential, elevated extracellular potassium ion concentration and stimulated rate	43

Conditions of the Experiment	Dose	Cardiovascular Effects	Reference
3.4:6 Sheep			
Hearts obtained from the slaughterhouse, cooled immediately after removal	range of doses 1×10^{-5} to 5×10^{-5} M	Dose-dependent shortening of the duration of action potential. No change in transmembrane resting potentials, upstroke velocities or amplitudes of action potential. Hypothesize that Droperidol partially blocks the sodium carrying system of the surface membrane	44
Hearts from slaughterhouse. Dissected Purkinje strands.	1-5×10^{-5} M	Dose-dependent decrease in action potential duration. Rate of rise decreased with no significant change in amplitudes. Resting potentials and membrane resistances were not changed.	110

Table 3.5: The Butyrophenones (Haloperidol and Azaperone)

Conditions of the Experiment	Dose	Cardiovascular Effects	Reference
3.5:1 Dogs - Haloperidol			
Anesthetized with Thiopental (20 mg/kg, IV) and alpha-chloralose (60 mg/kg, IV), positive pressure ventilation with room air, dT/dt of left ventricle measured with a Walton-Brodie strain gauge	range of doses	Alpha-adrenergic receptor blockade, less potent than chlorpromazine but more potent than thioridazine. Decreased aortic pressure and dT/dt. Increased conduction time and decreased conduction velocity in AV nodal tissue, HIS-Purkinje tissue and ventricular myocardium	8

Conditions of the Experiment	Dose	Cardiovascular Effects	Reference
3.5:2 Cats - Haloperidol			
Anesthetize with Chloralose (80 mg/kg, IV), halothane and nitrous oxide	1 mg/kg/day/ or for 23 days prior to experiment	Apparently caused greater modulation of central alpha-1- than of alpha -2-adrenoceptors. Increased mean aortic pressure, no change in heart rate. Increased response to bilateral carotid occlusion. No change from brachial nerve stimulation. No change to 30° head-up tilt induced fall in blood pressure, but increased duration of fall. No change in response to norepinephrine, Angiotensin II or Bradykinin.	111

Conditions of the Experiment	Dose	Cardiovascular Effects	Reference
3.5:3 Guinea Pigs - Haloperidol			
Animal heparinized prior to killing, right ventricular papillary muscle preparation	1×10^{-6} M	Prolongation of action potential, flattening of the repolarization phase and a 40% decrease in contractile force	**19**
	1×10^{-5} M	Decreased resting potential, action potential amplitude, maximum upstroke velocity of the action potential and contractile force	**19**
Isolated papillary muscle from right ventricle. Heparinized prior to killing	10^{-6} M	Prolongation of the action potential, flattening of repolarization phase and a 40% decrease in contractile force	**96**
Same	10^{-5} M	Decreased; resting potential, action potential amplitude, maximum upstroke velocity and contractile force	**96**

Conditions of the Experiment	Dose	Cardiovascular Effects	Reference
3.5:4 Horses - Azaperone			
Intact, awake	0.4 and .08 mg/kg, IM	No change in arterial pH, pCO_2 or pO_2, no change in plasma protein concentration, venous blood packed cell volume and Hb concentration decreased 5-10% for 4 hours. Heart rate increased for up to 60 min. and then there was a slight decrease in some individuals. Mean aortic pressure decreased for at least 4 hours. Cardiac output increased slightly 20 min. after administration.	**45**

Conditions of the Experiment	Dose	Cardiovascular Effects	Reference
Intact, awake	0.8 mg/kg, IM	Decreased mean aortic pressure for at least 4 hours, partially antagonized the pressor action of adrenaline (1.5 g/kg, IV). Assumed alpha-adrenoceptor blocking activity	32
Intact, awake	0.7 mg/kg, IM	Significant increase in heart rate, decrease in packed cell volume and increase in serum cortisol	30

Conditions of the Experiment	Dose	Cardiovascular Effects	Reference
3.5:5 Pigs - Azaperone			
Intact, awake	5 mg/kg, IM	After 15 minutes, mean aortic pressure decreased 35%, systemic vascular conductance increased 45%, cardiac output decreased 10%. Increased pulmonary blood volume flow, no change in brain blood flow, decreased left ventricular myocardial blood flow. Vascular conductance of skin decreased.	112

Table 3.6: The Benzodiazephines (Diazepam)

Conditions of the Experiment	Dose	Cardiovascular Effects	Reference
3.6:1 Dogs			
Intact, awake, 10-48 hours following ligation of the left anterior descending coronary artery	1 mg/kg, IV and oral	Decreased the frequency of ectopic beats by 80-98%, an immediate response with a duration of about 5 min. after the IV dose. About 1 hr. after the oral dose there was 4-6 hr. of protection. Mean aortic pressure decreased only after the IV dose	27

Conditions of the Experiment	Dose	Cardiovascular Effects	Reference
Intact, awake, previously instrumented	0.5, 1.0, and 2.5 mg/kg, IV	No change in heart rate, no change in mean aortic pressure, a 17% decrease in left ventricular dP/dt max at 1.0 and 2.5 mg/kg doses and a 10% increase in cardiac output with the 2.5 mg/kg dose. There were no changes in regional coronary blood flow, systemic or coronary vascular resistance, stroke volume or stroke work	46
Intact, awake, previously instrumented. Comparisons were made between Diazepam and the solvent used in the commercial preparation	1 mg/kg, IV	Drug: Increase in heart rate, no change in mean aortic pressure, increase in left circumflex coronary flow, decrease in coronary resistance, no change in cardiac output, systemic resistance or dF/dt, but a decrease in stroke volume. Solvent: Increase in heart rate, mean aortic pressure, left circumflex flow and no change in coronary resistance, cardiac output, stroke volume, systemic resistance or dF/dt	47
Direct perfusion of the A-V nodal artery *in situ*, anesthetized with Pentobarbital (30 mg/kg, IV) open chest, positive pressure ventilation Heparin (500 micro-g/kg). Dogs were vagotomized and sympathectomized.	300 micro-g to 3 mg intra-arterial into A-V nodal artery	Third degree A-V block, longer duration than 3° A-V block caused by acetylcholine. Not affected by loss of autonomic control	48
Intact, awake, previously instrumented	2 mg/kg, IV	There was an early increase in aortic blood pressure then a return to baseline at the same time there was a significant decrease in renal blood flow	79
Intact, awake	0.5 mg/kg, IV	No tranquilizing effect, frequently associated with excessive excitement. Heart rate increased.	113

Conditions of the Experiment	Dose	Cardiovascular Effects	Reference
Intact, awake	1 mg/kg, IV	Increased heart rate, decreased stroke volume, increased coronary blood flow, decreased coronary resistance	**114**
Acute, open thorax, anesthetized with Fluothane	0.1 mg/kg, intra-coronary artery bolus	Significant increase in coronary blood flow and decrease in coronary resistance (Same reaction to solvent vehicle for this substance.)	**114**
Intact, awake, acutely instrumented	0.5 mg/kg, IV	Increased heart rate, no change in mean aortic pressure, mean pulmonary arterial pressure, central venous pressure, cardiac output, stroke volume or peripheral resistance	**115**
Anesthetized with Thiopental (20 mg/kg, IV) maintained with enflurane in Oxygen at 0.97 ± 0.04% blood concentration. Vagotomy plus spinal block.	Cumulative dose to 3.0 mg/kg (0.1, 0.3, 0.6, 1.0 then 3.0 mg/kg)	After final dose, no change in heart rate, left ventricular dP/dt/P, cardiac index. Mean aortic pressure, peripheral resistance and peak LVdP/dt decreased.	**116**

Conditions of the Experiment	Dose	Cardiovascular Effects	Reference
3.6:2 Cats			
Anesthetized with Pentobarbital (35 mg/kg, IP), positive pressure ventilation with room air, Deslanoside (digitalis glycoside) toxicity induced arrhythmia (25 micro-g/kg every 15 min. until death). Diazepam in propyleneglycol solvent	7-10 mg, IV every 45 sec.	No apparent effect of diazepam noted, solvent seemed to worsen the arrhythmia. Pure Diazepam was not evaluated since they were unable to dissolve it in an aqueous solution. No oral treatment was evaluated.	**49**

Conditions of the Experiment	Dose	Cardiovascular Effects	Reference
Anesthetized with halothane & oxygen, decerebrated and immobilized with gallamine triethiodide. Spinal cord segments L_1-S_1 exposed and ventral roots of L_7 and S1 were cut and placed on recording electrodes	1 mg/kg, IV	Stimulation of the femoral venous afferents elicited inhibition which was enhanced almost to the point of complete reflex suppression of both flexor and extensor monosynaptic reflexes, i.e. enhanced inhibitory mechanisms associated with primary afferent depolarization	50

Conditions of the Experiment	Dose	Cardiovascular Effects	Reference
3.6:3 Rats			
Primary cultures of myocardial cells	4, 16, or 32 micro-g/ml for 1, 4 or 24 hours	After 1 hr., cultures exhibited dose-dependent tachycardia, longer durations produced either arrhythmias or arrest, pseudopodia formation and increased cytoplasmic granulation of the cells were observed. After 24 hrs., cell viability (i.e., leakage of lactic dehydrogenase) was greatly reduced, some leakage occurred at 4 hrs.	51
Exsanguinated, isolated right atrium preparation	10 micro-g/ml	Prevented arrhythmic contractions induced by electrical stimulation during spontaneous rhythmic contractions	18
Exsanguinated, isolated left atrium and papillary muscle preparations	10 micro-g/ml	Increased refractory period by 90.5% in the left atrium and by 54.5% in papillary muscles. Decreased maximum driving frequency of the left atrium by 25.1%	18

Conditions of the Experiment	Dose	Cardiovascular Effects	Reference
Same	0.1-10 micro-g/ml	Had little effect on the rate of spontaneous contractions but there was a concentration-dependent increase in force of the spontaneous contractions, up to 204.7% in the left atrium and 163.1% in papillary muscle	18
Same	20 micro-g/ml	Decreased contractile force of electrically driven preparations	18
Anesthetized with open-drop Enflurane, venous injections of varying concentrations of diazepam with lidocaine, sacrificed at 24, 48, 72, 96 hrs., and 5 and 10 days post infusion. Light microscopic evaluation	Range of doses	Diazepam resulted in marked inflammation with inflammatory edema and intramural polymorphonuclear cell infiltration. Some animals showed thrombosis and complete vein wall destruction. Diazepam vehicle and diluted diazepam produced similar lesions. Lidocaine and saline showed no lesions. Lidocaine added to the diazepam product did not provide protection.	52
Isolated right ventricle preparation from rats killed by a blow to the head	30-50 μM	Abolished abnormal rhythm from local injury to the right ventricle. Effectively reduced ectopic automaticity. Is a calcium ion dependent phenomena at least partially mediated by "peripheral" type Diazepam receptors rather than "central" type.	117
Same as above	Dose-response 10, 30, and 50 μM	Inhibitory effect on ventricular automaticity resulting from inhibition of adenosine uptake	118
Isolated atria from ether anesthetized rats	5, 10 and 50 μM (Diazepam) 10 and 30 μM (Clonazepam)	Reduced the chronotropic responses to noradrenaline through the interaction with the cAMP-linked chain of events following beta-adrenoceptor activation.	119

Conditions of the Experiment	Dose	Cardiovascular Effects	Reference
Isolated left and right atria and papillary muscle preparations	10 μg/ml	Arrhythmic contractions induced by threshold electrical stimuli in rhythmic spontaneous contractions of the right atrium were prevented. Increased refractory periods by 90.5% in left atria and 54.4% in papillary muscle. Decreased maximum driving frequency of the left atria by 25.1% but no effect on papillary muscle.	120
Same	0.1-10 μg/ml	No effect on rate of right atrial spontaneous contractions. Dose-dependent increase in force of contraction.	120
Same	20 μg/ml	Contractile force in left atrial and papillary muscle decreased.	120
Same	0.5-10 μg/ml	Dose-dependent increase in contractile force, 204.7% in left atrial and 163.7% in papillary muscle	120
Chloral hydrate anesthesia (400 mg/kg, IP)	0.2 mg/kg, IV 5 min. before giving 2 mg/kg bupivacaine	Increased the incidence of serious ventricular or supraventricular tachyarrhythmias	121

Conditions of the Experiment	Dose	Cardiovascular Effects	Reference
3.6:4 Mice			
Sedation, muscle relaxation and hyporeflexia dosage	5 gm/kg	No data given	53
Motor coordination (ED_{50})	2.6 mg/kg	No data given	53

Conditions of the Experiment	Dose	Cardiovascular Effects	Reference
3.6:5 Guinea Pigs			
Electrically driven ($2H_Z$) isolated left atrium prep. killed by a blow to the head and exsanguination. Stabilized for 30 min.	1×10^{-6} and 10^{-5} M	Significant dose-dependent potentiation of the negative inotropic actions of adenosine (reduction of isometric tension)	**54**
Blow to the head and exsanguination, 10 mg slices of left ventricle incubated in adenosine with tritiated adenosine marker for 20 min. Uptake of adenosine measured.	Range of concentrations	Resulted in inhibition of adenosine uptake but not as potent as dipyridamole, a known potent inhibitor of adenosine uptake. Theorized that coronary vasodilation caused by diazepam is due to potentiation of adenosine following inhibition of the nucleoside transport system	**55**

Conditions of the Experiment	Dose	Cardiovascular Effects	Reference
3.6:6 Rabbits			
Anesthetized with pentobarbital (30 mg/kg, IV) plus additional doses as required	0.5 and 1.0 mg/kg	No effect on the response of arterial pressure to carotid occlusion, i.e., no effect on carotid sinus baroreflex	**122**

Conditions of the Experiment	Dose	Cardiovascular Effects	Reference
3.6:7 Roosters			
Intact, awake, fed an atherosclerotic diet	0.2 mg/kg b.i.d./os over a 5 month period	Provided same protection against the development of the nucleoside transport system	**56**

Conditions of the Experiment	Dose	Cardiovascular Effects	Reference
3.6:8 Pigs			
Intact, awake, previously instrumented, spontaneously breathing. Given bupivacaine (2 mg/kg/min) until cardiovascular collapse	0.15 mg/kg, IV	Delayed onset of ventricular dysrhythmias, decreased incidence of clonic-tonic seizures, prevented increases in aortic pressure and heart rate. Did not affect the dose of bupivacaine or the blood concentration required to produce cardiovascular collapse.	123

Conditions of the Experiment	Dose	Cardiovascular Effects	Reference
3.6:9 Sheep & Cattle			
Chronic, instrumented, pregnant ewes	0.2 and 0.5 mg/kg, IV	Dose dependent increase in maternal heart rate and mean aortic pressure. An increase in fetal heart rate which lasted more than 1 hr., an up to 10% decrease in fetal mean aortic pressure. No change in arterial pO_2, pCO_2 or pH in either the ewe or the fetus	57
Cultured bovine adrenal chromaffin cells in presence of ouabain	Dose-response	Potentiated effects of GABA on catecholamine release and phosphoinositide metabolism	142

Table 3.7: The Benzodiazepines (Midazolam)

Conditions of the Experiment	Dose	Cardiovascular Effects	Reference
3.7:1 Dogs			
Intact, awake, previously instrumented	0.25, 1.0 and 10.0 mg/kg, IV	Heart rate increase 10-20% with all doses, mean aortic pressure decreased 10-20% with the 1 and 10 mg/kg doses, cardiac output increased 10-12% with all doses and left ventricular dP/dt max decreased 13-16% at the higher doses. There were no changes in regional coronary blood flow, systemic or coronary vascular resistance, stroke volume or stroke work	46
Intact, awake, previously instrumented 24 hrs. prior to the study	2, 4, and 10 mg/kg, IV	No change in heart rate or mean aortic pressures with all doses, pulmonary wedge pressure decreased at 2 & 4 mg/kg, no change at 10 mg/kg. Cardiac index decreased with all doses. Stroke volume and left ventricular stroke work index decreased with 2 mg/kg. No change in mean pulmonary artery pressure, pulmonary artery resistance increased at 2 mg/kg. Right ventricular stroke work index did not change. No change in arterial pO_2, pCO_2 or % saturation. Arterial pH decreased with 2 and 4 mg/kg doses. No change in venous pCO_2 or % saturation but venous pO_2 increased at 4 mg/kg and pH decreased at 4 and 10 mg/kg	58
Isolated, cross-perfused right atrial preparation	100-1000 µg direct injection into sinus node artery	Direct cardiac inhibition of Catecholamine release due to a tyramine-like action. Inhibition characterized by negative then positive chronotropy and positive, then negative, then positive inotropy	124

Conditions of the Experiment	Dose	Cardiovascular Effects	Reference
Halothane anesthetized @ 1 MAC and 50% $N_2O:O_2$, succinylcholine (2 mg/kg, IV) immediately following induction dose of Midazolam	10 mg/kg, IV	Less arrhythmogenic than Thiopentone, induced when tested to Dose-response of epinephrine-aminophylline	**143**
Intact, awake, previously instrumented	2, 4 & 10 mg/kg, IV	No change in HR, mean aortic pressure, peripheral resistance, mean pulmonary arterial pressure, right ventricular stroke work index; decrease in pulmonary wedge pressures at 2 & 4 mg/kg; decrease in cardiac index at all doses; @ 2 mg/kg decreased stroke volume, left ventricular stroke work index and increased pulmonary vascular resistance	**144**

Conditions of the Experiment	Dose	Cardiovascular Effects	Reference
3.7:2 Sheep			
Chronically instrumented pregnant ewes	0.5 mg/kg, IV	Increased maternal heart rate and mean aortic pressure	**57**
Same	0.2 mg/kg	Same as 0.5 mg/kg but less magnitude. No change in uterine blood flow with low dose but minimal increase with 0.5 mg/kg. Fetal heart rate increased with both doses, duration 1 hr., no change in arterial pO_2, pCO_2, or pH in either ewe or fetus	**57**

Conditions of the Experiment	Dose	Cardiovascular Effects	Reference
3.7:3 Pigs			
Intact, awake, previously instrumented, spontaneously breathing. Given bupivacaine (2 mg/kg/min) until cardiovascular collapse	0.06 mg/kg, IV	Delayed onset of ventricular dysrhythmias, decreased incidence of clonic-tonic seizure, prevented increases in blood pressure and heart rate. Did not affect the dose of bupivacaine or the blood concentration required to produce cardiovascular collapse	123

Table 3.8: The Rauwolfia Derivatives (Reserpine)

Conditions of the Experiment	Dose	Cardiovascular Effects	Reference
3.8:1 Dogs			
Previously instrumented, intact, awake dogs, challenged with Trimazosin (1 mg/kg/min for 7 min), peak effects seen 30-60 min after start of infusion	0.25 mg/kg/day, IM, for 3 days pretreatment	Blocked Trimazosin induced decreases in mean aortic pressure, left ventricular end-diastolic diameter and partially blocked the decrease in late diastolic coronary artery resistance	59
Intact awake measurements of heart rate and mean aortic blood pressure. After euthanasia measured arterial tissue levels of K^+Ca^{++}, norepinephrine levels	0.03 mg/kg orally for 6 weeks	Sustained decreased in mean aortic pressure and heart rate. Arterial tissue levels of K^+, Ca^{++} and Mg^{++} were decreased, Mg^{++} most affected. There was no change in arterial tissue Na+ levels but norepinephrine levels decreased and there was slight but significant increase in plasma Mg^{++} levels	60

Conditions of the Experiment	Dose	Cardiovascular Effects	Reference
Anesthetized with Pentobarbital (30mg/kg, IV), measured femoral vascular resistance using aortic blood pressure and femoral artery flow with an electromagnetic flowmeter	1 mg/kg, IM 24 hrs. prior to experiment	Calculated slope of a dose-response regression line for adenosine, nitroglycerin, acetylcholine and isoproterenol. Reserpine pretreatment increased the slopes, i.e. enhanced vasodilator responses	**61**
Anesthetized with Pentobarbital (25 mg/kg,IV), open chest, positive pressure ventilation, mapping of epicardial S-T segment changes for ischemic injury following acute occlusion of the LAD coronary	5 mg/kg, IP for 2 consecutive days prior to the experiment	Prevented changes in S-T segments produced by pyridylcarbinol. Showed that inhibition of lipolysis during coronary occlusion reduces ischemic changes only when myocardial stores of catecholamines are intact.	**63**
Anesthetized with Pentobarbital (30mg/kg,IV) positive pressure ventilation	0.3 mg/kg pretreatment 24 hrs prior to the experiment	Prevented time dependency of ventricular fibrillation threshold (VFT) to actual occurrence of ventricular fibrillation, i.e. this parameter is dependent upon local catecholamine release	**64**
Anesthetized with Pentobarbital (30mg/kg, IV) Heparin (500 units/kg IV), exsanguination and heart removal, trabeculae corneae isolated preparation	0.1 mg/kg,SC 48 and 24 hrs prior to experiment	Phenylephrine and tyramine dose response curves shifted downward and to the right, i.e. less inotropy at higher doses. Concluded that reserpine blocks the beta-adrenoceptors in ventricular myocardium which mediate inotropic responses	**62**
Anesthetized with Pentobarbital (25 mg/kg,IV), open chest positive pressure ventilation, mapping of epicardial S-T segment changes for ischemic injury following acute occlusion of the LAD coronary	5 mg/kg, IP for 2 consecutive days prior to the experiment	Prevented changes in S-T segments produced by pyridylcarbinol. Showed that inhibition of lipolysis during coronary occlusion reduces ischemic changes only when myocardial stores of catecholamines are intact	**63**

Conditions of the Experiment	Dose	Cardiovascular Effects	Reference
Anesthetized with Pentobarbital (30mg/kg, IV), positive pressure ventilation	0.3 mg/kg pretreatment 24 hrs prior to experiment	Prevented time dependency of ventricular fibrillation threshold (VFT) to actual occurrence of ventricular fibrillation, i.e. this parameter is dependent upon local catecholamine release	64
Anesthetized with Pentobarbital (30 mg/kg, IV), spiral strips from femoral artery, ventricle mounted in isometric tension with 2.5 g preload	1 mg/kg, IM 24 hrs. prior to experiment	Reserpine pretreatment did not alter contractile response to norepinephrine. Reserpine pretreatment made the preparation supersensitive to glyceryl trinitrate but not to adenosine or hydralazine	65
Anesthetized with Pentobarbital (30mg/kg, IV), open chest, positive pressure ventilation, 2 stage LAD ligation with distal artery injected with 3% agar (no collateral circulation)	3 mg/kg, IV 24 hrs. prior to the experiment	No change in aortic flow, decrease in heart rate, aortic pressure, systemic resistance, left ventricular end-diastolic pressure and left ventricular dp/dt max	66
Anesthetized with Pentobarbital (50 mg/kg, IP), exsanguination isolated smooth muscle prep	0.5 mg/kg, 20-24 hours prior to experiment	Following contraction with PGF_2, relaxation produced by electrical stimulation was blocked	67
Anesthetized with Pentobarbital (50 mg/kg, IP), exsanguination isolated arterial helically cut segments from basilar and middle cerebral arteries, intrarenal interlobar branches of the mesenteric and femoral arteries	0.5 mg/kg, IP, for 20-24 hrs pre-experiment	Abolished ouabain induced contractions of the peripheral, but not the cerebral, arteries. (beta-adrenergic effects)	68

Conditions of the Experiment	Dose	Cardiovascular Effects	Reference
Intact, awake, trained	0.1 mg/kg, SQ daily for 15 days	Significant and decrease in resting aortic pressure and heart rate. The alpha-2-mediated pressure response to norepinephrine was decreased. Clonidine induced marked pressure effects after treatment. Increased numbers of platelet alpha-2 adrenoceptors. Concluded that reserpine pretreatment induces vascular alpha-2-adrenergic super sensitivity and an up-regulation in platelet alpha-2-adrenoceptors.	125
Thiopental Anesthetized (20 mg/kg)	0.03 mg/kg/day for 6 weeks	Sustained decreases in mean aortic pressure and heart rate. Arterial tissues contained less K^+, Ca^{++} and Mg^{++}. No change in Na. Arterial norepinephrine significantly decreased. Slight but significant increase in plasma Mg^{++}, no change in plasma levels of other cations. Changes in Mg^{++} linked to vascular tone and/or sensitivity	126
Isolated mesenteric artery	1.0 mg/kg pretreatment o.i.d. for 4 days, i.p.	Contraction of the isolated mesenteric artery induced by electrical transmural stimulation consists of an adrenergic component (the latter mediated via post synaptic P2- purinoceptors)	127

Conditions of the Experiment	Dose	Cardiovascular Effects	Reference
3.8:1 Dogs (Continued)			
Previously instrumented, intact, awake dogs, challenged with Trimazosin (1 mg/kg/min for 7 min), peak effects seen 30-60 min. after start of infusion	0.25 mg/kg/day, IM, for 3 days pre-treatment	Blocked Trimazosin induced decreases in mean aortic pressure, left ventricular end-diastolic diameter and partially blocked the decrease in late diastolic coronary artery resistance	**59**
Intact, awake measurements of heart rate and mean aortic blood pressure. After euthanasia measured arterial tissue levels of K^+, Ca^{++}, $Mg+$, Na^+ and norepinephrine levels	0.03 mg/kg orally for 6 weeks	Sustained decrease in mean aortic pressure and heart rate. Arterial tissue levels of K^+, Ca^{++}, and Mg^{++} were decreased, Mg^{++} most affected. There was no change in arterial tissue Na^+ levels but norepinephrine levels decreased and there was a slight but significant increase in plasma Mg^{++} levels	**60**
Anesthetized with Pentobarbital (30 mg/kg, IV), measured femoral vascular resistance using aortic blood pressure and femoral artery flow with an electromagnetic flowmeter	1 mg/kg, IM 24 hrs. prior to experiment	Calculated slope of a dose-response regression line for adenosine, nitroglycerin, acetylcholine, and isoproterenol. Reserpine pretreatment increased the slopes, i.e. enhanced vasodilator responses.	**61**
Anesthetized with Pentobarbital (30mg/kg, IV) Heparin (500 units/kg/IV), exsanguination and heart removal, trabeculae corneae isolated preparation	0.1 mg/kg, SC 48 and 24 hrs. prior to experiment	Phenylephrine and tyramine dose response curves shifted downward and to the right, i.e., less inotropy at higher doses. Concluded that reserpine blocks the beta-adrenoceptors in ventricular myocardium which mediate inotropic responses	**62**

Conditions of the Experiment	Dose	Cardiovascular Effects	Reference
Anesthetized with Pentobarbital (25 mg/kg, IV), open chest, positive pressure ventilation, mapping of epicardial S-T segment changes for ischemic injury following acute occlusion of the LAD coronary	5 mg/kg, IP for 2 consecutive days prior to the experiment	Prevented changes in S-T segments produced by pyridylcarbinol. Showed that inhibition of lipolysis during coronary occlusion reduces ischemic changes only when myocardial stores of catecholamines are intact	63
Anesthetized with Pentobarbital (30 mg/kg, IV), positive pressure ventilation	0.3 mg/kg pretreatment 24 hrs. prior to experiment	Prevented time dependency of ventricular fibrillation threshold (VFT) to actual occurrence of ventricular fibrillation, i.e., this parameter is dependent upon local catecholamine release	64
Anesthetized with Pentobarbital (30 mg/kg, IV), spiral strips from femoral artery, ventricle mounted in isolation chamber, measured isometric tension with 2.5 g preload	1 mg/kg, IM 24 hrs. prior to experiment	Reserpine pretreatment did not alter contractile response to norepinephrine. Reserpine pretreatment made the preparation supersensitive to glyceryl trinitrate but not to adenosine or hydralazine	65
Anesthetized with Pentobarbital (30 mg/kg, IV), open chest, positive pressure ventilation, 2 stage LAD ligation with distal artery injected with 3% agar (no collateral circulation)	3 mg/kg, IV 24 hrs. prior to the experiment	No change in aortic flow, decrease in heart rate, aortic pressure, systemic resistance, left ventricular end-diastolic pressure and left ventricular dP/dt max	66
Anesthetized with Pentobarbital (50 mg/kg, IP), exsanguination isolated smooth muscle prep	0.5 mg/kg, 20-24 hours prior to experiment	Following contraction with PGF_2, relaxation produced by electrical stimulation was blocked	67
Anesthetized with Pentobarbital (50 mg/kg, IP), exsanguination, isolated arterial helically cut segments from basilar and middle cerebral arteries, intrarenal interlobar branches of the renal artery, distal portions of the mesenteric and femoral arteries	0.5 mg/kg, IP, for 20-24 hrs. pre-experiment	Abolished ouabain induced contractions of the peripheral, but not the cerebral, arteries (beta-adrenergic effects)	68

Conditions of the Experiment	Dose	Cardiovascular Effects	Reference
Intact, awake, trained	0.1 mg/kg, SQ daily for 15 days	Significant decrease in resting aortic pressure and heart rate. The alpha-2-mediated pressor response to norepinephrine was decreased. Clonidine induced marked pressor effects after treatment. Increased numbers of platelet alpha-2-adrenoceptors. Concluded that Reserpine pretreatment induces vascular alpha-2-adrenergic supersensitivity and an up-regulation in platelet alpha-2-adrenoceptors.	125
Thiopental anesthetized (20 mg/kg)	0.03 mg/kg/day/os for 6 weeks	Sustained decreases in mean aortic pressure and heart rate. Arterial tissues contained less K^+, Ca^{++} and Mg^{++}. No change in Na^+. Arterial norepinephrine significantly decreased. Slight but significant increase in plasma Mg^{++}, no change in plasma levels of other cations. Changes in Mg^{++} linked to vascular tone and/or reactivity.	126
Isolated mesenteric artery	1.0 mg/kg pretreatment o.i.d. for 4 days IP	Sympathetic contraction of the isolated mesenteric artery induced by electrical transmural stimulation consists of an adrenergic and a purinergic component (the latter mediated via post synaptic P_2-purinoceptors).	127

Conditions of the Experiment	Dose	Cardiovascular Effects	Reference
3.8:2 Cats			
Anesthetized with Pentobarbital (30mg/kg, IP), heparinized (5,000 units, IV Langendorf type isolated heart prep	1 mg/kg, IV 24 hrs prior to experiment	Failed to block increase in blood pressure and increase in inotropy initiated by infusion of angiotensin I or angiotensin II	69

Conditions of the Experiment	Dose	Cardiovascular Effects	Reference
Anesthetized with Pentobarbital (35 mg/kg/IP), exsanguinated, posterior communicating cerebral artery removed and cylindrical segments mounted in an organ bath	3 mg/kg, IP, pretreatment	Pretreatment failed to modify the dose response curve to 5-HT except in the lowest range. This indicates that vasoconstriction caused by 5-HT, in the posterior communicating cerebral artery of the cat, is primarily due to direct stimulation of tryptaminergic receptors	70
Pentobarbital anesthesia (30mg/kg, IP, isolated organ preparation of electrically driven right ventricular papillary muscles	5 mg/kg, IP, pretreated 15-18 hours before the experiment	Reserpine failed to block the positive inotropic effects of ammonium vanadate (50-1000 micro-M)	71

Conditions of the Experiment	Dose	Cardiovascular Effects	Reference
3.8:2 Cats (Continued)			
Anesthetized with Pentobarbital (30 mg/kg, IP), heparinized (5,000 units, IV) Langendorff type isolated heart prep	1 mg/kg, IV 24 hrs. prior to experiment	Failed to block increase in blood pressure and increase in inotropy initiated by infusion of angiotensin I or angiotensin II	69
Anesthetized with Pentobarbital (35 mg/kg, IP), exsanguinated, posterior communicating cerebral artery removed and cylindrical segments mounted in an organ bath	3 mg/kg, IP pretreatment	Pretreatment failed to modify the dose response curve to 5-HT except in the lowest range. This indicates that vasoconstriction caused by 5-HT, in the posterior communicating cerebral artery of the cat, is primarily due to direct stimulation of tryptaminergic receptors	70
Pentobarbital anesthesia (30 mg/kg, IP) isolated organ preparation of electrically driven right ventricular papillary muscles	5 mg/kg, IP, pretreated 15-18 hours before the experiment	Reserpine failed to block the positive inotropic effects of ammonium vanadate (50-1000 micro-M)	71

Conditions of the Experiment	Dose	Cardiovascular Effects	Reference
Anesthetized with Pentobarbital (35 mg/kg, IP), exsanguinated, isolated pial arteries from the circle of Willis	3 mg/kg, 24 hrs. prior to experiment	Reserpine produced a significant decrease in the outflow of tritiated noradrenaline induced by 5-HT	72

Conditions of the Experiment	Dose	Cardiovascular Effects	Reference
3.8:3 Rats			
Killed by a blow to the head, left atrial preparation	1.0 mg/kg, i.e., daily for 7 days pretreatment	Brown but not white adipocyte beta-adrenoceptors innervated	128
Biochemical analysis of cardiac membrane beta-adrenoceptors	2.5 mg/kg/day pretreatment	Induced either an increase or decrease in cardiac beta-adrenoceptor density and coupling, dependent on the dose and the time at which the beta-adrenoceptors were measured after treatment.	129
In vitro rat tail artery preparation	Pretreatment with 3.2 and 2 mg/kg, IP Reserpine @ days 3, 2 and 1 prior to experiment	Pretreatment with reserpine potentiates alpha-2 but not alpha-1 adrenoceptor-mediated responses. Probably due to changes in calcium ion influx.	130

Conditions of the Experiment	Dose	Cardiovascular Effects	Reference
3.8:4 Rabbits			
Killed by a blow to the head, isolated strips of left atrium	5 mg/kg pretreatment 24 hours before study	Markedly depressed the potentiation of contraction by tyramine, there was no norepinephrine fluorescence found histochemically	39

Conditions of the Experiment	Dose	Cardiovascular Effects	Reference
Isolated saphenous artery	3 mg/kg 48 hrs. plus 5 mg/kg 24 hrs., IP, pretreatment	Substantial contractions produced by stimulation of sympathetic nerves despite a 95.7% decrease in noradrenaline content of the tissue. Responses not significantly affected by an alpha-1 antagonist but desensitization of P_2-purinoceptors abolished the response. Norepinephrine containing nerves were not observed. Potencies of ATP and histamine not significantly affected but there was a slight supersensitivity to norepinephrine	131

Conditions of the Experiment	Dose	Cardiovascular Effects	Reference
3.8:5 Sheep			
Intact, awake, previously instrumented adult females and newborn lambs	10 micro-g/kg b.i.d., IM	Adrenergic neuronal depletion, usually required 7-10 days of this treatment until there was no response to a tyramine challenge	73

Conditions of the Experiment	Dose	Cardiovascular Effects	Reference
3.8:6 Goats			
Arterial segments	0.02 mg/kg/day for 3 days	Contraction produced by electrical stimulation was significantly decreased compared to non-reserpine treated controls	74
Killed by IV injection of 30 ml of a saturated solution of KCl, brain removed, middle cerebral arteries dissected out, cylindrical segments in an organ bath preparation	0.02 mg/kg/day for 3 days prior to the experiment	Resulted in significant decrease in contractions produced by 5-HT	75

Conditions of the Experiment	Dose	Cardiovascular Effects	Reference
Killed with IV injection of KCl, isolated arteries from the Circle of Willis, fluorometric determination of norepinephrine tissue concentrations	0.02 mg/kg/day for 3 days before experiment	Controls 2.10 micro-g/gm tissue, reserpine pretreatment, unable to detect, i.e. < 0.1 micro-g/g of tissue	76

Conditions of the Experiment	Dose	Cardiovascular Effects	Reference
3.8:7 Monkeys			
Anesthetized with Pentobarbital (50 mg/kg, IP), exsanguination, isolated arterial, helically cut segments from the basilar and middle cerebral arteries, intra-renal interlobar branches of the renal artery and distal portions of the mesenteric and femoral arteries	0.5 mg/kg, IP for 20-24 hrs. pre-experiment	Abolished ouabain induced contractions of the peripheral but not the cerebral arteries	77

Conditions of the Experiment	Dose	Cardiovascular Effects	Reference
3.8:8 Guinea Pigs			
Cervical dislocation heart removal, isolated atrial preparation	5 mg/kg, SC 24 hours before the experiment	Prevented release of catecholamines from cardiac sympathetic nerve terminals and prevented increases in myocardial contractile force induced by hydroxylated metabolites of chlorpromazine	20
Isolated ductus-arteriosus from fetuses taken by cesarian section from dams anesthetized with urethane	Range of concentrations in organ bath	Blocked response to transmural electrical stimulation, i.e., adrenergic mediated response	78

Conditions of the Experiment	Dose	Cardiovascular Effects	Reference
Cerebral dislocation, exsanguination, right ventricular strips in tissue chamber, electrical stimulation	0.1 and 0.03 mg/kg/day for 7 days pretreatment	Inotropic supersensitivity, nonspecific, preceded by norepinephrine depletion, no direct toxic effects, no increase in beta-adrenoceptor activity, dependent on mechanism(s) at or distal to adenylate cyclase activation.	132

Table 3.9: Xylazine HCl and Detomidine

Conditions of the Experiment	Dose	Cardiovascular Effects	Reference
3.9:1 Dogs - Xylazine			
Twenty minutes after a dose of xylazine the animals were anesthetized with thiamylal and halothane and then given an epinephrine challenge	1.1 mg/kg	Serious ventricular arrhythmias, including ventricular fibrillation, were induced with much smaller doses of epinephrine in the xylazine pretreated group compared to an identically anesthetized, but non-premedicated controls	27
Anesthetized with Thiamylal (10 mg/kg, IV) maintained with chloralose (50 mg/kg) and urethane (350 mg/kg) initial IV bolus, followed by small IV boluses of 5% chloralose and 35% urethane to effect, as needed. Positive pressure ventilation was provided. The spleen was exteriorized.	0.01, 0.1 and 1 mg/kg, IV	There was a dose-dependent decrease in splenic weight which was significant at the 1 mg/kg dose. Alpha-adrenergic blockade prevented the splenic contractile response to xylazine but beta-blockade had no effect. There was a decrease in heart rate and in splenic arterial flow. The mean, systolic and diastolic aortic pressures all decreased at the 0.1 and 1 mg/kg doses. At 1 mg/kg central venous pressure increased.	81

Conditions of the Experiment	Dose	Cardiovascular Effects	Reference
Xylazine preanesthesia then pentobarbital IV	2.2 mg/kg, IM, Xylazine 14 mg/kg, IV 10 min. after Xylazine	No change in arterial pH or $PaCO_2$ until +120 min., then pH increased and $paCO_2$ decreased. Were able to block these effects with Atropine (0.045 mg/kg, IM) pretreatment.	133
Intact, awake	1.0 mg/kg, IV	Decreased heart rate, cardiac output, left ventricular work, respiratory rate, minute ventilation, physiologic dead space, oxygen transport, mixed venous pO_2 and oxygen concentration. There was an increase in mean arterial pressure, central venous pressure, peripheral resistance, tidal volume and oxygen utilization ratio.	134
Anesthetized with 4-5% Isoflurane by mask, intubated, maintained at 1.8% (1.5 MAC)	1.1 mg/kg, IV	Three minutes after infusion heart rate decreased, mean aortic pressure increased. These responses were blocked by Yohimbine (alpha-2 adrenoceptor antagonist). There was no change in the epinephrine induced arrhythmia dose.	135
Intact, awake, previously instrumented	1.1 mg/kg, IV	No change in pulse pressure, stroke volume, arterial pH, PaO_2 or $PaCO_2$; decreased heart rate, cardiac output; initial increase in aortic pressure followed by a decrease and an increase in peripheral resistance	145
	2.2 mg/kg, IM	No change in mean aortic pressure, systemic resistance, arterial pH, PaO_2 or $PaCO_2$; decreased cardiac output and heart rate	

Conditions of the Experiment	Dose	Cardiovascular Effects	Reference
3.9:2 Cats - Xylazine			
Pentobarbital (30 mg/kg, IP) more as required	1 mg/kg, IV	Decreased heart rate, contractility and cardiac output. Increased left ventricular end diastolic pressure, myocardial, renal and GI blood flow rates.	**136**

Conditions of the Experiment	Dose	Cardiovascular Effects	Reference
3.9:3 Horses - Xylazine			
Intact awake, not instrumented	2.0 mg/kg IM	No change in heart rate or packed cell volume, slight decrease in plasma cortisol	**30**
Intact, awake, pain free, previously instrumented	1.1 mg/kg, IV	Decrease in heart rate, cardiac output and respiratory rate, increase in central venous pressure, mean aortic pressure increased than decreased, no change in arterial pO_2, pO_2, or pH	**31**
Intact, awake, acutely instrumented. Catheters were placed using local anesthesia. There was a 20-30 min. wait for stabilization before any measurements were made.	1.1 mg/kg, IV	This dose reduced the amount of guaifenesin needed to produce lateral recumbency. There was a decrease in heart rate, respiratory rate, cardiac output and arterial pO_2. Central venous pressure increased but there was no change in aortic or pulmonary artery pressures.	**82**
Intact awake, acute instrumentation using only local anesthesia	1.1 mg/kg, IV	There was a decrease in heart rate, respiratory rate and cardiac output, central venous pressure increased and there was an increase followed by a decrease in mean aortic pressure. There was no change noted in arterial pCO_2, pO_2 or pH.	**31**

Conditions of the Experiment	Dose	Cardiovascular Effects	Reference
Intact, awake, instrumented	1.1 mg/kg, IV 2.2 mg/kg, IM	Decreased heart rate, cardiac output, cardiac index and both positive and negative dP/dt. Increased AV block, peripheral resistance. No change in stroke volume or ejection fraction.	137
Intact, awake, pretreated with acepromazine (0.1 mg/kg, IV)	0.4 mg/kg, IV 20 min. after acepromazine	Decreased heart rate, respiratory rate and arterial pO_2, increased diastolic aortic pressure	104

Conditions of the Experiment	Dose	Cardiovascular Effects	Reference
3.9:3 Horses - Detomidine			
Intact, awake	10 µg/kg, IV	No change in mean aortic pressure, heart rate, PaO_2 or $PaCO_2$	138
Intact, awake	10 µg/kg, IV	Decreased heart rate, cardiac output, increased second degree heart block, alpha-2 adrenoceptor agonist.	139
Intact, awake	0.01, 0.02 mg/kg, IV 0.04 mg/kg, IM	Decreased heart rate, packed cell volume, cardiac output, cardiac index, and both positive and negative LV dP/dt. No change in stroke volume or ejection fraction. Increased AV block. At 0.02 mg/kg IV initial increase in blood pressure.	137

Conditions of the Experiment	Dose	Cardiovascular Effects	Reference
3.9:4 Sheep - Xylazine			
Intact, awake, monitored the ECG	0.1 to 0.2 mg/kg, IM	There were no changes in the ECG noted	83

Conditions of the Experiment	Dose	Cardiovascular Effects	Reference
3.9:5 Calves - Xylazine			
Intact, awake, previously instrumented	0.22 mg/100 kg, IM	There was a decrease in heart rate, cardiac output, aortic pressure, and left ventricular dP/dt max. Stroke volume initially decreased and then returned to baseline within 15 min. Systemic resistance, left ventricular end-diastolic pressure, left ventricular end-diastolic volume and left ventricular residual volume were all increased. There was no hypertensive response noted in these animals.	**84**
Intact, awake	0.7 mg/kg	Decreased heart rate from approx. 83 to approx 50 b/min. and stayed depressed for at least 60 minutes of measurement	**140**
Intact, awake, previously instrumented	0.22 mg/100 kg, IM	Decreased heart rate, cardiac output, mean aortic pressure, left ventricular dP/dt max; stroke volume initially increased then decreased to baseline; increased systemic resistance, LVEDP and LV end-diastolic diameter	**146**

Conditions of the Experiment	Dose	Cardiovascular Effects	Reference
3.9:6 Monkey (macaca mulatta)- Xylazine			
Intact, instrumented under Thiamylal anesthesia just prior to the experiment but allowed to regain consciousness	0.6 mg/kg, IM	There were no changes seen in respiratory rate, arterial pH, pO_2, pCO_2 or venous pO_2. There were significant decreases in mean aortic pressure and heart rate within 30 minutes.	**85**

References

1. Booth, N.H. Introduction to drugs acting on the central nervous system, section 4 in Veterinary Pharmacology and Therapeutics, 5th ed., ed. by N.H. Booth and L.E. McDonald, The Iowa State University Press, Ames, Iowa, 1982.

2. Parker, J.L., Adams, H.R. The influence of chemical restraining agents on cardiovascular function: a review. *Lab Anim Sci*, 28(5):575-583, 1978.

3. Elkayan, U., Frishman, W., Cardiovascular effects of phenothiazines, *Am Heart J*, 100(3):397-401, 1980.

4. Kohn, C.W. Preoperative management of the equine patient with an abdominal crisis. *Vet Clin N America (Lg Anim Prac)*, 1(2):289-311, 1979.

5. Pugh, D.M. Observations of certain effects of promazine, chlorpromazine and chlorprothixene following intravenous injection into conscious dogs. *Vet Anaes, Great Britain, Ireland*, 8:35-40, 1981.

6. Goldberg, S.J., Linde, L.M., Wolfe, R.R., Griswold, W., Momma, K. The effects of meperidine, promethazine and chlorpromazine on pulmonary and systemic circulation. *Am Heart J*, 77:214-221, 1969.

7. Turner, D.M., Ilkin, J.E., Rose, R.J., Warren, J.M. Respiratory and cardiovascular effects of five drugs used as sedatives in the dog. *Aust Vet J*, 50(6): 260-267, 1974.

8. Brannon, M.D., Riggs, J.J., Hageman, W.E., Pruss, T.P. A comparison of the cardiovascular effects of haloperidol, thioridazine and chlorpromazine HCl. *Arch Int Pharmacodyn Ther*, 244(1):48-57, 1980.

9. Kitazawa, M., Sugiyama, S., Ozawa, T., Miyazaki, Y., Kotaka, K. Mechanism of chlorpromazine-induced arrhythmia--arrhythmia and mitochondrial dysfunction. *J Electrocardiol*, 14(3):219-24, 1981.

10. Caroni, P., Reinlib, L., Carafoli, E. Charge movements during the Na^+-$Ca2^+$ exchange in heart sarcolemmal vesicles. *Proc Natl Acad Sci USA*, 77(11):6354-8, 1980.

11. Beckman, J.K., Owens, K., Knauer, T.E., Weglicki, W.B. Hydrolysis of sarcolemma by lysosomal lipases and inhibition by chlorpromazine. *Am J Physiol*, 242(4):H652-6, 1982.

12. Aminoff, M.J., Jaffe, R.A., Sampson, S.R., Vidruk, E.H. Effects of droperidol on activity of carotid body chemoreceptors in cat. *Br J Pharmacol*, 63(2):245-250, 1978.

13. Dhalla, N.S., Lee, S.L., Takes, S., Panagia, V., Bhayana, V. Effects of chlorpromazine and imipramine on rat heart subcellular membranes. *Biochem Pharmacol*, 29:629-633, 1980.

14. Cooper, M., Wyllie, J.H. Some properties of 5-hydroxytryptamine receptors in the hindquarters of the rat. *Br J Pharmacol*, 67(1):79-85, 1979.

15. Chien, K.R., Peau, R.G., Farber, J.L. Ischemic myocardial cell injury. Prevention by chlorpromazine of an accelerated phospholipid degradation and associated membrane dysfunction. *Am J Pathol Dec*, 97(3):505-29, 1979.

16. Aronson, C.E., Serlick, E.R. Effects of chlorpromazine on the isolated perfused rat heart. *Toxicol Appl Pharmacol*, 39(2):157-76, 1977.

17. Bell, F.P., Hubert, E.V. Effect of chlorpromazine on rat arterial lipid synthesis *In Vitro, Lipids*, 17(10):672-675, 1982.

18. Sugimoto, J., Nagata, M., Ikeda, Y. The effects of diazepam on rat isolated heart muscle. *Clin Exp Pharmacol Physiol*, 5:655-663, 1978.

19. Arlock, P., Gullberg, B., Sven-Olle, R.O. Cardiac electrophysiology of four neuroleptics: melperone, haloperidol, thioridazine and chlorpromazine. *Naunyn-Schmiedebergs Arch Pharmacol*, 304:27-36, 1978.

20. Temma, K., Akera, T., Brody, T.M. Hydroxylated chlorpromazine metabolites: positive inotropic action and the release of catecholamines. *Mol Pharmacol*, 13(6):1076-85, 1977.

21. Itoh, T., Kuriyama, H., Suzuki, H. Effects of chlorpromazine on the electrical and mechanical properties of intact and skinned muscle cells of guinea-pig mesenteric artery. *Br J Pharmacol*, 75(3):513-23, 1982.

22. Bell, F.P., Hubert, E.V. Membrane-active agents. Effect of various anesthetics and chlorpromazine on arterial lipid metabolism. *Atherosclerosis*, 39(4):517-25, 1981.

23. Tuganowski, W. The influence of adenylate cyclase inhibitors on the spontaneous activity of the cardiac pacemaker. *Arch Int Pharmacodyn Ther*, 225(2):275-86, 1977.

24. Burton, K.P., Hagler, H.K., Willerson, J.T., Buja, L.M. Abnormal lanthanum accumulation due to ischemia in isolated myocardium: effect of chlorpromazine. *Am J Physiol*, 241(5):H714-23, 1981.

25. Asano, M., Suzuki, Y., Hidaka, H. Effects of various calmodulin antagonists on contraction of rabbit aortic strips. *J Pharmacol Exp Ther*, 220(1):191-6, 1982.

26. Barron, J.T., Barany, M., Barany, K., Storti, R.V. Reversible phosphorylation and dephosphorylation of the 20,000-dalton light chain of myosin during the contraction-relaxation-contraction cycle of arterial smooth muscle. *J Biol Chem*, 10:255(13):6238-44, 1980.

27. Muir, W.W., Werner, L.L., Hamlin, R.L. Antiarrhythmic effects of diazepam during coronary artery occlusion in dogs. *Am J. Vet Res*, 36(8)1203-1206, 1975.

28. Peres-Gomes, F., Ribeiro, J.A. Modification of the cardiotoxic effects of ouabain by acepromazine, tetrodotoxin and magnesium sulphate. *Pharmacol* 18(2):80-90, 1979.

29. Rezakhani, A., Edjtehadi, M., Szabuniewicz, M. Prevention of thiopental and thiopental/halothane cardiac sensitization to epinephrine in the sheep. *Can J Comp Med*, 41(4):389-395, 1977.

30. Mackenzie, G., Snow, D.H. An evaluation of chemical restraining agents in the horse. *Veterinary Record*, 101(2):30-33, 1977.

31. Muir, W.W., Skarda, R.T., Sheehan, W. Hemodynamic and respiratory effects of a xylazine-acetylpromazine drug combination in horses. *Am J Vet Res*, 40(11):1518-1522, 1979.

32. Serrano, L., Lees, P. The applied pharmacology of azaperone in ponies. *Res Vet Sci*, 20(3):316-323, 1976.

33. Arndt, J.O., Mameghani, F. The effects of etomidate, fentanyl and dehydrobenzperitol on baroreflex function. A study on dog's carotid sinus reflex. *Anaesthesist*, 29(4):200-207, 1980.

34. Muldoon, S.M., Janssens, W.J., Verbeuren, T.J., Vanhoutte. Alpha-adrenergic blocking properties of droperidol on isolated blood vessels of the dog. *Br J Anaesth*, 49:211-216, 1977.

35. Perez-Medina, T., Garcia-Barreto, D., Hernandez-Canero, A. Experimental HIS bundle escape rhythms. *Cor Vasa*, 20:129-134, 1978.

36. Toda, N., Hatano, A. Antagonism by droperidol of dopamine-induced relaxation in isolated dog arteries. *Eur J Pharmacol*, 57(2-3):231-238, 1979.

37. Hyatt, M., Muldoon, S.M., Rorie, D.K. Droperidol, a selective antagonist of postsynaptic alpha-adrenoceptors in the canine saphenous vein. *Anesthesiol*, 53(4):281-286, 1981.

38. van Nueten, J.M., Reneman, R.S., Janssen, P.A. Specific alpha-adrenoceptor blocking effect of droperidol on isolated smooth muscle. *Eur J Pharmacol*, 44(1):1-8, 1977.

39. Satoh, M., Kaya, K., Yamanaka, I., Kasama, A., Yanagisawa, M. Droperidol, its alpha-adrenergic blocking action on the aortic strip and inhibitory action on norepinephrine uptake of the adrenergic terminal of the left atrial strip of the rabbit. *Tohoku J Exp Med*, 124:65-72, 1978.

40. Garcia-Barreto, D., Perez, A., Hernandez, K. Inhibiting effect of droperidol compared with verapamil on the myocardial fiber calcium exchange determined by a simple physiological procedure. *Arch Int Pharmacodyn Ther*, 229(2):213-218, 1977.

41. Dorticas, F.R., Garcia-Barreto, D. Electrophysiological effects of droperidol on sinoatrial nodal fibers. *Arch Int Pharmacodyn Ther*, 240(1):137-142, 1979.

42. Brodde, O.E., Meyer, F.J., Schemuth, W., Freistuhler, J. Demonstration of specific vascular dopamine receptors mediating vasodilation on the isolated rabbit mesenteric artery. *Naunyn-Schmiedebergs Arch Pharmacol*, 316(1):24-30, 1981.

43. Grant, A.O., Hondeghem, L.M., Katzung, B.G. Effects of droperidol on depolarization-induced automaticity, maximum upstroke velocity (Vmax) and the kinetics of recovery of Vmax in guinea pig ventricular myocardium. *J Pharmacol Exp Ther*, 205(1):193-203, 1978.

44. Hauswirth, O. Effects of droperidol on sheep Purkinje fibers. *Naunyn-Schmiedebergs Arch Pharmacol Exp Path*, 261:133-142, 1968.

45. Lees, P., Serrano, L. Effects of azaperone on cardiovascular and respiratory functions in the horse. *British J of Pharm*, 56(3):263-269, 1976.

46. Jones, D.J., Stehling, L.C., Zauder, H.L. Cardiovascular responses to diazepam and midazolam maleate in the dog. *Anesthesiology*, Nov:51(5):430-4, 1979.

47. Bloor, C.M., Leon, A.S., Walker, D.E. Coronary and systemic hemodynamic effects of diazepam (valium) in the unanesthetized dog. *Res Commun Chem Pathol Pharmacol*, 6(3):1043-1051, 1973.

48. Nakajima, T., Kaneshiro, S., Yatabe, Y., Azumi, T., Iwasaki, H. Negative dromotropic effect of diazepam on the AV node of dog heart in situ. *Arch Int Pharmacodyn Ther*, 241(1):153-64, 1979.

49. Pearl, D.S., Quest, J.A., Gillis, R.A. Effect of diazepam on digitalis-induced ventricular arrhythmias in the cat. *Toxicol Appl Pharmacol*, 44(3):643-52, 1978.

50. Thompson, F.J., Barnes, C.D., Wald, J.R. Interactions between femoral venous afferents and lumbar spinal reflex pathways. *J Auton Nerv Syst*, 6(2):113-26, 1982.

51. Acosta, D., Chappell, R. Cardiotoxicity of diazepam in cultured heart cells. *Toxicology*, 8(3):311-7, 1977.

52. Graham, C.W., Pagano, R.R., Katz, R.L. Thrombophlebitis after intravenous diazepam--can it be prevented? *Anesth Analg (Cleve.)*, 56(3):409-13, 1977.
53. Brogden, R.N., Heel, R.C., Speight, T.M., Avery, G.S. Clobazam: A review of its pharmacological properties and therapeutic use in anxiety. *Drugs*, 20(3):161-78, 1980.
54. Clanachan, A.S., Marshall, R.J. Potentiation of the effects of adenosine on isolated cardiac and smooth muscle by diazepam. *Br J Pharmacol*, 71(2):459-66, 1980.
55. Barker, P.H., Clanachan, A.S. Inhibition of adenosine accumulation into guinea pig ventricle by benzodiazepines. *Eur J Pharmacol*, 78(2):241-4, 1982.
56. Patel, D.J., Wong, H.Y.C., Newman, H.A.J., Nightingale, T.E., Frasinel, C., Johnson, F.B., Patel, S., Coleman, B. Effect of Valium (Diazepam) on Experimental Atherosclerosis in roosters. *Artery*, 10(4):237-149, 1982.
57. Conklin, K.A., Graham, C.W., Murad, S., Randall, F.M., Katz, R.L., Cabalum, T., Lieb, S.M., Brinkman, C.R. 3rd. Midazolam and diazepam: maternal and fetal effects in the pregnant ewe. *Obstet Gynecol*, 56(4):471-4, 1980.
58. Reves, J.G., Mardis, M., Strong, S. Cardiopulmonary effects of midazolam. *Ala J Med Sci*, 15(4):347-351, 1978.
59. Macho, P., Vatner, S.F. Effects and mechanism of action of trimazosin on coronary and left ventricular dynamics in conscious dogs. *J Pharmacol Exp Ther*, 217(2):333-9, 1981.
60. Komatsu, Y., Constantopoulos, G., Gutkowska, J., Rojo-Ortega, J.M., Genest, J. Effects of reserpine on water, cation and norepinephrine contents of cardiovascular tissues of normotensive dogs. *Can J Physiol Pharmacol*, 55(2):206-211, 1977.
61. Cauvin, C.A., Devia, C.J., Kirkendol, P.L. Effect of reserpine pretreatment on *in vivo* femoral arterial responses to vasodilator agents. *J Pharmacol Exp Ther,* 216(3):447-52, 1981.
62. Endoh, M., Shimizu, T., Yanagisawa, T. Characterization of adrenoceptors mediating positive inotropic responses in the ventricular myocardium of the dog. *Br J Pharmacol*, 64(1):53-61, 1978.
63. Kjekshus, J.K. Effect of inhibition of lipolysis on acute myocardial injury during coronary occlusion in normal and reserpinized dogs. *Acta Med Scand*, (Supp. 2). 645:85-9, 1981.
64. Winkle, R.A., Jaillon, P., Griffin, J.C., Schnittger, I. Time dependency of ventricular fibrillation thresholds determined using trains of stimuli. *Am J Physiol*, 239(4):H457-H463, 1980.
65. Cauvin, C.A., Devia, C.J., Kirkendol, P.L. Effect of reserpine on relaxant responses of canine femoral arterial strips. *Clin Exp Pharmacol Physiol*, 9:511-514, 1982.
66. Kedem, J., Zurovski, Y., Miller, H., Battler, A. Effect of reserpine upon the haemodynamic course of recovery following experimental myocardial infarction. *Arch Int de Physiol et de Bioch*, 88:427-436, 1980.
67. Toda, N., Hayashi, S. Responses of canine coronary arteries to transmural electrical stimulation and nicotine. *Eur J Pharmacol*, 80(1):73-81, 1982.
68. Toda, N. Mechanisms of ouabain-induced arterial muscle contraction. *Am J Physiol*, 239(2):H199-205, 1980.
69. Cross, R.B., Chalk, J., South, M., Liss, B. The action of angiotensin on the isolated perfused cat heart. *Life Sci*, 29(9):903-8, 1981.
70. Marin, J., Salaices, M., Marco, E.J., Gomez, B., Lluch, S. Analysis of the contractile effect of 5-hydroxytryptamine on the isolated posterior communicating artery of the cat. *J Pharma Pharmacol*, 31(7):456-9, 1979.
71. Scholz, H., Hackbarth, Il, Schmitz, W., Wetzel, E. Effect of vanadate on myocardial force of contraction. *Basic Res Cardiol*, 75(3):418-22, 1980.
72. Marin, J., Salaices, M., Sanchez, C.F. Release of [3H] noradrenaline induced by 5-hydroxytryptamine from cat pial arteries. *J Pharm Pharmacol*, 31(12):818-21, 1979.
73. Woods, J.R., Dandarino, A., Nuwayhid, B., Brinkman, C.R., Assali, N.S. Cardiovascular reactivity of neonatal and adult sheep to autonomic stimuli during adrenergic depletion. *Biol Neonate*, 34:112-120, 1978.
74. Marin, J., Salaices, M. Vasoconstriction of the isolated communicating cerebral artery induced by field electrical stimulation. *Revista Espanola de Fisiologia*, 35:353-358, 1979.
75. Marin, J., Salaices, M., Gomez, B., Lluch, S. Noradrenergic component in the vasoconstriction induced by 5-hydroxytryptamine in goat cerebral arteries. *J Pharm Pharmacol*, 33(11):715-9, 1981.
76. Conde, M.V., Marin, J., Salaices, M., Marco, E.J., Gomez, B., Lluch, S. Adrenergic vasoconstriction of the goat middle cerebral artery. *Am J Physiol*, 235(2):H131-5, 1978.
77. Toda, N. Mechanisms of ouabain-induced arterial muscle contraction. *Am J Physiol*, 239(2):H199-205, 1980.

78. Bodach, E., Coceani, F., Dumbrille, A., Okpako, D.T., Olley, P.M. The response of the isolated ductus arteriosus to transmural stimulation and drugs. *Br J Pharmacol*, 71(2):419-27, 1980.

79. Priano, L.L. Comparative renal vascular effects of thiopental, diazepam, Actamine and halothane. *Anesthesiol*, 57(3), A34, 1982.

80. Knight, A.P., Sylzazine, J. *J Am Vet Med Assoc*, 176(5):454-455, 1980.

81. Hubbell, J. A., Muir, W.W. Effect of Xylazine hydrochloride on canine splenic weight: an index of vascular capacity. *Am J Vet Res*, 43(12):2188-2192, 1982.

82. Hubbell, J.A., Muir, W.W., Sams, R.A. Guaifenesin: cardiopulmonary effects and plasma concentrations in horses. *Am J Vet Res*, 41(11):1751-1755, 1980.

83. Freire, A.C., Gontigo, R.M., Pessoa, J.M., Souza, R. Effect of xylazine on the electrocardiogram of the sheep. *Br Vet J*, 137(6):590-595, 1981.

84. Campbell, K.B., Klavano, P.A., Richardson, P., Alexander, J.E. Hemodynamic effects of xylazine in the calf. *Am J Vet Res*, 40(12):1777-1780, 1979.

85. Reutlinger, R.A., Karl, A.A., Vinal, S.I., Nieser, M.J. Effects of ketamine HCl-xylazine combination on cardiovascular and pulmonary values of the rhesus macaque. *Am J Vet Res*, 41(9):1453-1457, 1980.

86. Pugh, D.M. Observations on certain effects of promazine chlorpromazine and chlorprothixene following intravenous injection into conscious dogs, *Proc Assoc of Vet Anaesthesiologists of Great Britain and Ireland*, 8: 35-40, 1981.

87. Turner, D.M., Ilkins, J.E., Rose, R.J., Warren, J.M. Respiratory and Cardiovascular Effects of Fine Drugs used as Sedatives in the Dog., *Aust Vet J*, 50: 260-265, 1974.

88. Lathers, C.M., Lipka, L.J. Chlorpromazine: Cardiac Arrhythmogenicity in the Cat. *Life Sciences*, 38: 521-538, 1986.

89. Lipka, L.J., Lathers, C.M., Roberts, J. Does chlorpromazine produce cardiac arrhythmia via the central nervous system? *So J Clin Pharmacol*, 1988 Nov. 28 (11) 968-983.

90. Dhalla, N.S., Lee, S.L., Takeo, S., Ponagia, V., Bhayana, V. Effects of Chlorpromazine and Imipramine on Rat Heart Subcellular Membranes, *Biochem Pharmacol*, 29: 629-633, 1980.

91. Sugimoto, J., Nagata, M., Ikeda, Y. The effects of Diazepam on Rat Isolated Heart Muscle, *Clin Exp Pharmacol Physiol*, 5: 655-663, 1978.

92. Bell, F.P., Hubert, E.V. Effects of Chlorpromazine on Rat Arterial Lipid Synthesis, *in vitro, Lipids*, 17(10): 672-675, 1982.

93. Okumura, K. Ogawa, K. Satake, T. Effects of trifluoperazine and Chlorpromazine on calcium-repleted injury in isolated ventricle strips. *So Basic Res Cardiol*, 80(5) 556-563, 1985.

94. Liu, J.J., Yang, Y.C., Tan, S.J. Three correlations between extracellular calcium concentration and myocardial cell injury induced by drugs, *So Life Sci*, 40 (22): 2175-2182, 1987.

95. Clergue, M., Riou, B., Le Carpentier, Y. Inotropic and lusitropic effects of chlorpromazine on rat left ventricular papillary muscle, *J Pharm Exp Ther*, 253 (1): 296-304, 1990.

96. Arlock, P. Gullberg, B., Olsson, S-O. R. Cardiac Electrophysiology of Four Neuroleptics: Melperone, Haloperidol, Thioridazine and Chlorpromazine, *Naunyn-Schmiedebergs Arch Pharmacol*, 304: 27-36, 1978.

97. Ogata, N., Nishimura, M., Narahashi, T., Kinetics of chlorpromazine block of sodium channels in single guinea pig cardiac myocytes, *So J Pharmacol Exp Ther*, 248(2): 605-613, 1989.

98. Nedergaard, O.A., Abrahamsen, J. Effects of chlorpromazine on sympathetic neuroeffector transmission in the rabbit isolated pulmonary artery and aorta. *So Br J Pharmacol*, 93 (1): 23-34, 1988.

99. Rabkin, S.W. Effects of chlorpromazine and trifluoperazine on choline metabolism and phosphatidylcholine biosynthesis in cultured chick heart cells under normoxic and anoxic conditions. *Biochem Pharmacol*, 38 (14):2349-2355, 1989.

100. Farner, T.B., Haskins, S.C., Patz, J.D. Cardiopulmonary effects of acepromazine and of the subsequent administration of detamine in the dog, *Am J Vet Res*, 47 (3): 631-635, 1986.

101. Farver, T.B., Haskins, S.C., Patz, J.D. Cardiopulmonary effects of acepromazine and of the subsequent administration of ketamine in the dog. *Am J Vet Res*, 47 (3):631-635, 1986.

102. Dyson, D.H., Allen, D.G., Inginsen, W., Pascol, P.J. Evaluation of Acepromazine, Meperidine, Atropine Premedication followed by thiopental anesthesia in the cat. *Am J Vet Res*, 52(4):419-422, 1988.

103. Dyson, D.H., Pascoe, P.J. Influence of preinduction methoxamine, lactated Ringer solution, or hypertonic saline solution infusion or postinduction dobutamine infusion on anesthetic-induced hypotension in horses. *Am J Vet Res*, 51(1):17-21, 1990.

104. Nilsfors, L., Kuart, C., Kallings, P., and Carlson, J. Cardiorespiratory and sedative effects of a combination of allpromazine, xylazine and methadone in the horse, *Equine Vet* I, Vol C, 364-367, 1988.

105. Lochner A, Van Niekerk I, Kotze J.C. Normothermic ischaemic cardiac arrest of the isolated perfused rat heart: Effects of trifluoperazine and lysolecithin on mechanical and metabolic recovery. *Basic Res Cardiol*, 80(4):363-376, 1985.

106. Perez-Medina, T., Garcia-Barreto, D., Hernances-Canero, A. Experimental His Bundle Escape Rhythms, *Cor Vasa*, 20:129-134, 1978.

107. Muldoon, S.M., Janssens, W.J., Verbeuren, J.J., Vanhoutte, P.M. Alpha-Adrenergic blocking properties of Dropenitol on Isolated Blood Vessels of the Dog, *Br J Anesth*, 49:211-216, 1977.

108. Montiel, C. Artalejo, A.R., Bermejo, P.M., Sanchez-Garcia, P. A dopaminergic receptor in adrenal medulla as a possible site of action for the droperidol-evoked hypertensive response. *Anesthesiology*, 65(5):474-479, 1986.

109. Satoh, M., Kiays, K, Yamamka, J., Kasama, A., Yanagisaiva, M. Droperidol, Its Alpha-Adrenergic Blocking Action on the Aortic Strip and Inhibitory Action on Norepinephrine Uptake of the Adrenergic Terminal of the Left Atrial Strip of Rabbit, *Tohoku J Exp Med*, 124:65-72, 1978.

110. Hauswirth, O. Effects of Droperidol on Sheep Purkinje Fibers, *Nauyn-Schmiedebegs Arch Pharmacol U Exp Path*, 261: 133-142, 1968.

111. Bentley, G.A., Copeland, I.W. The Effect of chronic haloperidol treatment on some cardiovascular parameters in cats., *Br J Pharmacol*, 86 (3):737-741, 1985.

112. Van Woerkens, L.J., Duncker, D.J., Huigen, R.J., Van der Giessen, W.J., Verdouw, P.D. Redistribution of cardiac output caused by opening of arteriovenous anastomoses by a combination of azaperone and metomidate. *Br J Anaesth*, 65 (3):393-399, 1990.

113. Haskins, S.C., Farver, T.B., Patz, J.D. Cardiovascular changes in dogs given diazepam and diazepam, Aetamine, *Am J Vet Res*, 47 (4):795-798, 1986.

114. Bloor, C.M., Leon, A.S., Walker, D.E. Coronary and Systemic Hemodynamic Effects of Diazepam (Valium) in the Unanesthetized Dog, *Res Commun in Chem Path Pharmacol*, 6 (3):1043-1051, 1973.

115. Haskins, S.C., Farver, T.B., Patz, J.D. Cardiovascular changes in dogs given diazepam and diazepam, Ketamine, *Am J Vet Res*, 47(4):795-798, 1986.

116. Flacke, J.W., Davis, L.J., Flacke, W.E., Bloor, B.C., Van Etten, A.P. Effects of fentanyl and diazepam in dogs deprived of autonomic tone., *Anesth Analg*, 64 (11):1053-1059, 1985.

117. Ruiz, F., Hernandez, J., Perez, D. The effect of diazepam on ventricular automaticity induced by local injury. Evidence of involvement of "peripheral type" benzodiazepine receptors. *So J Pharm Pharmacol*, 41(5):306-310, 1989.

118. Ruiz, F., Hernandez, J., Ribeiro, J.A. Theophylline antagonizes the effect of diazepam on ventricular automaticity. *Eur J Pharmacol*, 155(3):205-209, 1988.

119. Elgoyhen, B., Adler, Graschinsky, E. Diminution by benzodiazepines of the chronotropic responses to noradrenaline in rat isolated atria., *Eur J Pharmacol*, 164(3):467-478, 1989.

120. Kobinger, W., Pichler, L. Adrenoceptor subtypes in cardiovascular regulation, *J Cardiovasc Pharmacol*, 4:581-585, 1982.

121. Gregg, R.V., Turner, P.A., Densen, D.D., Stuebing, R.C., Sehlhorst, C.S., Forsberg, T. Does diazepam really reduce the cardiotoxic effects of intravenous bupivacaine?, *Anesth Analg*, 67(1):9-14, 1988.

122. Sakamoto, M., Ohsumi, H., Yamazaki, T., Okumura, F. Effects of diazepam on the carotid sinus baroreflex control of circulation in rabbits. *Acta Physiol Scand*, 139(2):281-287, 1990.

123. Bernards, C.M., Carpenter, R.L., Rupp, S.M., Brown, D.L., Morse, B.V., Morell, R.C. Thompson, G.E. Effect of midazolam and diazepam premedication on central nervous system and cardiovascular toxicity of bupivacaine in pigs, *Anesthesiology*, 70(2):318-323, 1989.

124. Saegusa, K., Furukawa, Y., Ogiwara, Y., Takeda, M., Chiba, S. Pharmacologic basis of responses to midazolam in the isolated, cross-perfused, canine right atrium., *Anesth Analg*, 66(8):711-718, 1987.

125. Estan, L., Senard, J.M., Tran, M.A., Montastruc, J.L., Berlan, M. Reserpine induces vascular alpha 2-adrenergic supersensitivity and platelet alpha 2-adrenoceptor up-regulation in dog, *Br J Pharmacol*, 101(2):329-336, 1990.

126. Komatsu, Y., Constantopoulos, G., Gutkowska, J., Rojo-Ortega, J.M., Genest, J. Effects of reserpine on water, cation, and norepinephrine contents of cardiovascular tissues of normotensive dogs, *Can J Physiol Pharmacol*, 55 (2):206-211, 1977.

127. Muramatsu, I. The effect of reserpine on sympathetic, puringergic neurotransmission in the isolated mesenteric artery of the dog: a pharmacological study, *So Br J Pharmacol*, 91(3):467-474, 1987.

128. Grassby, P.F., Arch, J.R., Wilson, C., Broadley, K.J. Beta-adrenoceptor sensitivity of brown and white adipocytes after chronic pretreatment of rats with reserpine, *Biochem Pharmacol*, 36(1):155-162, 1987.

129. Cros, G.H., Chanez, P.O., McNeill, J.H., Serrano, J.J. Short and long term effects of reserpine on rat cardiac beta-adrenoceptors, *Gen Pharmacol*, 20(3):277-284, 1989.

130. Abe, K., Saito, H., Matsuki, N. Potentiation by treatment with reserpine of alpha 2-adrenoceptor, mediated contractions of rat tail artery, *Eur J Pharmacol*, 171(1):59-67, 1989.

131. Warland, J.J., Burnstock, G. Effects of reserpine and 6-hydroxydopamine on the adrenergic and puringergic components of sympathetic nerve responses of the rabbit saphenous artery, *Br J Pharmacol*, 92(4):871-880, 1987.

132. Tenner, T.E. Jr., Young, J., Riker, B.J., Ramanadham, S. Nonspecific supersensitivity induced by reserpine in guinea pig cardiac ventricle tissue, *J Pharmacol Exp Ther*, 246(1):1-6, 1988.

133. Hsu, W.H. Effects of atropine on Xylazine-pentobarbital anesthesia in dogs: Preliminary Study, *Am J Vet Res*, 46(4):856-858, 1985.

134. Haskins, S.C., Patz, J.D., Farner, T.B. Xylazine and Xylazine ketamine in dogs, *Am J Vet Res*, 47(3):636-641, 1986.

135. Tranquilli, W.J., Thurmon, J.C., Benson, G.J. Alterations in epinephrine-induced arrhythmogenesis after xylazine and subsequent yohimbine administration in isoflurane-anesthetized dogs, *Am J Vet Res*, 49(7):1072-1075, 1988.

136. Fosse, R.T., Grona, K., Stavgeland, L., Lekven, J. Anesthetic interaction in cardiovascular research models: Effects of Xylazine and pentobarbital in cats, *Am J Vet Res*, 48(2):211-218, 1987.

137. Wagner, A.E., Muir, W.W., Hinchchiff, K.W. Cardiovascular effects of xylazine and detomidine in horses, *Am J Vet Res*, 52(5):651-657, 1991.

138. Clarke, K.W., and Paton, B.R. Combined use of detornidine with opiates in the horse, *Am Vet J*: 49:331-334, 1988.

139. Virtanen R, Ruskoaho, H., Nyma, L. Pharmacological evidence for the involvement of alpha-2-adrenoceptors in the sedative effect of detomidine, a novel sedative analgesic, *J Vet Pharmacol Ther*, 8:30-37, 1985.

140. Thompson, J.R., Kersting, K.W., Hsu, W.H. Antagonistic, effects of atipamezole on xylazine induced sedation, bradycardia, and ruminal atony in calves, *Am J Vet Res*, 52(8):1265-1268, 1991.

141. Booth, N.H. Nonnarcotic Analgesics Chp. 16 in Veterinary Pharmacology and Therapeutics ed. by N.H. Booth and L.E. McDonald, 6th ed. Iowa State University press, Ames, Iowa, 1988.

142. Negishi, M., Ito, S. Involvement of phosphoinositide metabolism in GABA-induced catecholamine release from cultured bovine adrenal chromaffin cells, *Biochem Pharmacol*, 40:2719-2725, 1990.

143. Lina, A.A., Dauchot, P.J., Anton, A.H. Epinephrine-aminophylline-induced arrhythmias after midazolam or thiopentone in halothane-anaesthetized dogs, *Can J Anaesth*, 38:1037-1042, 1991.

144. Reves, J.G., Mardis, M., Strong, S. Cardiopulmonary effects of midazolam, *Ala J Med Sci*, 15:347-351, 1978.

145. Klide, A.M., Calderwood, H.W., Soma, L.R. Cardiopulmonary effects of xylazine in dogs, *Am J Vet Res*, 36:931-935, 1975.

146. Campbell, K.B., Klavano, P.A., Richardson, P., Alexander, J.E. Hemodynamic effects of xylazine in the calf, *Am J Vet Res*, 40:1777-1780, 1979.

4. Cardiovascular effects of other drugs commonly used in cardiovascular research

Neuromuscular Blocking Agents

All anesthetic agents have been shown to have some effect on the cardiovascular system, there has therefore been a conscious and sustained effort by investigators to minimize these effects. This has been done by reducing dosages, increasing the use of narcotic analgesics, whose deleterious cardiovascular effects are less than those of the general anesthetics, and by the use of neurolept analgesia regimens. Under these circumstances, voluntary and/or involuntary muscular movement can be a problem. To combat this undesirable movement and to be able to control ventilation and blood gases without having the animal trying to breath against the system, a variety of neuromuscular blocking agents have been used. These agents can be classified into two types: 1) Competitive or nondepolarizing agents, which compete with acetylcholine for available cholinergic receptors at the post-synaptic membrane. The prototype for this kind of agent is d-tubocurarine. Metocurine iodide, gallamine, pancuronium and alcuronium chloride are other examples of competitive blockers.   Newer agents include; fazadinium, atracurium and vecuronium. 2) Depolarizing agents which interfere with acetylcholine-mediated depolarization of the post-synaptic membrane constitute the second group of neuromuscular blockers.   Examples of this type of agent are succinylcholine chloride and decamethonium bromide.[1]

Not all of these agents have been systematically investigated for their cardiovascular effects. As might be expected there are also conflicting reports. Gallamine, pancuronium and alcuronium chloride have been reported to have vagolytic effects with slight increases in heart rate and cardiac output in cats, while others have reported no change in these parameters in dogs.[1] Ruminants are known to be extremely sensitive to these agents and it is extremely important to reduce the dosage in these species, especially if the animal is to be allowed to recover. When given as a rapid intravenous bolus injection in dogs, d-tubocurarine has been shown to induce a transient hypotension.[1] During thiobarbiturate anesthesia in dogs, injection of pancuronium resulted in a slight increase in heart rate, blood pressure and cardiac output. These effects were blocked by atropine.[1] Atracurium and vecuronium were reported to have negligible effects on arterial blood pressure in dogs.[1] Gallamine has been shown to have no effect on sympathetic nerve function but to have vagolytic properties. It induces a tachycardia without modification of the carotid arterial pressure.[2]

Succinylcholine was tested in unanesthetized and/or nontranquilized horses. At recommended doses, there was an initial decrease in heart rate followed by an increase in heart rate. There were atrioventricular conduction disturbances and extrasystoles. There have been reports of suspected myocardial damage. It has been shown that autonomic nervous system blocking agents will substantially modify all of these effects in horses.[1] This leads us to believe that many of these effects may be due to a catecholamine response, especially in horses, when the animal is losing, or no longer has, control over its skeletal muscles. When ventilation is provided in anesthetized dogs or horses, succinylcholine evokes minimal changes.[1] Lower doses of succinylcholine increase the arrhythmogenicity of epinephrine during light anesthesia with halothane in dogs and increases susceptibility to digitalis toxicity in horses.[1]

Table 4.1: Cardiovascular effects of skeletal muscle relaxants:

Conditions of the experiment	Dose	Cardiovascular effects	Reference
4.1:1 Gallamine-dogs			
Induction with halothane maintained on 1.0-1.5% halothane	0.4 mg/kg,IV	No change in cardiac output, cardiac index, heart rate, stroke volume, central venous pressure or mean aortic pressure	**11**
5-8% halothane induction, chloralose (40 mg/kg,IV)	0.27-1.57 mg/kg,IV	Slight increase in phasic aortic flow, stroke volume and cardiac output. Slight reduction in blood pressure and peripheral resistance. Results probably the effect of cardiovagal block	**24**
Anesthetized with pentobarbital-Na (30 mg/kg,IV)	Dose-response	Inhibited the chronotropic and dromotropic responses in a dose-dependent manner to direct sympathetic stimulation of atrioventricular and sinoatrial areas. Binding properties of muscarinic receptors on SA node different from those on the AV node	**15**

4.1:2 Gallamine-cats Conditions	Dose	Cardiovascular Effects	Reference
Isolated atrial and right ventricular papillary muscle preparations from cats anesthetized with pentobarbital (30 mg/kg,IP), also in situ measurements of ventricular contractility on cats anesthetized with pentobarbital (70 mg/kg,IP) using strain gauge arches attached to the right ventricle	Dose-response	Increased heart rate and increased right ventricular contractile force	3
4-8% halothane induction, maintained with chloralose (60-80 mg/kg,IV)	Dose-response	No significant change in blood pressure or heart rate. Significant increase in percent inhibition of vagal response	12

4.1:3 Gallamine-Guinea Pigs, Conditions	Dose	Cardiovascular Effects	Reference
Killed by a blow to the head, hearts removed, isolated, electrically driven left atrial preparation	Dose-response	Increase in heart rate and in contractile force, the effects were blocked by reserpine pretreatment which indicates a possible catecholamine mediated mechanism	3
Isolated atrial preparation	Dose-response	Presynaptic antimuscarinic effect by inhibiting muscarinic receptors located on the axon terminals of sympathetic neurons thereby enhancing norepinephrine release. Could account for gallamine-induced tachycardia	28

4.1:4 Gallamine-Sheep	Dose	Cardiovascular Effects	Reference
Lambs, anesthetized with thiopentone (12.5 mg/kg,IV), maintained with halothane and nitrous oxide	2 mg/kg followed by 1 mg/kg,IV	No change in heart rate, mean aortic pressure, left ventricular end-diastolic pressure, cardiac output, stroke volume or peripheral resistance	13
Fetal lambs, chronically instrumented and monitored in utero	10-20 mg total dose	Fetal oxygen consumption decreased 17%, decreased umbilical oxygen extraction. No change in umbilical blood flow. Increased umbilical arterial (14%) and venous (18%) pO_2 values	14
4.1:5 Gallamine-Rats			
Minced cardiac tissue from decapitated rats	Dose-response	Dose-response curves for inhibition of adenylate cyclase activity by a muscarinic agonist were shifted to the right. Effect could be explained by allosteric antagonism	26
Frozen hearts, binding studies	Dose-response	High affinity for M_2-muscarinic receptors	25
4.1:6 Gallamine-Cattle			
Heart tissue, binding studies	Dose-response	Dissociation from cardiac muscarinic receptors was slowed by the gallamine. This is cited as further evidence that gallamine interacts with muscarinic receptors in a non-competitive manner because of binding to the allosteric site modulating in a negative cooperative way the binding to the first receptor site	27
4.1:7 Gallamine-Chickens			
Frozen hearts, binding studies	Dose-response	High affinity for atypical muscarinic receptors present in chicken myocardium	25

4.2:1 d-Tubocurarine-Dogs, Conditions	Dose	Cardiovascular Effects	Reference
Halothane anesthesia (1.2% MAC), epinephrine infusion (2.5 μg/kg/min) until PVC's initiated, instrumented, positive pressure ventilation	0.1 mg/kg, IV	No change in heart rate but a significant increase in the arrhythmogenic dose of epinephrine required	4
Anesthetized with a minimal dose of thiopentone, maintained on oxygen and nitrous oxide at 2 atmospheres	0.352 and 0.704 mg/kg, IV	Decreased mean aortic pressure at 5 minutes post-injection. Decreased cardiac output, heart rate and stroke volume. Small transient fall in central venous pressure	23
5-8% halothane induction, chloralose (40 mg/kg, IV)	0.1-0.45 mg/kg, IV	Decreased phasic aortic flow, aortic blood pressure, stroke volume, heart rate, cardiac output and peripheral resistance, all probably due to blockade of sympathetic ganglia and histamine release	24
Anesthetized with thiopental (35 mg/kg, IV) + additional doses during instrumentation, NO_2 (2 L/min) + O_2 (1 L/min). Lactated Ringer's + Fentanyl (8-20 μg/kg/hr, adjusted to maintain stable anesthesia).	0.288 mg/kg + Pancuronium (0.048 mg/kg), IV bolus	Decreased central venous and arterial pressures at 2 min, increased heart rate at 2 and 5 min. After 10 min all parameters returned to baseline. No changes in pulmonary arterial pressures, stroke volume, cardiac output or resistance	29
4.2:2 d-Tubocurarine-Cats			
4-8% halothane inductions with chloralose (60-80 mg/kg, IV)	Dose-response	Decreased blood pressure and heart rate. Increased % inhibition of vagal response. The latter was dose-dependent.	12

4.2:3 d-Tubocurarine-Rabbits	Dose	Cardiovascular Effects	Reference
Isolated atrial preparation	Dose-response	Dose-dependent decrease in contractility but it was found to be due to the benzyl alcohol or 4-chloro-3 methyl creosol used as preservatives in the commercial preparations	5
Isolated left atrial preparations	Concentration response, 9 doses from 4.31×10^{-7} M to 5.36×10^{-4} M	Negative inotropic effects related to myocardial Ca^{++} exchange using the commercial product but the pure crystalline preparation produced increased inotropy. Concluded that antibacterial preservatives in the preparation are responsible for the negative inotropic effects	6
Newborn rabbits (6-10 days), pentobarbital,IP. Tracheal cannulation and positive pressure ventilation	0.2 mg/kg every 30 min, IV (total dose = 0.8 mg/kg)	Increased renal vascular resistance, decreased GFR and renal blood flow	30
4.2:4 d-Tubocurarine-Sheep			
Fetal lambs, previously instrumented in utero, intact, awake	3.0 mg/kg, IV (1.2 ml/min for 5 min)	Decreased heart rate and mean arterial pressure. Saline control no effect. Opposite effect than that seen with Pancuronium in the same preparation	31

Conditions	Dose	Cardiovascular Effects	Reference
1-3 day old lambs, intact, awake, local anesthesia only. Spontaneous respiration versus spontaneous resp. with hypoxia versus mechanical ventilation with room air versus mechanical ventilation with room air and muscle paralysis	0.3 mg/kg, IV	Total body oxygen consumption decreased in hypoxic lambs but no effect on normoxic. Increased level of hypoxic pulmonary vasoconstriction but does not interfere with hypoxia-induced redistribution of blood flow	32
4.2:5 d-Tubocurarine-Guinea pig			
Ventricular papillary muscle preparation. Depolarized in high potassium-barium Tyrode's with field stimulation to measure the slow action potential, a measure of the calcium current	3 mg/ml with and without chlorobutanol (5 mg/ml). The latter is an antimicrobial preservative	Depressed amplitude and duration at 0 mV and dV/dt of the action potential as well as contractile tension. Found to be due to the preservative chlorobutanol, no effect from crystalline Tubocurarine on these measures	33
Isolated, crystalloid perfused hearts	bolus injection of 1 mg into the coronary perfusate	Released 4.6 ± 1.6% of the total cardiac histamine. Increased heart rate and contractility	34

4.3:1 Succinylcholine-Dogs, Conditions	Dose	Cardiovascular Effects	Reference
Halothane anesthesia (1.28% MAC) instrumented, positive pressure ventilation, epinephrine infusion (2.5 µg/kg/min) until PVC's were produced	0.25 mg/kg	Significant decrease in arrhythmogenic dose of epinephrine, pretreatment with atropine significantly increased the arrhythmogenic dose of epinephrine required.	4

Conditions	Dose	Cardiovascular Effects	Reference
Pentobarbital (30 mg/kg, IV), Fentanyl (100 µg/kg, IV (n=6) and 400 µg/kg, IV (n=5)	2 mg/kg, IV	Significantly shortened R-R intervals in both high and low fentanyl dose groups. Unpaced HIS-ventricle intervals not changed. No significant effect on AV nodal effective or functional refractory periods or on retrograde ventricular effective refractory periods.	**15**
Induction with halothane, maintained on 1.0-1.5 %	0.4 mg/kg, IV	Small but significant early (1 min) increases in heart rate and blood pressure. No change in cardiac output, cardiac index, stroke volume, total peripheral resistance or central venous pressure	**11**
5-8 % halothane induction, chloralose (40 mg/kg, IV)	0.03-0.240 mg/kg, IV	Slight increase in phasic aortic flow, stroke volume and cardiac output which lasted 3-8 min. Slight reduction in peripheral resistance. Minimal changes of aortic pressure and cardiac contractility, heart rate unchanged	**11**
Pentobarbital (30 mg/kg, IV), Fentanyl (100 & 400 µg/kg)	2 mg/kg, IV	Partially reversed action of Fentanyl on R-R intervals, AV nodal conduction and refractory periods and ventricular refractory periods	**35**
Halothane or enflurane anesthesia with hypoxia of hypoxic hypercarbia	0.3 mg/kg, IV	Induces arrhythmias by sympathetic stimulation. Halothane sensitizes the myocardium to these succinylcholine-induced arrhythmias more than does enflurane	**37**
4.3:2 Succinylcholine-Cats, Conditions			
Isoflurane anesthesia, 2 groups; normal intracranial pressure and increased intracranial pressure	2 mg/kg, IV	Increased intracranial pressure in both groups	**36**

4.3:3 Succinylcholine- Horses	Dose	Cardiovascular Effects	Reference
Rapid IV thiopentone (10 mg/kg, IV) halothane/oxygen or ether/oxygen	0.2 mg/kg, IV	Increased $PaCO_2$, arterial bicarbonate, sodium and potassium levels. Decreased arterial pH and PaO_2. Increased blood pressure and heart rate	16
Same	0.4 mg/kg, IV	Dose-dependent increase in heart rate and blood pressure. Effects were diminished, but not abolished by positive pressure ventilation. Effects were blocked by hexamethonium and partially blocked by propranolol.	16
4.3:4 Succinylcholine- Cattle			
Intact, awake, previously instrumented calves	0.5 and 1.0 mg/kg, IM	Apnea leading to asphyxia with increased blood pressure and bradyarrhythmias caused by massive catecholamine release	17
4.3:5 Succinylcholine- Pigs			
Anesthetized with Desflurane or Isoflurane 1.2 MAC	1 and 2 mg/kg	No cardiovascular effects noted	37
Instrumentation with Xylazine (2 mg/kg) and Ketamine (20 mg/kg), IM. Anesthetized with 250 µg Fentanyl (IV bolus) + 25 µg/kg/hr	0.2 mg/kg, IV	Decreased intracranial pressure early then a rise, decreased mean aortic pressure, decreased cerebral perfusion pressure	38
Azaperone (2 mg/kg), 3-4% halothane, α-chloralose (200 mg/kg) + 33 mg/Kg/hr, IV	0.6 mg/kg, IV	No cardiovascular effects noted	37

4.3:6 Succinylcholine- Rabbits	Dose	Cardiovascular Effects	Reference
Modified Langendorff, isolated heart prep. Also in vivo study in rabbits anesthetized with α-chloralose (150 mg/kg, IV), positive pressure ventilation with 100% O_2, slight hypercapnia	Dose-response	In vitro, decrease heart rate, initial increase in left ventricular pressure and left ventricular dP/dt followed by a decrease in these parameters. Reserpine pretreatment resulted in nodal and/or ventricular ectopic beats	7
Same	Dose-response	In vivo; immediate decrease in heart rate, a decrease then an increase in left ventricular pressure and dP/dt, no arrhythmias except when given succinyldicholine and succinylmonocholine in combination	7

4.4:1 Pancuronium- Dogs, Conditions	Dose	Cardiovascular Effects	Reference
Positive pressure ventilation, normocapnia, normothermia, endocardial ECG, halothane anesthesia (1.25%, end-tidal)	0.1 mg/kg, IV	No change in HIS-Purkinje or ventricular conduction, increase in heart rate, AV nodal conduction decreased. No change in atrial refractory period or AV nodal functional refractory period	8
Pentobarbital (30 mg/kg, IV), Fentanyl (100 µg/kg, n=6) and (400 µg/kg, n=5), IV	0.1 mg/kg, IV	Significantly shortened R-R interval and both Atrial-HIS and paced Atrial-HIS intervals in both high and low fentanyl dose groups. Significantly prolonged AV nodal effective and functional refractory periods in both groups. Retrograde ventricular effective refractory period was shortened only in high dose group.	15

4.4:1 Pancuronium- Dogs, Conditions	Dose	Cardiovascular Effects	Reference
Previously instrumented, closed chest, anesthetized with Thiopental (12 mg/kg, IV), maintained with 1% halothane + 70% nitrous oxide	0.01 and 0.1 mg/kg, IV	Increased blood pressure and heart rate at high dose. Increased blood pressure and dQ/dt at low dose. No change in left ventricular end-diastolic pressures, LV dP/dt or dQ/dt at high dose. No change in heart rate, LVEDP or LVdP/dt at low dose	18
Minimum dose Thiopentone + nitrous oxide/oxygen at 2 atmospheres	0.088 and 0.176 mg/kg, IV	Slight increase in mean arterial pressure, small increase in cardiac output, and transient decrease in central venous pressure	23
Induction with Thiopental (35 mg/kg) + 5-10 mg/kg Fentanyl + 8-20 μg/kg/hr	0.1 mg/kg, IV bolus	Decreased right and left filling pressures and depressed arterial and pulmonary vascular resistance.	41
Pentobarbital (30 mg/kg, IV), Fentanyl (100 and 400 μg/kg)(2 different groups)	0.1 mg/kg, IV	Partially reversed effects of Fentanyl on R-R intervals, AV nodal conduction and AV nodal and ventricular refractory periods	35
Isolated myocardial tissue, binding assay for muscarinic receptors	10^{-8} to 10^{-3} M	Direct inhibition of binding to cardiac muscarinic receptors	42
4.4:2 Pancuronium-Cats			
4-8% halothane induction, maintain with chloralose (60-80 mg/kg, IV)	Dose-response	No change in blood pressure or heart rate. Increased percent inhibition of vagal response	12
4.4:3 Pancuronium-Horses			
Induced with 5% sodium Thiamylal, intubated, halothane in oxygen	0.125 ± 0.017 mg/kg, IV	Increased blood pressure and heart rate. No dysrhythmias noted	19
Serum cholinesterase determinations	Log doses	non-competitive inhibitor of serum cholinesterases	20

4.4:4 Pancuronium-Cattle, Conditions	Dose	Cardiovascular Effects	Reference
Calves, halothane anesthesia, masked then intubated	43 ± 9 µg/kg, IV	No change in heart rate or blood pressure	21
Purified erythrocyte acetylcholinesterase	Log doses	Noncompetitive inhibitor of erythrocyte cholinesterases	20
4.4:5 Pancuronium-Sheep			
Newborn lambs, intact, awake	0.1 mg/kg, IV +0.1 mg/kg/hr constant infusion	Transient increases in blood pressure (32%), No change in any of the parameters of cerebral blood flow or cerebral metabolic rate of O_2 and glucose consumption	22
Fetal lambs, previously instrumented in utero, no anesthesia	0.5 mg/kg, IV (1.2 ml/min for 5 min)	Increased heart rate, increased mean aortic blood pressure, no effect from saline control injection. This was the opposite of the effects caused by d-tubocurarine	31
1-3 day old lambs, intact, awake, compared spontaneous respiration normoxia, hypoxia, mechanical ventilation with room air and mechanical ventilation with room air and muscle paralysis	0.1 mg/kg, IV	Decreased total body oxygen consumption in hypoxic but not normoxic lambs. Increased level of hypoxic pulmonary vasoconstriction but did not interfere with hypoxia-induced redistribution of blood flow	32

Conditions	Dose	Cardiovascular Effects	Reference
Neonatal lambs, Pentobarbital (20 mg/kg, IP) + 15% of initial dose/hr + local anesthesia with 0.5% Lidocaine. Succinylcholine (2 mg/kg + 2 mg/kg/hr, IV), mechanical ventilation. Response to acetylcholine (2 mg/kg, IV)	0.1 mg/kg, IV bolus	No change in arterial pO_2, pCO_2, pH, pulmonary resistance, heart rate or mean aortic pressures. No changes in acetylcholine-induced bradycardia	43
4.4:6 Pancuronium-Pigs, Conditions			
Tranquilized with Azaperone (2 mg/kg), 3-4% halothane, α-chloralose (200 mg/kg + 33 mg/kg/hr, IV)	ED_{90} and 3 X ED_{90}	Increased mean aortic pressure and heart rate	39
Tranquilized with Azaperone (2 mg/kg), 3-4% halothane, α-chloralose (200 mg/kg + 33 mg/kg/hr, IV)	ED_{90} and 3 X ED_{90} of Org 6368 (17-desacetoxy analog)	Increased mean aortic pressure, no change in heart rate	39
4.4:7 Pancuronium-Rabbits			
Isolated left atrium	4-20 μg/ml, Dose-response	No change in isometric contraction	44
Isolated Langendorff perfused heart	3 mg/l in perfusate	Blocked acetylcholine-induced bradycardia	44

Conditions	Dose	Cardiovascular Effects	Reference
Newborn rabbits (6-10 days), Pentobarbital, IP, tracheal cannulation and positive pressure ventilation	0.1 mg/kg + 0.05 mg/kg every 30 min, total dose=0.25 mg/kg	No change in GFR or renal blood flow, increased renal vascular resistance	30
Isolated left atria, rabbits killed by a blow to the head	4-20 µg/ml, Dose-response (Pipecuroniu mlong-acting-steroidal molecule similar to pancuronium actually used)	No change in isometric contractions	44
Isolated, crystalloid perfused hearts, response to 1 µg acetylcholine-induced bradycardia	2 mg/l in perfusate (Pipecuron-ium)	Did not block acetylcholine-induced bradycardia	44
4.4:8 Pancuronium-Guinea pig, Conditions			
Isolated atrial preparation	Dose-response	Presynaptic antimuscarinic (atropine-like) effect. Inhibits muscarinic receptors on the axon terminals of sympathetic neurons thereby enhancing norepinephrine release	28
4.4:9 Pancuronium-Rat			
Cultured cardiomyocytes	0.34 µM	No significant effect on creatine phosphokinase leakage	45

4.5:1 Atracurium-Dogs, Conditions	Dose	Cardiovascular Effects	Reference
Induction with thiopental (35 mg/kg + 5-10 mg/kg), Fentanyl (8-20 µg/kg/hr)	0.4 mg/kg, IV bolus	Decreased right and left filling pressures and aortic pressure	41

Conditions	Dose	Cardiovascular Effects	Reference
Conscious beagles (n=4)	2 mg/kg, IV	Increased heart rate 41 ± 10.2 beats/min within 1 min, lasted 75 min. Increased heart rate 50 b/min at 45 min and 40 b/min at 60 min.	46
Thiopentone (20 mg/kg) + halothane (0.5-1%) (n=3)	2 mg/kg then 7.8 mg/kg/hr for 30 min then 2.04 mg/kg/hr for 210 min (Actually used Laudanosine-metabolite of atracurium). Same as previous	Decreased both blood pressure and heart rate	46
4.5:3 Atracurium-Horses			
Halothane anesthetized ponies	0.11±0.01 mg/kg,IV + 0.052 mg/kg in 2 to 4 additional doses	No changes in heart rate, aortic pressure, arterial pH, pO_2 or pCO_2	48
Anesthetized with Thiamylal Na (10 mg/kg, IV), Guaifenesin (100 mg/kg, IV) (1 horse with Xylazine 0.3 mg/kg & butorphanol 0.01 mg/kg, IV) Maintained with halothane (1.0±0.05% end-tidal concentration)	Dose-response, 0.07±0.01 + 0.04±0.003 mg/kg (4 doses)	No cardiovascular changes measured	49
4.5:4 Atracurium-Pigs			
Anesthetized with Desflurane or Isoflurane (1.2 MAC)	0.6 mg/kg	No cardiovascular effects	37

Conditions	Dose	Cardiovascular Effects	Reference
Instrumentation with Xylazine 2 mg/kg), Ketamine (20 mg/kg) or anesthetized with Fentanyl (250 µg bolus + 25 µg/kg/hr, IV)	0.6 mg/kg, IV	No effect on heart rate, mean aortic pressure, intracranial pressure, or cranial perfusion pressure	38
Anesthetized with Isoflurane or Desflurane (1.2 MAC)	1 and 2 mg/kg, IV	No cardiovascular effects	37
4.5:5 Atracurium-Rabbits			
Isolated heart, Langendorff preparation	6 µg/L in perfusate	Significantly inhibited the negative chronotropic effects of an acetylcholine injection	50
4.5:6 Atracurium-Chickens, Conditions			
Isoflurane anesthetized	0.15, 0.25, 0.35 or 0.45 mg/kg, IV	Dose-independent decrease in heart rate; increase in systolic aortic pressure; no change in mean or diastolic aortic pressure; no change in blood gases	178

4.6:1 Vecuronium-Dogs, Conditions	Dose	Cardiovascular Effects	Reference
Induction with thiopental (35 mg/kg + 5-10 mg/kg, IV), Fentanyl (8-20 µg/kg/hr, adjusted as required)	0.1 mg/kg, IV bolus	Minimal changes in cardiovascular parameters measured	41

Conditions	Dose	Cardiovascular Effects	Reference
Intact, awake, previously instrumented	0.1 mg/kg, IV + Sufentanil (25 µg/kg, IV) + Diltiazem (0.3 mg/kg, IV +Propranolol (1.0 mg/kg, IV)	Bradyarrhythmias, 2 cases of asystole out of 19 dogs	**51**
Isolated myocardium, tissue-binding assay for muscarinic receptors	10^{-8} to 10^{-3} M, Dose-response	Direct inhibition of binding to cardiac muscarinic receptors but weaker than pancuronium	**42**
Induction with Thiopental (35 mg/kg + 5-10 mg/kg/hr), Fentanyl (8-20 µg/kg/hr)	0.4 mg/kg, IV bolus (RGH-4201)	Increased heart rate, increased cardiac output, decreased both arterial and pulmonary resistances	**41**
Halothane anesthesia	Dose-response (ORG 9616 and ORG 9991)	Decreased aortic pressure and increased heart rate at higher doses (5 times ED_{90})	**52**
Halothane anesthesia	Dose-response (ORG 9426)	No cardiovascular effects measured	**52**
4.6:2 Vecuronium-Cats, Conditions			
Anesthetized with pentobarbital (33 mg/kg, IP), Acepromazine (0.6 mg/kg, IP)	80 µg/kg, IV bolus	No change in heart rate, mean aortic pressure or cerebral perfusion pressure	**53**
Anesthetized with α-chloralose (80 mg/kg) and Pentobarbital (5 mg/kg), IP	Dose-response (ORG-7617 and ORG-9616)	Blocked heart rate response to vagal stimulation at high doses. Decrease in mean aortic pressure more pronounced with ORG-7617. ORG-9616 increased heart rate slightly	**54**

Conditions	Dose	Cardiovascular Effects	Reference
Anesthetized with α-chloralose (80 mg/kg) and Pentobarbital (5 mg/kg), IP	Dose-response (ORG-9426)	Blocked bradycardia produced by vagal stimulation only in doses larger than those necessary to produce neuromuscular blockade. Small decrease in mean aortic pressure at high doses	55
4.6:3 Vecuronium-Pigs			
Anesthetized with Azaperone (2 mg/kg, IM), Masked with 3-4% halothane, α-chloralose (200 mg/kg + 33 mg/kg/hr, IV)	Dose-response (ORG-9426)	Blocked the bradycardia produced by vagal stimulation only in doses 4.4 times greater than the dose required to produce neuromuscular blockade	55
Anesthetized with Azaperone (2 mg/kg, IM), 3-4% halothane then α-chloralose (200 mg/kg + 33 mg/kg/hr, IV), positive pressure ventilation	Dose-response (ORG-7617 and ORG-9616)	Blocked heart rate response to vagal stimulation at doses higher than those necessary to cause neuromuscular blockade. Decreased mean aortic pressure more pronounced with ORG-7617. ORG-9616 increased heart rate slightly.	54
Instrumentation with Xylazine (2 mg/kg), Ketamine (20 mg/kg), IM, Anesthetized with Fentanyl (250 μg + 25 μg/kg/hr)	0.2 mg/kg, IV	No effect on heart rate, mean aortic pressure, intracranial pressure or cranial perfusion pressure	36
Tranquilized with Azaperone (2 mg/kg, IM), Anesthetized with Fentanyl (250 μg + 25 μg/kg/hr), IV	ED_{90} and 3 X ED_{90}	Decreased mean aortic pressure, no change in heart rate	39

4.6:4 Vecuronium-Rabbits, conditions	Dose	Cardiovascular effects	Ref
Isolated Langendorff perfused heart preparation	2.5 µg/L in perfusate	Did not enhance negative chronotropic effects of acetylcholine injection	50
Same as above	3 mg/L in perfusate	Did not block acetylcholine-induced bradycardia	44
4.6:5 Vecuronium-Rats			
Cultured cardiomyocytes	0.32 µM	No significant effects on creatine phosphokinase leakage	45
Anesthesia with halothane or Isoflurane 0.6 X MAC or 0.75 MAC. Tail clamp as noxious stimulus	1.0 mg/kg, IV	No effect on increases in heart rate and mean aortic pressure caused by noxious stimulus at either concentration of anesthesia	56

4.7:1 Alcuronium-Cats			
4-8 % halothane induction, maintained with chloralose (60-80 mg/kg, IV)	Dose-response	Decreased blood pressure, no change in heart rate. Increased percentage inhibition of vagal response	18
4.8:1 Fazadinium-Cats			
4-8 % halothane induction, maintained with chloralose (60-80 mg/kg, IV)	Dose-response	Decreased blood pressure, no change in heart rate. Increase in percent inhibition of vagal response	41
4.9:1 Metocurine-Dogs			
Induction with Thiopental (35 mg/kg + 5-10 mg/kg, IV) plus Fentanyl (8-20 µg/kg/hr)	0.3 mg/kg, IV bolus	Decreased right and left filling pressures and decreased both arterial and pulmonary vascular resistance	41

Non-Steroidal Anti-Inflammatory and Analgesic Agents

The use of intact, awake, previously instrumented animals, and an awareness of the necessity to alleviate pain whenever possible, has resulted in an increase in use of the non-steroidal anti-inflammatory/analgesics, especially post-operatively. As should be apparent by now few, if any, xenobiotic agents are without some cardiovascular effects. Acetylsalicylic acid, for example, has been shown to exert a protective effect on myocardial necrosis induced by catecholamine infusion in dogs and rats.[9] The mechanism of this catecholamine blocking effect has not been elucidated. These agents have also been shown to decrease the incidence of arrhythmias and ventricular fibrillation and to significantly increase survival rates in dogs with coronary occlusion.[10] These effects are not related to platelet inhibitory actions, but seem to reinforce the catecholamine blockade concept.

A rank order of potency for inhibition of responses to norepinephrine has been established using isolated, perfused, mesenteric blood vessels from rats.[132] The potency is: meclofenamate > flufenamate = diclofenac > indomethacin > fenbufen > phenylbutazone > ibuprofen > ketoprofen > naproxen > paracetamol. The latter is a pure cyclo-oxygenazae inhibitor.

The following tables summarize the documented cardiovascular effects of a number of different anti-inflammatory/ analgesic agents, by species:

Table 4.10: Cardiovascular effects of the salicylates

Conditions of the experiment	Dose	Cardiovascular effects	Reference
4.10:1 Aspirin-Dogs			
Anesthetized with pentobarbital (30-40 mg/kg, IV), positive pressure ventilation, open thorax, acute instrumentation, response to coronary artery occlusion	3 mg/kg and 30 mg/kg, IV	Significant increase in epicardial collateral flow from 5 min after post-treatment occlusion to 4 hours later. There was no change in heart rate or mean aortic pressure	58

Conditions	Dose	Cardiovascular Effects	Reference
Induction with thiopental (15 mg/kg, IV), anesthesia with α-chloralose (100 mg/kg, IV), positive pressure ventilation, acute instrumentation	50 mg/kg + 50 mg/hr (ASA)	Without acetylsalicylic acid (ASA) cardiac output increased about 25-40%, with ASA cardiac output increased about 40-100%	**59**
Previously instrumented, closed chest, anesthetized with halothane (0.75%), succinylcholine in a continuous drip and positive pressure ventilation	50 mg/kg, IV single bolus (lysine acetylsalic-ylate, approx. 1/2 potency of ASA)	Increased cardiac output and stroke volume, decreased heart rate, central venous pressure and systemic resistance. All effects were blocked by propranolol (0.5 mg/kg, IV)	**60**
Thiopental anesthesia (no dose given), positive pressure ventilation, nitrous oxide in O_2, acute instrumentation, infusion of thrombin (200-300 NIH units/min, for 2 min, into right atrium)	1 g ASA, IV before thrombin infusion	ASA prevented most of the increase in pulmonary arterial pressure and tracheal insufflation pressure. There was no effect on the fall in platelet counts. ASA inhibited the acute pulmonary reaction to thrombin but this was probably not due to inhibition of platelet aggregation. The increase in femoral blood flow caused by local infusion of thrombin (4-10 NIH U/min) was not inhibited by ASA	**61**
Anesthetized with morphine (3 mg/kg, IM), phenobarbital (20 mg/kg, IV), positive pressure ventilation, coronary occlusion with a balloon catheter, treated versus untreated	600 mg/dog/day/ os for 7 days pre-experiment	No significant differences between the 2 groups in; left ventricular function or the extent of injury as judged by ECG mapping. There was a significant decrease in the incidence of ventricular fibrillation in treated dogs (5% vs 39%). There was a significant increase in plasma free fatty acid in the untreated group	**62**
Isolated and perfused heart preparation, no description of anesthesia given	10 mg, ASA intracoronary	Decrease in contractile force, decrease in coronary blood flow and no change in heart rate	**63**

Conditions	Dose	Cardiovascular Effects	Reference
Isolated strips of coronary artery	10^{-4} M, ASA	Produced contractions which were significantly inhibited by calcium free solution, diltiazen, nifedipine, phospholipase A_2, arachidonate and PGE	63
Isolated helical strips of coronary, cerebral and mesenteric arteries. Dogs were anesthetized with pentobarbital (50 mg/kg, IP), then killed by exsanguination	No dose given	Did not alter the relaxant effect of ADP, adenosine or adenine. This suggests that vasoactive prostaglandins are not involved in the contraction caused by these perturbations	64
Anesthetized with morphine (2 mg/kg, SQ), urethane (200 g) & α-chloralose (20 g),IV	5,10,20 & 25 mg, intracoronary injections	Reduced coronary blood flow in a dose-dependent manner. Doses of 10-25 mg inhibited reactive hyperemia following 15 sec coronary occlusions	65
Anesthetized with Pentobarbital (30 mg/kg, IV), ventilated with 40-60% O_2, acute lower left lung preparation	1 mM, IV	Increased resting lobar vascular resistance 4 times, no change in ratio of pre- to post-capillary resistance	66
Adult dogs (2-4 years), Chloralose anesthesia (100 mg/kg + additional doses as needed), tested for arrhythmia sensitivity to ischemia by balloon inflation + IV epinephrine (0.05 - 0.1 µg/kg/min)	30 mg b.i.d. for 1 week prior to the study	Decreased effects of ischemia on arrhythmia sensitivity	67
4.10:2 Aspirin-Cats			
Anesthetized with pentobarbital (30 mg/kg, IV), acute instrumentation, coronary ligation model	50 mg/kg/os, pretreatment	There was no effect on hemodynamics or on the time course of response to coronary ligation	68

Conditions	Dose	Cardiovascular Effects	Reference
Anesthetized with pentobarbital (30 mg/kg, IP), gallamine (0.3 mg/kg), positive pressure ventilation, open thorax, acute instrumentation	7 mg/kg, IV	Significant increase in refractory period, no significant changes in diastolic threshold. This probably contributes to the antiarrhythmic action reported by others	10
Anesthetized with thiamylal (25 mg/kg, IV), halothane anesthesia (2%), acute instrumentation	650 mg/os/hr prior to the experiment	Platelet counts were decreased in untreated versus treated cats. There was inhibition of adenosine diphosphate-induced platelet aggregation. There was an increase in collateral circulation following aortic occlusion in the aspirin treated cats	69
Pentobarbital anesthesia (30 mg/kg, IV), isolated aortic strips	1×10^{-4} to 1×10^{-3} M	No effect	68
4.10:3 Aspirin-Rats			
Fresh, isolated thoracic aorta preparations	5,10,15 & 20 mg/ml	Did not significantly affect the production of PGI_2 by these tissues. Inhibition was seen with 200 mg/ml (approx. 40 X the maximum therapeutic blood concentration in man	7
given 40 mg/kg isoproterenol SQ, sacrificed after 24 hrs	mg/kg & 50 mg/kg/os	No preservation of creatine kinase activity, no protection against isoproterenol induced hypertrophy or increase in cyclic AMP levels. There was a decrease in plasma prostaglandins at 50 mg/kg but not at the lower dose	71
Isolated, perfused rat hearts. Rats were heparinized and then killed by decapitation	5 mM (sodium salicylate and ASA)	There was a glycogenolytic effect and an increase in the levels of phosphorylase A	72

Condition	Dose	Cardiovascular effects	Reference
Killed by decapitation while under light ether anesthesia, isolated perfused heart preparation	0.1 to 3.2 mM (sodium salicylate & ASA)	There were negative chronotropic and antilipolytic effects. In lower concentrations there was a decrease in the release of lactate dehydrogenase from the heart, associated with the decrease in heart rate. A significant increase in lactate production was accompanied by an increased uptake of glucose from the medium and increased coronary flow. In the presence of epinephrine, sodium salicylate only decreased heart rate. Equimolar doses of ASA did not mimic the sodium salicylate effects	9
Rats killed by decapitation, isolated perfused heart preparations	50 & 100 µg/ml in perfusate	There was no effect on the degree of increase in coronary pressure caused by adrenochrome (an oxidation product of epinephrine)	73
Pentothal (35 mg/kg, IP)	Dose-response, compared same doses IV, per os or directly into duodenum	IV- slightly more effective in inhibiting platelet thromboxane B_2 than aortic 6-keto-prostaglandin ORAL- 5 X more effective on platelet versus aortic cyclooxygenase activity	74
Intact, spontaneously hypertensive rats (SHR) anesthetized with pentobarbital (30 mg/kg)	100 mg/kg, IP, b.i.d. for 1 day then 2 hours prior to blood pressure measurements	Increased blood pressure in SHR, no change in heart rate. Found differences in prostanoid formation between male and female rats	75
Anesthetized rats, 21-32 weeks old, SHR, Pentobarbital (60 mg/kg, IP), IV injection of BM 13177 (60 mg/kg)(a selective TxA_2 receptor antagonist)	pretreatment with aspirin (100 mg/kg)	BM 13177 induces decreased aortic pressure and heart rate in male but not in female SHR, ASA pretreatment attenuated this response	76

4.10:4 Aspirin-Rabbits	Dose	Cardiovascular Effects	Reference
Intact, endothelial injury and rehealing	ASA, 13.5 mg/kg/day + 15 mg/kg/day dipyridamole /os pretreatment	Treated groups showed retarded endothelial regrowth by 66% at 4 days, post-injury. Regrowth was retarded 22% at 7 days and 28% at 14 days post-injury	77
Anesthetized with thiopental (30 mg/kg, IV), isolated aortic and pulmonary arterial strips	1 mg/kg, IV pretreatment with ASA	There was a strong inhibition of synthesis of both PGI_2 and thromboxane A_2. The inhibitory effect was maximal from 4-12 hours and back to baseline at 48 hrs	78
Anesthetized with urethane (25%, IP, no dose given), a central ear artery preparation	Dose-response	There was a significant potentiation of the vasoconstrictor response to norepinephrine (almost doubled). Prior treatment of the preparation with either normetnephrine or deoxycorticosterone reduced the potentiation effect. Authors concluded that ASA potentiates both the *in vitro* and *in vivo* catecholamine response	8
Killed by a blow to the head and exsanguinated. Intracellular recordings from SA nodal cells and atrial muscle fibers	300-500 μM ASA and 30-100 μM 5-bromo salicylate	Dose-dependent decrease in frequency of SA nodal discharge. Depolarization and shortening of the action potential duration. Higher concentrations of 5-Bromo caused a dose-dependent reduction in action potential amplitude, overshoot and Vmax. Both agents reversibly decreased the rate of rise of the "slow response" elicited by increased K^+ concentration and isoprenaline. Increased Ca^{2+} concentration had no effect on the salicylate response. Suggested that the salicylates have an effect on the slow inward current	79

4.10:5 Aspirin-Sheep	Dose	Cardiovascular effects	Reference
Chronically instrumented, intact, awake, pregnant (3rd trimester)	100 mg/min from 0-10 min, then 5 mg/min from 10-40 min	No significant effects on uterine blood flow, maternal heart rate, maternal mean aortic pressure, fetal paO$_2$, fetal mean aortic pressure or fetal heart rate	**80**
Fetal lambs (125-130 days gestation), instrumented in utero, measurements made 24 hrs later	55-90 mg/kg/os into the fetal stomach	Pulmonary arterial pressure increased in the fetus after 58 min, resistance across the ductus arteriosus increased. The difference in pressure between the fetal pulmonary artery and aorta increased. The proportion of combined fetal ventricular output distributed to the placenta, adrenals, heart and lungs increased while that to the brain, liver, intestine, kidney and upper and lower body decreased	**81**
Thin slices of isolated ventricular myocardium	Dose-response (10-20 mM)	Glycoside-induced shortening of the action potential duration was blocked. Salicylate alone produced a small prolongation of the action potential duration	**82**
Isolated Purkinje fiber, voltage clamp technique	Dose-response	There were reversible changes in the resting potential and in action potential duration. The threshold current for initiating an action potential by an intracellular electrode was reversibly increased. The activation curve for the pacemaker potassium current is shifted in a hyperpolarizing direction	**83**
Isolated Purkinje fiber preparation	10 mM (in bath)	Reversibly reduces contractility	**173**
Intact, awake, previously instrumented, treadmill exercise	10 & 100 mg/kg, IV	Slight increase in resting pulmonary arterial resistance, no effect on exercise-induced decrease in pulmonary arterial resistance. Same response with both doses	**84**

4.10:6 Aspirin-Cattle	Dose	Cardivascular effects	Reference
Cultured pulmonary artery endothelial and smooth muscle cells	1 mM	No effect on metabolism of ADP by the endothelial cells	85
In vitro biosynthesis of hexosamine-containing substances in heart valves	1.5×10^{-2} M	Biosynthesis of mucopolysaccharide, especially galactosamine-containing substances, was inhibited	86
4.10:7 Aspirin-Pigs			
Pentobarbital (30 mg/kg, IV)	40 mg/kg	No change in renal blood flow, no change in GFR, decreased renal PGE_2 excretion	87
4.10:8 Aspirin-Guinea Pigs			
Isolated atrial preparation	Dose-response	Reduces the duration of the action potential	82
Isolated heart-lung preparations, perfused with homologous RBC's suspended in 1.5 vol. of Tyrode with 6% Dextran. Anesthetized with ethylurethane (1 g/kg, IP) and then surgical removal of the heart and lungs	0.11 mg/ml of blood	Delayed and attenuated bronchoconstriction, increased pulmonary vascular resistance and heart failure which occurred rapidly without salicylate in these preparations	88
4.10:9 Aspirin-Primates (Cynomolgus)			
Intact animals fed an atherogenic diet	81 mg/ monkey/day	No effect on plasma cholesterol levels or on the amount of aortic atherosclerosis. *In vitro* platelet aggregation to arachidonic acid was almost completely suppressed. There was a reduced amount of coronary atherosclerosis	89
Intact, awake, atherosclerotic diet fed	50 mg/kg/os, daily	No effect on arterial uptake of plasma LDL and cholesterol and no protection against atherosclerosis	89

Table 4.11: Cardiovascular effects of indothmethacin:

Conditions of the experiment	Dose	Cardiovascular effects	Reference
4.11:1 **Indomethacin-Dogs**			
Intact, awake, experiments done 2 days after instrumentation	2 mg/kg, IV	Increased mean aortic pressure 5%, cardiac output decreased 24%, heart rate decreased 10%, stroke volume decreased 18%. There were no changes in blood flow to bone, heart, spleen, kidney or brain. There was a significant decrease in blood flow to the skin, stomach, and small intestine. There was a 41% increase in systemic resistance	**90**
Intact, awake, previously instrumented	20 mg/kg, IV	Decreased heart rate, no effect on left ventricular pressure, renal blood flow, coronary blood flow or any of the other measured parameters	**91**
Anesthetized with pentobarbital (35-40 mg/kg, IV), positive pressure ventilation, acute instrumentation, pericardiotomy	10 mg/kg, IV	Reduced the cyclical reduction of flow in the partially constricted coronary artery. This reduction was eliminated with PGI_2	**92**
Anesthetized with pentobarbital (30 mg/kg, IV), acute instrumentation, closed thorax	10 mg/kg, slowly administered IV in divided doses over a 25 min period	There was a marked decrease in mesenteric blood flow, an increase in aortic pressure and no change in celiac blood flow	**93**
Isolated heart-lung preparation	1 mg intracoronary	Decreased coronary flow, no change in heart rate or myocardial contractile force	**94**
Isolated left circumflex coronary artery helical strip preparation	10^{-8} to 10^{-5} M dose-response	Dose-dependent contractions increase. The mechanism for this was thought to be via inhibition of the intramural synthesis of vasodilating prostaglandins	**94**

Condition	Dose	Cardiovascular effects	Reference
Anesthetized with pentobarbital (30 mg/kg, IV), isolated coronary artery helical strips	3×10^{-8} and 3×10^{-7} g/ml	Resulted in an increase in contractions	95
Isolated lateral saphenous vein preparation, studied the response to bradykinin and norepinephrine	10^{-6} M	Responses to bradykinin were markedly enhanced while there was no change in the response to norepinephrine	96
Puppies 1-27 days old, anesthetized with Pentobarbital (20 mg/kg, IV)	0.3 mg/kg, IV	In newborn dogs this dose had no effect on cardiac output or an flow distribution except the later was decreased in 3 or 8 puppies less than 3 days old	97
Anesthetized with Pentobarbital (30 mg/kg, IV), ventilated with 40-60% O_2, acute lower left lung lobe preparation	40 µM, IV	Increased resting lobar vascular resistance by $36 \pm 8.3\%$, decreased ratio of pre- and post-capillary resistance. RA/Rv from 1.9 ± 0.3 to 1.1 ± 0.2	66
Pentobarbital anesthetized vs awake	5 mg/kg, IV	Active, flow-independent pulmonary vasoconstriction in both conscious and pentobarbital anesthetized dogs, but magnitude increased greatly in pentobarbital anesthetized	98
Coronary artery vascular rings, anesthetized with pentobarbital (30 mg/kg, IV) then exsanguinated	10^{-5} M	Dose-response to serotonin was shifted to the right	99

4.11:2 Indomethacin-Cats	Dose	Cardiovascular effects	Reference
Anesthetized with pentobarbital (30 mg/kg + supplemental doses as needed), spontaneous breathing, acute instrumentation, autologous blood perfused mesenteric and hindquarter vascular bed preparations	1 and 2.5 mg/ml concentration used but no dose given, IV	Prevented mesenteric vasodilator responses to nitroglycerin, responses to bradykinin were increased. The same effects were seen in the hindquarter prep. There was an increase in vascular resistance in both vascular beds and a decrease in systemic vasodepressor responses to arachidonic acid	100
Isolated papillary muscle preparation	10 µM, 0.25, 0.5 & 1.0 mM	Decreased action potential duration at 50 and 100% repolarization at all concentrations. There was no change in resting membrane potential or action potential amplitude	101
Anesthetized with pentobarbital (30 mg/kg, IV), acute instrumentation, coronary ligation model	Pretreated with 9 mg/kg/os the 60 min after the surgical preparation 180 µg/hr, IV infusion	There was no effect on myocardial infarction. There was a significantly higher mean aortic pressure in the indomethacin treated versus the vehicle treated cats with myocardial infarction but the infarction itself resulted in a significant decrease in mean aortic pressure. There was no direct effect of indomethacin on hemodynamics	68
Pentobarbital anesthetized (30 mg/kg, IV), isolated aortic strips	10^{-6} to 10^{-4} M	Increased developed tension	68
Pentobarbital (30 mg/kg, IP) + additional doses as needed. By-passed isolated small intestine (mesenteric artery) preparation with flow controlled	Dose-response	Mesenteric vasoconstriction, dose-dependent	102

4.11:3 Indomethacin-Rats, Conditions	Dose	Cardiovascular Effects	Reference
Isolated, *in situ*, perfused superior mesenteric artery preparations, prepared under ether anesthesia, perfused with a non-blood cell perfusate. Studied the ability to block effects of pressor agents	1 to 64 µg/ml, dose-response	Was able to block pressor effects of norepinephrine, angiotensin II, arginine vasopressin, histamine, serotonin, calcium ions and potassium ions	**103**
Ether anesthesia, perfused mesenteric bed preparation used a peristaltic flow inducer	10 µg/ml added to the perfusate	Attenuated the norepinephrine-induced vascular response. There was no effect on captopril responses	**104**
Rats killed by decapitation, isolated perfused heart prep.	1 & 10 µg/ml in perfusate	The higher dose attenuated the degree of coronary pressure increase caused by adrenochrome (an oxidation product of epinephrine)	**73**
Intact, awake, measured cerebral blood flow at 15, 30, 60 & 90 min following indomethacin injection	10 mg/kg, IP	Decreased cerebral blood flow during entire period of observation, no change in mean aortic pressure or arterial blood gases	**105**
Isolated heart, killed by a blow to the head, Langendorff preparation with isometric contractions	300 µg/min infusion	Decreased myocardial contractility and decreased calcium ion induced increases in contractility. No effects on changes in perfusion pressure or coronary flow caused by calcium ion infusion	**106**
Exercised-trained and non-exercise-trained controls, isoproterenol induced myocardial necrosis	4 mg/kg	Decreased myocardial creatine kinase in exercise-trained but not in controls. A marker for prostacyclin was not altered by exercise but was decreased by indomethacin pretreatment	**107**

Condition	Dose	Cardiovascular effects	Reference
Sodium methohexitone anesthesia (60 mg/kg, IP), supplemented as needed for initial instrumentation, reanesthetized in 7 days with same at 40 mg/kg, IP for more instrumentation, recovered, measured as intact awake	5 mg/kg + 5 mg/kg/hr	No effect on renal vasodilations caused by endothelin-3 and sarafotoxin-56b-, Endothelin-1 caused early renal vasodilation only after indomethacin. Early vasoconstrictor effects on mesenteric bed only seen with indomethacin pretreatment. Indomethacin caused mesenteric constriction	108
Endurance exercise-trained vs controls, anesthetized with ether, hearts rapidly removed, isolated Langendorff type prep.	50 μM	Inhibited the endurance exercise training-induced potentiation of the coronary flow response to hypoxia	109
4.11:4 Indomethacin-Rabbits			
Isolated ear arteries, electrically stimulated nerve to cause contractions	1.5×10^{-6} M	Potentiated the constrictor responses evoked by nerve stimulation	1
Conscious, previously instrumented	0 mg/kg, IV	Reduced blood flow in the stomach wall, jejunum and brain. Increased hepatic artery flow and reduced blood flow in the retina, no significant effects in a number of other tissues studied	111
Conscious, previously instrumented	10 mg/kg, IV + 50 μg/kg/min for 30 min	Increased mean aortic pressure only during norepinephrine, Angiotensin II or arginine vasopressin infusions. No cardiovascular effects when administered by itself at these rates	112

4.11:5 Indomethacin- Sheep	Dose	Cardiovascular effects	Reference
Isolated coronary artery strips	2.8 μmol/L and 28 μmol/L	The lower dose had no effect on basal tone, the X 10 dose increased tension in 50% of the preparations tested. With acetylcholine used as a spasmogen, oscillations in induced tone and relaxations produced by arachidonic acid were abolished by 2.8 and 7 mol/L respectively. Blocks prostacyclin synthesized and released in the presence of ACh and arachidonic acid	113
Isolated neonatal lamb mesenteric and renal artery preparations. Studied the constrictor response to electrical field stimulation	1 μM (358 ng/ml)	Increased baseline tension, vasoconstrictor responses were increased 144 ± 55% in mesenteric vessels and 70 ± 11% in renal vessels. The potentiating effects of indomethacin were completely reversed when PGI_2 was added to the baths	114
Halothane anesthesia	10 mg/kg/hr for 3 hrs	Increased lymphatic clearance of protein from the lungs, mechanisms of this response not related to a loss of endothelial integrity, more likely related to the hemodynamic effects	115
Fetal lambs, chronically instrumented	0.33 ± 0.07 mg/kg of fetal weight	Nearly a two fold increase in vascular resistance of both the ductus venosus and the fetal liver	116
Intact, awake, previously instrumented	0.2 mg/kg, IV	Measurements of intracranial blood flow velocities before and 60 min after indomethacin injection, decreased significantly. Did not change response to hypercapnia	117

4.11:6 Indomethacin-Goats,	Dose	Cardiovascular effects	Reference
Intact, awake, chronically instrumented with flowmeter transducer on the external pudic artery, induced mastitis	3 mg/kg, IV	There was a small effect on the biphasic flow pattern caused by the induced mastitis with a partial suppression of the second peak of the flow response	118
4.11:7 Indomethacin-Pigs			
Sedated with ketamine, anesthetized with pentobarbital (no dose given), positive pressure ventilation, acute instrumentation, open thorax. Studied responses to leukotriene injections	6 mg/kg, IV	The dose-dependent decrease in coronary flow caused by injection of leukotriene was not blocked by indomethacin	119
Newborn, intact, awake, previously instrumented	5 mg/kg, IV	During high mean airway pressures from a ventilator (30 cm water) decrease in cerebral blood flow within 10 min, MVO_2 maintained by increased extraction	120
Newborn, intact, awake, previously instrumented	5 ± 1 mg/kg, IV	Decreased cerebral blood flow by 18-28% with no change in cardiac output, mean aortic pressure or blood gases. With hypoxia/hypercapnia decreased cerebral blood flow. Crossed the blood-brain barrier enough to inhibit prostanoid release into cerebrospinal fluid	121
Newborn, 4-5 days old, intact, awake	0.2 mg/kg and 5 mg/kg, IV	Lower dose decreased cerebral blood flow approx. 20% in hypotensive piglets (60-34 mmHg). Decreased cerebral MVO_2,modest changes compared to 5 mg/kg effects which decrease severely and result in coma	122

Conditions	Dose	Cardiovascular Effects	Reference
Newborn, 4-5 days old, intact, awake	5 ± 1 mg/kg, IV	Decreased cerebral blood flow and cerebral hyperemia in response to asphyxia, without affecting blood flow to any other systemic organ	123
1-3 day old, previously instrumented, 2.5-3 hrs after halothane anesthesia	3 mg/kg, IV	Decreased cerebral blood flow by 39%	124
4.11:8 Indomethacin-Guinea Pigs			
Heart removed under light ether anesthesia, isolated and perfused hearts, at constant volume	1.4×10^{-6} M	Increased coronary vascular resistance by 15%, without changing contractility of the myocardium. The indomethacin caused increase in coronary resistance was not affected by pretreatment with reserpine and/or phenoxybenzamine and propranolol but was prevented completely by the previous treatment with PGE_2 (1.4×10^{-7} M)	125
Anesthetized with urethane (1.5-1.75 g/kg, IP)	0.1-2.0 mg/kg	Increased aortic pressure and firing rate in the carotid sinus nerve	126
Isolated thoracic inferior vena cava	100 µM	Shape change of endothelial cells in response to histamine, bradykinin, PGE_2 or leukotrienes is partially blocked, possibly by reduction of the amount of intracellular calcium ion available for shortening of endothelial cell contractile proteins	127

Table 4.12: Cardiovascular effects of Dipyridamole:

Conditions of the experiment	Dose	Cardiovascular Effects	Reference
4.12:1 Dipyridamole-Dogs			
Anesthetized with pentobarbital (30 mg/kg, IV), positive pressure ventilation, acute instrumentation, open thorax	25-100 µg, intra-coronary infusion	No change in mean aortic pressure, an increase in coronary flow and no change in either epicardial or endocardial pO_2	**128**
Anesthetized with chloralose (140 mg/kg) and urethane (1.4 g/kg), IV, models of iatrogenic coronary artery stenosis	0.08 mg/kg/min, IV	Increased myocardial blood flow in all cases. A redistribution of coronary transmural flow occurs in non- or mildly-stenosed regions (endo to epi steal). Absolute decrease in endothelial flow in regions distal to severe stenosis	**133**
Conscious, previously instrumented	0.25 mg/kg, IV 3 min prior to second of 2 LAD occlusions	Adversely affected the extent af myocardial ischemia in the collateral-dependent zone	**134**
Isolated mesenteric vein preparation from dogs anesthetized with pentobarbital (40 mg/kg, IV)	10^{-6} M	Inhibited both the excitatory function potential and the slow depolarization evoked by perivascular nerve stimulation. No change in post junctional membrane potential. Suggests inhibition did not involve either endogenous adenosine or prejunctional α-autoregulation mechanisms. Results suggest that dipyridamole decreases norepi. directly and also indirectly vie activation of catechol-o-methyltransferase, with no alteration of monoamine oxidase activity or the uptake mechanisms for norepi into nerve terminals	**135**

4.12:2 Dipyridamole-Cats	Dose	Cardivascular effects	Reference
Adult cats, ketamine (2 mg/kg, IM), acepromazine (1 mg/kg, IM), pentobarbital (30 mg/kg, IV + 12-25 mg/hr as needed	0.4 mg/kg/min, IV infusion	Marked reduction in coronary resistance with major component accounted for by dilation of microvessels	136
4.12:3 Dipyridamole-Rats			
Left ventricular papillary muscles, myocardial capillary stereological studies	4 mg/kg, IP, b.i.d. for 6 weeks	Length-density of myocardial capillaries increased 5%, surface density of capillaries increased 8%, 3-dimensional capillary fiber ratio increased 6%	137
4.12:4 Dipyridamole-Mice			
Anesthetized with urethane (no dose given), IV sodium fluorescein, platelet aggregation induced by illumination with a UV lamp	1, 10, 25 & 50 mg/kg	There was no effect on *in vivo* platelet aggregation whereas aspirin prevented same	129
4.12:5 Dipyridamole-Rabbits			
Conscious, previously instrumented	0.25 mg/kg, IV	Increased blood flow to cerebral cortex, caudate nucleus, putamen, hippocampus, thalamus. Also increased tissue pO_2 in the caudate nucleus but no change in other measured portions of the brain	138
Aortic vascular rings	1-100 µM, dose-response	No significant stimulation of PGI_2 release	139
Same as above	10-100 µM, pretreatment	Prolonged the transient stimulation of PGI_2 release induced by mechanical de-endothelialization (partial protection of cyclooxygenase against oxidative self-inactivation	139

Condition	Dose	Cardiovascular effects	Reference
Platelets and isolated aortic segments	1-30 μM	Potentiated anti-aggregating activity of NO, clearly enhanced dilations induced by exogenous NO	**140**
4.12:6 Dipyridamole-Cattle			
Cultured pulmonary artery endothelial and smooth muscle cells	10 μM	Found to increase the concentration of adenosine near thrombus sites, possibly by preventing the intracellular uptake of adenosine	**85**
Cultured endothelial and aortic smooth muscle cells	1-100 μM	Nitric oxide (NO) induction of significant stimulation of PGI_2 release	**139**
4.12:7 Dipyridamole-Pigs			
Intact, awake, miniature pigs, exercising	1 mg/kg, IV	At 11.2 Km/hr treadmill running produced increases in blood flow only in myocardial, respiratory and slow-twitch skeletal muscle. At maximum exercise (17.6 Km/hr) dipyridamole decreased aortic blood pressure and increased vascular conductance in all muscles studied	**141**
4.12:8 Dipyridamole-Primates (Cynomolgus)			
Intact, awake, atherosclerotic diet fed	10 mg/kg/os daily	no effect on arterial uptake of plasma LDL or cholesterol. No protection against atherosclerosis	**89**

Table 4.13: Cardiovascular effects of Meclofenamate:

Conditions of the experiment	Dose	Cardiovascular effects	Reference
4.13:1 Meclofenamate- Dogs			
Anesthetized with pentobarbital (30 mg/kg, IV), trachea intubated, acute instrumentation, closed thorax	10 mg/kg, slow IV in divided doses over a 25 min period	There was a marked decrease in mesenteric blood flow, an increase in aortic pressure but no change in celiac blood flow	93
Intact, awake, conscious	2 mg/kg, IV + 2 mg/kg/hr, IV	Osmotic arginine vasopressin serum concentrations were reduced by cyclo-oxygenase blocking activity	130
Coronary artery vascular rings, anesthetized with pentobarbital (30 mg/kg, IV) then exsanguinated	10^{-6} M	Dose-response to serotonin shifted to the left	9
l (30 mg/kg, IV), ventilated with 40-60% O_2, acute lower left lung lobe preparation	5 µM, IV	Increased resting lobar vascular resistance by $36 \pm 8.3\%$ and ratio of pre- and post-capillary resistance from 1.9 ± 0.3 to 1.1 ± 0.2	66
4.13:2 Meclofenamate- Cats			
Anesthetized with pentobarbital (30 mg/kg, IV), acute instrumentation, coronary ligation model	2 mg/kg/os, pretreatment	No effect on hemodynamics or on the time-course of response to myocardial infarction	68
Isolated aortic strips, anesthetized with pentobarbital (30 mg/kg, IV)	1×10^{-6} to 1×10^{-5} M	No effects observed	68

4.13:3 Meclofenamate-Pigs	Dose	Cardiovascular effects	Reference
Pentobarbital anesthetized (30 mg/kg, IV), pretreatment with salicylate (40 mg/kg)	2 mg/kg	When given after the salicylate decreased renal blood flow but no change in GFR	**87**
4.13:4 Meclofenamate-Guinea Pigs			
Intact, awake, chronic hypoxia for 6 weeks	2 mg/kg, IV + 2 mg/kg/hr, IV	Phenylephrine challenge increased peripheral resistance with meclofenamate in chronic hypoxic animals, no effect in normoxic. Dose-response to Angiotensin II the same in both groups, with and without meclofenamate	**131**
Same animals as above, killed with an overdose of pentobarbital and aortic strips harvested	10^{-6} g/ml	Dose-response to phenylephrine shifted to the left in the chronic hypoxic	**131**

Table 4.14: Cardiovascular effects of other non-steroidal anti-inflammatory/analgesic agents:

Conditions of the experiment	Dose	Cardiovascular effects	Reference
4.14:1 Sulfinpyrazone-Dogs			
Anesthetized with α-chloralose (100 mg/kg, IV + 50 mg/kg as needed), positive pressure ventilation, acute instrumentation, coronary occlusion model	30 mg/kg, IV bolus	There was a significant increase in the ventricular fibrillation threshold, an increase in the mid-diastolic threshold and an increase in effective refractory period. No changes in heart rate or mean aortic pressure. Afforded significant protection during coronary occlusion but there was no effect on the ventricular fibrillation threshold after reperfusion	**142**

Condition	Dose	Cardiovascular effects	Reference
Anesthetized with pentobarbital (30-40 mg/kg, IV), positive pressure ventilation, open thorax, acute instrumentation, response to coronary occlusion	30 mg/kg, IV	There was a significant increase in flow to the ischemic epicardium from 5 min after pretreatment occlusion to 5 min after post-treatment occlusion. There was a significant increase in epicardial collateral flow from 5 min after post-treatment occlusion to 4 hrs later. There was no change in HR or mean aortic pressure	58
anesthetized with methohexital and chloralose (no doses given), positive pressure ventilation, open thorax, acute instrumentation	1) 20-40 mg intracoronary 2) 10-300 mg, intra-femoral	1) Small doses resulted in a transient increase in coronary flow, no change in left ventricular pressure, aortic pressure or LV dP/dt. Larger doses resulted in a significant increase in coronary flow with a transient decrease in left ventricular pressure and LV dP/dt 2) There was a dose-dependent increase in femoral blood flow	143
Same as above	10 & 20 mg/min to total of 500 mg, IV infusions	There was an inconsistent change in coronary flow at 27.8 µg/ml plasma concentration which is comparable to therapeutic concentrations in man	143
Anesthetized with pentobarbital (30 mg/kg, IV), hearts removed, isolated Purkinje fiber prep	10^{-6}, 10^{-5} & 10^{-4} M in perfusate	Rate of rise of the action potential (AP) phase 0, AP duration and effective refractory period were not altered significantly. Neither the AP phase 4 slope nor the mean cycle length of spontaneously firing Purkinje fibers were affected	144
4.14:2 Sulfinpyrazone-Rats			
Pretreatment of 14 days then given 40 mg/kg isoproterenol SQ, the animals were sacrificed 24 hrs later	100 mg/kg/os	There was significantly preserved myocardial creatinine kinase activity and a decrease in cardiac hypertrophy. No suppression of increased cAMP levels but a decrease in plasma prostaglandins	145

Condition	Dose	Cardiovascular effects	Reference
Intact, awake, prolonged unpredictable stress-induced morphological changes in the coronary circulation	1) 8 mg/kg/day prophylactic admin. from the onset 2) 8 mg/kg/day after 30 days of stress treatment	Stress induced changes included dilation of venules, DAS positive staining deposits in venules (platelet aggregation) and endothelial lining breakdown in arterioles. Treatment did no prevent but decreased the incidence of morphological change from stress	**145**
Spontaneously beating and electrically stimulated isolated rat atrial prep. Hearts excised under light ether anesthesia	Dose-response	Increasing doses decreased the spontaneous atrial frequency, prolonged the sinus node recovery time after overdrive pacing, slightly increased the electrical threshold for excitation and decreased the contractile force	**146**
4.14:3 Flunixin-meglumine-Horses			
Halothane anesthesia, isolated, autoperfused intestinal segments	1.1 mg/kg, IV bolus	Increased mean aortic pressure and increased intestinal vascular resistance at 10 min. Jejunal blood flow decreased at 60 min post-injection. A-VO$_2$ difference of intestine unchanged. Oxygen consumption unchanged	**57**
Intact, awake ponies	1 mg/kg, IV, 2.2 mg/kg, IM	No changes in heart rate, aortic pressure, respiratory rate, central venous pressure or blood gases	**1,148**
Induced with glyceryl guiacolate (5%), to effect, intubated, halothane anesthesia. Acute instrumentation, shock induced by 0.2 mg of *E coli* endotoxin, blood flow measured with microspheres	1.1 mg/kg, IV, 5 min after injection of endotoxin	Prevented endotoxin induced decreases in blood flow to brain, stomach, small intestine, large intestine, pancreas, skeletal muscle, skin, heart and lung. Did not prevent general tissue damage, decreased lactoacidosis, significant decrease in platelet counts. Some evidence that Flumixin blocked brain damage from endotoxin	**149,175**

4.14:4 Tolectin (tolmetin)-Dogs	Dose	Cardiovascular effects	Reference
Anesthetized with thiopental (20 mg/kg, IV), maintained with α-chloralose (60 mg/kg, IV), spontaneous breathing, acute instrumentation	10 mg/kg, IV	No change in mean aortic pressure, heart rate, or ECG. No autonomic effects observed	150
4.14:5 Fluriprofen-Goats			
Intact, awake, chronic instrumentation of the external pudic artery flow, induced mastitis	2 mg/kg, IV	Partial suppression of the second peak of the flow response to induced mastitis	118
4.14:6 Suprofen-Goats			
Same as above	3 mg/kg, IV	Same as above	118
4.14:7 Ibuprofen-Rabbits			
Isolated, Langendorff perfused heart prep	50, 140 & 289 µg/ml concentration in perfusate	50 µg/ml: 1/2 max coronary vasodilator response 140 µg/ml: coronary vasodilation equivalent to that caused by hypoxia. 280 µg/ml: decreased contractile function, no change in myocardial lactate extraction, suggests a direct effect	151

Antibiotics

With more and more work being done on intact, previously instrumented animals, another possible pitfall awaits the unwary investigator. Post-operatively, the experimental animals will often require antibiotic therapy. A number of antibiotics have been shown to have adverse effects on the cardiovascular system. The aminoglycosides, which include neomycin, streptomycin, dihydrostreptomycin, kanamycin and gentamicin, have been reported to decrease cardiac output, aortic pressure and left ventricular contractility and to increase heart rate.[152] Penicillin and penicillin related agents have been associated with myocardial depression, conduction abnormalities and vasodilating effects in many species, possibly related to effects on calcium ion transport.[152,153] Chloramphenicol and the tetracyclines have been reported to cause myocardial depression[152] as have erythromycin and vancomycin.[154] Tables 4.15 through 4.17 summarize the cardiovascular effects of some of the antibiotics and the circumstances under which this information was obtained.

Another note of caution. We have found that the vehicle in which the xenobiotic is suspended or dissolved may be the culprit in some instances. Adverse cardiovascular effects to propylene glycol, for example, have been well documented.[155] Other vehicles may also result in apparent responses to the parenteral agent being administered.

Table 4.15: Cardiovascular effects of the aminoglycoside antibiotics:

Conditions of the experiment	Dose	Cardiovascular Effects	Reference
4.15:1 Neomycin-Dogs			
Anesthetized with pentobarbital (28-35 mg/kg, IV, to effect), acute instrumentation, positive pressure ventilation, 20-30 min after instrumentation allowed for "stabilization"	21 mg/kg, IV & 28 mg/kg, IV	Dose-dependent decrease in heart rate and mean aortic pressure	1
Pentobarbital, isolated vascular smooth muscle preparations from the aorta, femoral, carotid, renal, superior and terminal mesenteric and the coronary arteries	reincubation with 0.7 to 3.5 mM	Dose-dependent inhibition of contractile responses	157
4.15:2 Neomycin-Cats			
Anesthetized with pentobarbital (28-35 mg/kg, IP), acute instrumentation, positive pressure ventilation, 20-30 min "stabilization"	3.5, 7 & 14 mg/kg, IV	Dose-dependent decrease in heart rate and mean aortic pressure	156

4.15:3 Neomycin-Rabbits	Dose	Cardiovascular effects	Reference
Killed by air embolus injected into an ear vein, aortic strips from the thoracic aorta, isolated preparation	7.0 mM	Acts to prevent re-uptake or rebinding of calcium ions at a portion of the superficial cellular sites or stores in the aortic smooth muscle. Inhibited contractile responses to 80 mM potassium ions	158
4.15:4 Neomycin-Primates			
Anesthetized with pentobarbital (28-35 mg/kg, IP), acute instrumentation, positive pressure ventilation	14, 21 & 35 mg/kg	Dose-dependent decrease in heart rates and mean aortic pressures. In baboons, there was a dose-dependent decrease in LV dP/dt, RV dF/dt, cardiac output, heart rate and aortic pressures. Maximum effects seen in 2-5 min with return to baseline in next 30-60 min. Effects were rapidly reversed by calcium chloride infusion	156
Anesthetized with pentobarbital (28-35 mg/kg, IP + more as needed)	14, 28 & 56 mg/kg, IV	Dose-dependent decrease in aortic pressure, cardiac output, LV dP/dt, dF/dt and heart rate. When the heart rate was held constant, the other parameters were still depressed	159
4.15:5 Streptomycin-Dogs			
Intact, anesthetized with pentobarbital (no dose given)	2 g, IM	Cardiac output decreased 26%, mean aortic pressure decreased 22% 1 hr after administration	154
Anesthetized with pentobarbital (30 mg/kg, IV), open thorax, acute instrumentation, bilateral vagotomy on 5 of 6, contractile force measured with strain gauge arch	2.5, 10 & 40 mg/kg, IV	Dose-dependent depression of cardiovascular function	154
Isolated heart-lung preparations	Approx 3 g	Severe heart failure, effects seemed to be due to calcium ion transport	160
Isolated hindlimb preparation	5 mg/kg	Decreased vascular resistance, approx. 30%	154

Condition	Dose	Cardiovascular effects	Reference
Anesthetized with pentobarbital (28-35 mg/kg, IV, to effect), acute instrumentation, positive pressure ventilation, 20-30 min "stabilization"	32 & 40 mg/kg, IV	Dose-dependent decrease in heart rate and mean aortic pressure	**156**
4.15:6 Streptomycin-Cats			
Same as previous	8 & 20 mg/kg, IV	Same as previous	**156**
Isolated heart preparation (Langendorff)	5 g to 50 mg	Dose-dependent decrease in LV pressure and LV dP/dt	**154**
4.15:7 Streptomycin-Primates			
Anesthetized with pentobarbital (28-35 mg/kg, IP), acute instrumentation, positive pressure ventilation	16, 24 & 40 mg/kg (baboon), 4, 8 & 16 mg/kg (squirrel)	Dose-dependent decrease in heart rate and mean aortic pressure	**156**
5.15:8 Kanamycin-Dogs			
Anesthetized with pentobarbital (30 mg/kg, IV), open thorax, acute instrumentation	333 mg, IV	Decreased LV dP/dt 16.3 ± 1.6%, strain gauge force transducer on right ventricle showed a decrease in developed tension of 21.4 ± 4.0%	**154**
Isolated hindlimb preparation	33 mg, intra-arterial	Decreased vascular resistance by about 30%	**154**
4.15:9 Kanamycin-Cats			
Anesthetized with pentobarbital (28-35 mg/kg, IP), acute instrumentation, positive pressure ventilation, 20-30 min "stabilization"	8, 16 & 32 mg/kg, IV	Dose-dependent decrease in heart rate and mean aortic pressure	**157**
Isolated heart preparation	5 g to 50 mg	Dose-dependent decrease in LV pressure and LV dP/dt	**154**

4.15:10 Gentamicin-Dogs	Dose	Cardiovascular effects	Reference
Isolated right ventricular trabeculae (ventricular muscle)	10^{-4} to 10^{-2} M, Dose-response	Decreased developed tension, near abolition at 10^{-2} M (negative inotropy)	**161**
Anesthetized with pentobarbital (30 mg/kg, IV), isolated, blood perfused, papillary muscle, SA and A-V nodal preparations (All perfused via the normal coronary distribution, with constant perfusion pressure)	0.3 - 100 µmol, intra-arterial	Increased coronary blood flow in all preparations, i.e. vasodilation. Decreased contractility in both paced and spontaneously beating papillary muscle. Decreased sinus rate of SA node, increased A-V conduction time, in large doses produced 3rd degree A-V block, prolonged A-V conduction times and reduced amplitude of ventricular bipolar electrograms	**162**
4.15:11 **Gentamicin-Rats**			
Killed by decapitation, isolated, electrically driven, left atrial appendage prep	0.0156-0.25 mM	Concentration-dependent decrease in myocardial contractile tension. Were able to antagonize the effect with increased calcium ion concentration in the bath	**163**
Cultured cardiocytes	200 nmol (0.8 X 10^{-3} to 8.0 X 10^{-3} M)	Decreased contraction amplitude by 50% and decreased action potential overshoot by 20%. No change in action potential duration or maximum diastolic potential	**164**
4.15:12 **Gentamicin-Guinea Pigs**			
Isolated left atrial prep	Dose-response	Dose-dependent decrease in cellular calcium ion concentrations by 10-20% and decreased contractility 40-90%	**165**
4.15:13 **Gentamicin-Primates**			
Anesthetized with pentobarbital (28-35 mg/kg, IP + more as needed), acute instrumentation	14, 28 & 56 mg/kg, IV	Dose-dependent decrease in aortic pressures, cardiac output, LV dP/dt, RV dP/dt and heart rate	**159**

Condition	Dose	Cardiovascular effects	Reference
Anesthetized with pentobarbital (28-35 mg/kg, IP), acute instrumentation, positive pressure ventilation)	8, 18, 26 mg/kg, IV (rhesus), 18, 26 & 43 mg/kg, IV (squirrel)	Dose-dependent decrease in heart rate and mean aortic pressure	**156**
4.15:14 Sisomicin-Guinea Pigs			
Isolated left atrial prep	Dose-response	Dose-dependent decrease in intracellular calcium ion concentrations by 10-20%, decrease in contractility 40-90%	**165**
4.15:15 Dibekacin-Guinea Pigs			
Same as above	Same	Reduced intracellular calcium by 10-20%, contractility reduced 40-90%	**165**

Table 4.16: Cardiovascular effects of penicillin and penicillin-type antibiotics:

Conditions of the experiment	Dose	Cardiovascular effects	Reference
4.16:1 Penicillin-Dogs			
Anesthetized with pentobarbital (30 mg/kg, IV), open thorax, acute instrumentation (only 2 dogs studied)	No dose cited	No changes in LV dP/dt, RV developed tension (measured with strain gauge) or mean aortic pressure	**154**
Isolated heart-lung prep	750-1000 mg (potassium penicillin G)	Decreased cardiac output, myocardial depression and ventricular arrhythmias, apparently effected calcium ion transport mechanisms	**160**
Isolated hindlimb preparation	1×10^5 units	No change in vascular resistance	**152**
4.16:2 Penicillin-Horses			
Awake, previously instrumented	20,000 IU/kg, IV	Decreased mean aortic pressure, no change in heart rate, respiratory rate, central venous pressure, pulmonary arterial pressure or blood gases	**166**

Condition	Dose	Cardiovascular effects	Reference
Anesthetized with Guaifenesin (50 mg/kg, IV) + Thiamylal Na (4 g/kg, IV), Preanesthetized with Xylazine (2.2 mg/kg), maintained with halothane (2-3 vol%)	20,000 IU/kg, IV	Decreased mean aortic and diastolic pressures which stayed depressed for 10 min following IV administration	**166**
4.16:3 Ampicillin-Dogs			
Isolated hindlimb prep	50 mg	Decreased vascular resistance about 30%	**152**
4.16:4 Oxacillin-Dogs			
Isolated hindlimb prep	50 mg	Decreased vascular resistance about 30%	**153**
4.16:5 Lincomycin-Dogs			
Preanesthetized with atropine (0.5 mg), anesthetized with thiopental (100 mg, IV), maintained with halothane (0.5%) in nitrous oxide, positive pressure ventilation	100-900 mg/kg	Decreased aortic pressure and resulted in severe ventricular arrhythmias	**167**
4.16:6 Cephalothin-Dogs			
Isolated hindlimb prep	100 mg	Decreased vascular resistance about 30%	**153**

Table 4.17: Cardiovascular effects of other antibiotics:

Conditions of the experiment	Dose	Cardiovascular effects	Reference
4.17:1 Erythromycin-Dogs			
Anesthetized with pentobarbital (30 mg/kg, IV), open thorax, acute instrumentation (only 2 dogs studied)	No dose given	Decreased LV dP/dt, decreased developed tension (strain gauge), decreased mean aortic pressure	**154**
Isolated hindlimb prep	15 mg	Decreased vascular resistance about 30%	**153**
Anesthetized with pentobarbital (30 mg/kg, IV), Purkinje fiber false tendon, isolated in tissue bath	Dose-response, 10, 50 & 100 mg/l	No response at low dose, substantial alterations at high dose; long QT resulting from increased action potential duration, decreased Vmax was concentration dependent	**168**
4.17:2 Vancomycin-Dogs,			
Anesthetized with pentobarbital (30 mg/kg, IV), open thorax, acute instrumentation (only 2 dogs studied)	No dose given	Decreased LV dP/dt, decreased developed tension as measured with a strain gauge arch on the RV, decreased mean aortic pressure	**154**
Isolated hindlimb prep	5 mg/kg	Decreased vascular resistance about 30%	**153**
4.17:3 Vancomycin-Cats			
Isolated heart prep	5 g to 50 mg	Dose-dependent decrease in LV pressure and LV dP/dt	**154**
4.17:4 Colymycin-Dogs			
Anesthetized with pentobarbital (30 mg/kg, IV), open thorax, acute instrumentation (only 2 dogs studied)	No dose given	Decreased LV dP/dt and rate of developed tension from strain gauge on RV, decreased mean aortic pressure	**154**

4.17:5 Chloramphenicol- Dogs	Dose	Cardiovascular effects	Reference
Anesthetized with pentobarbital (30 mg/kg, IV), open thorax, acute instrumentation (only 2 dogs)	No dose given	No changes in LV dP/dt, RV dT/dt or mean aortic pressure	**1**
Anesthetized with pentobarbital (30 mg/kg, IV), open thorax, acute instrumentation (only 2 dogs)	3 mg/kg/os 2 hrs prior to anesthesia; 50 mg/kg, IM, 2 hrs prior, 50 mg/kg, IM, immediately prior; 1-3 μg/kg/hr, 0.1-0.3 and 1-3 mg/kg/hr, slow IV infusion during anesthesia; 25 mg/kg, IM then 25 mg/kg/os b.i.d. for 4 days	All doses and routes of administration increased the duration of anesthesia	**169**
Anesthetized with pentobarbital (33 mg/kg, IV)	30 mg/kg, IM, 1 hr prior to anesthesia; 33 mg/kg, IV immediately prior to anesthesia	Increased the duration of anesthesia	**170**
Isolated heart-lung preparation	100-200 mg	Decreased cardiac output, increased atrial pressures, caused myocardial depression by effects on calcium ion transport	**160**
Isolated hindlimb prep	100 mg	Decreased vascular resistance by about 30 %	**154**

Condition	Dose	Cardiovascular effects	Reference
Anesthetized with pentobarbital (30 mg/kg, IV), drug compared with equal volume injections of vehicle (2% benzyl alcohol, 28% distilled water and 40% polyethylene glycol	50 mg/kg, rapid IV (60 mg/sec)	Severe decrease in mean aortic pressure and heart rate due to chloramphenicol, not vehicle. Direct vascular smooth muscle effects plus possible central nervous system effects	172
4.17:6 Chloramphenicol-Cats			
Anesthetized with pentobarbital (32 mg/kg, IP)	30 mg/kg, IM, 15 min prior to anesthesia, 35 mg/kg, IV, about 10 min after anesthesia	Prolonged the duration of anesthesia	170
Isolated heart preparation	5 µg to 50 mg	Dose-dependent decrease in LV pressure and LV dP/dt	154
4.17:7 Tetracyclines-Dogs			
Anesthetized with pentobarbital (30 mg/kg, IV) open thorax, acute instrumentation	250 mg, IV	Decreased LV dP/dt, decreased dT/dt on RV and decreased mean aortic pressure	154
Isolated heart-lung preparation	350 mg (chlor-tetracycline), 600 mg (tetracycline)	Increased atrial pressures, cardiac output decreased until eventual failure from myocardial depression, probably a result of effects on calcium ion transport	160
Isolated hindlimb prep	25 mg	Decreased vascular resistance about 30%	154
4.17:8 Tetracyclines-Cats			
Isolated heart prep	5 µg to 50 mg	Dose-dependent decrease in LV pressure and LV dP/dt	154

4.17:9 Tetracyclines- Cattle	Dose	Cardiovascular effects	Reference
Intact, awake, previuosly instrumented	11.2 mg/kg, IV (2 calves); 22.4 mg/kg, IV (2 calves); 56 mg/kg, IV (1 calf) (oxy-tetracycline)	Decreased heart rate to asystole, increased pulmonary arterial resistance, increased renal arterial resistance, found effects were due to the propylene glycol vehicle, not the oxytetracycline	171
Intact, awake, previously instrumented	20 mg/kg, IV at 1 ml/sec	No effects from aqueous preparation both propylene glycol and polyvinylpyrrolidone vehicles resulted in decreased cardiac function	155
4.17:10 Tetracyclines- Horses			
Intact, awake (14 hours total), also injected vehicle alone at same infusion rates and volumes	0.18-0.44 mg/kg, IV; 3 & 6.6 mg/kg, IV at different infusion rates	Apparent infusion rate dependent atrial tachycardia, signs of discomfort, collapse and death, apparently from atrial, progressing to ventricular, tachy-arrhythmias. No clear evidence of ventricular fibrillation but was presumed. Apparent increase in aortic pressure. Vehicle alone resulted in no significant changes	173
4.17:11 Macrolide antibiotic (LY281389)-Dogs			
Morphine sulfate (1.0 mg/kg, SQ), Na methohexital (5 mg/kg) and α-chloralose (80 mg/kg), IV	Doses ≥ 200 μg/kg	Increased mean aortic pressure, decreased P-R interval, no change in cardiac output, pulmonary artery wedge pressure, pulmonary arterial pressure, femoral flow, QRS interval, Q-T interval, stroke volume, stroke work index, pulmonary or systemic vascular resistance	176
4.17:12 Cyclosporine-Rats			
Conscious, previously instrumented	20 mg/kg	Decreased renal blood flow (RBF) & renal vascular resistance (RVR)	177
Same	10 mg/kg	no change in RBF or RVR	176

Condition	Dose	Cardiovascular effects	Reference
Same	20 mg/kg, IP or 7 days	No change in RBF or RVR but increased plasma renin activity and urinary 6-keto-PGF$_{1\alpha}$ excretion (Latter effect seen under all 3 dose circumstances)	176
4.17:13 Cefazolin-Horses			
Awake, previously instrumented	11 mg/kg	No change in mean aortic pressure, heart rate, respiratory rate, central venous pressure, pulmonary arterial pressure or blood gases	166
Anesthetized with guafenesin (50 mg/kg) + Thiamylal (4 g/kg), IV, Preanesthesia with Xylazine (2.2 mg/kg), maintained with halothane	2-3 vol %	No change in mean aortic pressure, heart rate, respiratory rate, central venous pressure, pulmonary arterial pressure or blood gases	166

References

1.   Adams, H.R. Cholinergic Pharmacology: neuromuscular blocking agents. Chp 9 in Veterinary Pharmacology and Therapeutics, 6th ed, ed. by Booth and McDonald, Iowa State University Press, 1988.

2.   Montasture, J.L., Montasture, R. Naloxone and acute neurogenic hypertension in anaesthetized dogs, *Arch de Farmacol y Toxicol*, 8:45-48, 1982.

3.   Brown, B.R., Crout, J.R. The sympathomimetic effect of gallamine on the heart, *J Pharmacol Exp Ther*, 172:266-273, 1970.

4.   Tucker, W.K., Munson, E.S. Effects of succinylcholine and d-tubocurarine on epinephrine-induced arrhythmias during halothane anesthesia in dogs, *Anesthesia*, 42:41-44, 1975.

5.   Carrier, O. Jr., Murphy, J.D. The effects of d-tubocurarine and its commercial vehicles on cardiac function, *Anesthesia*, 33:627-634, 1970.

6.   Dowdy, E.G., Holland, W.C., Yamanaka, I. *et al.* Cardioactive properties od d-tubocurarine with and without preservatives, *Anesthesia*, 34:256-261, 1971.

7.   Ohmura, A., Wong, K.C., Shaw, L. Cardiac effects of succinyldicholine and succinylmonocholine, *Can Anaesth Soc J*, 23:567-573, 1976.

8.   Kreul, J.F., Atlee, J.L. Pancuronium enhances atrioventricular conduction in anesthetized dogs, *Anesthes*, 51 (3 suppl.):S86, 1979.

9.   Tutterova, M., Mosinger, B., Vavrinkova, H. The effect of sodium salicylate and epinephrine on the release of lactate dehydrogenase from isolated rat heart, *Acta Biol Med Ger*, 39(4):433-443, 1980.

10. Kwiatkowska-Patzer, B., Herbaczynska-Cedro, K. Low dose of acetylsalicylic acid prolongs refractory periods in normal cat myocardium, *Arzneimittel-Forsch*, 31(6):959-961, 1981.

11. Evans, A.T., Anderson, L.K., Eyster, G.E., Sawyer, D.C. Cardiovascular effects of gallamine triethiodide and succinylcholine chloride during halothane anesthesia in the dog, *Am J Vet Res*, 38(3):329-331, 1977.

12. Hughes, R., Chapple, D.J. Effects of non-depolarizing neuromuscular blocking agents on peripheral autonomic mechanisms in cats, *Br J Anaesth*, 48:59-67, 1976.

13. Wyse, R.K., Silove, E.D., Godley, M.L., Welham, K.C. Cardiovascular effects of neuromuscular blockade during induced hypothermia, *Clin Exp Pharmacol Physiol*, 11(2):181-189, 1984.

14. Rurak, D.W., Gruber, N.C. The effect of neuromuscular blockade on oxygen consumption and blood gases in the fetal lamb, *Am J Obstet Gynecol*, 145(2):258-262, 1983.

15. Royster, R.L., Keeler, D.K., Haisty, W.K., Johnston, W.E., Prough, D.S. Cardiac electrophysiologic effects of fentanyl and combinations of fentanyl and neuromuscular relaxants in pentobarbital-anesthetized dogs, *Anesth Analg*, 67(1):15-20, 1988.

16. Lees, P., Tavernor, W.D. The influence of suxamethonium on cardiovascular and respiratory function in the anaesthetized horse, *Br J Pharmac*, 36:116-131, 1969.

17. Button, C., Bertschinger, H.J., Mulders, M.S. Haemodynamic and neurological responses of ventilated and apnoeic calves to succinyldicholine, *J S Afr Vet Assoc*, 52(4):283-288, 1981.

18. Reitan, J.A., Warpinski, M.A. Cardiovascular effects of pancuronium bromide in mongrel dogs, *Am J Vet Res*, 36(9):1309-1311, 1975.

19. Manely, S.V., Steffey, E.P., Howitt, G.A. Cardiovascular and neuromuscular effects of pancuronium bromide in the pony, *Am J Vet Res*, 44:1349-1353, 1983.

20. Barzu, T., Cuparencu, B., Cardan, E. The anticholinesterase activity of pancuronium bromide (Pavulon), *Biochem Pharmac*, 23:166-168, 1974.

21. Hildebrand, S.V., Howitt, G.A. Neuromuscular and cardiovascular effects of pancuronium bromide in calves anesthetized with halothane, *Am J Vet Res*, 45(8):1549-1552, 1984.

22. Belik, J., Wagerle, L.C., Delivoria-Papadopoulos, M. Cerebral blood flow and metabolism following pancuronium bromide in newborn lambs, *Pediatr Res*, 18(12):1305-1308, 1984.

23. Smith, G., Proctor, D.W., Spence, A.A. A comparison of some cardiovascular effects of tubocurarine and pancuronium in dogs, *Br J Anaesth*, 42:923-927, 1970.

24. Hughes, R. Haemodynamic effects of tubocurarine, gallamine and suxamethonium in dogs, *Brit J Anaesth*, 42:923-934, 1970.

25. Michel, A.D., Delmendo, R.E., Lopez, M., Whiting, R.L. On the interaction of gallamine with muscarinic receptor subtypes, *Euro J Pharmacol*, 182:335-345, 1990.

26. Ehlert, F.J. Gallamine allosterically antagonizes muscarinic receptor-mediated inhibition of adenylate cyclase activity in the rat myocardium, *J Pharmacol Exp Therap*, 247(2):596-602, 1988.

27. Roffel, A.F., Elzinga, C.R.S., Meurs, H., Zaagsma, J. Allosteric interactions of three muscarine antagonists at bovine tracheal smooth muscle and cardiac M_2 receptors, *Euro J Pharmacol*, 172:61-70, 1989.

28. Kobayashi, O., Nagashima, H., Duncalf, D., Chaudhry, I.A., Harsing, L.G. Jr., Foldes, F.F., Goldiner, P.L., Vizi, E.S. Direct evidence that pancuronium and gallamine enhance the release of norepinephrine from the atrial sympathetic nerve by inhibiting prejunctional muscarinic receptors, *J Auton Nervous Syst*, 18:55-60, 1987.

29. Hackett, G.H., Jantzen, A.H., Earnshaw, G., Siddiqui, S.A. Cardiovascular effects produced by a combination of d-tubocurarine and pancuronium in dogs, *Acta Anaesth Belg*, 37:259-266, 1986.

30. Gouyon, J.B., Torrado, A., Guignard, J.-P. Renal effects of d-tubocurarine and pancuronium in the newborn rabbit, *Biol Neonate*, 54:218-223, 1988.

31. Chestnut, D.H., Weiner, C.P., Thompson, C.S., McLaughlin, G.L. Intravenous administration of d-tubocurarine and pancuronium in fetal lambs, *Am J Obstet Gynecol*, 160:510-513, 1989.

32. Cameron, C.B., Gregory, G.A., Rudolph, A.M., Heyman, M.A. Cardiovascular effects of d-tubocurarine and pancuronium in newborn lambs during normoxia and hypoxia, *Pediatr Res*, 20(3):246-252, 1986.

33. Arimura, H., Ikemoto, Y., Ito, T., Yoshitake, J. Lack of effects of d-tubocurarine and pancuronium on the slow action potential of the guinea pig papillary muscle, *Can Anaesth Soc J*, 32(5):484-490, 1985.

34. Ali, H., Gristwood, R.W., Pearce, F.L. Some studies on the release of histamine from mast cells treated with d-tubocurarine, *Agents and Actions* 18:71-73, 1986.

35. Leiman, B.C., Katz, J., Butler, B.D. Mechanisms of succinylcholine-induced arrhythmias in hypoxic or hypoxic:hypercarbic dogs, *Anesth Analg*, 66(12):1292-1297, 1987.

36. Thiagarajah, S., Sophie, S., Lear, E., Azar, I., Frost, E.A. Effect of suxamethonium on the ICP of cats with and without thiopentone pretreatment, *Br J Anaesth*, 60(2):157-160, 1988.

37. Weiskopf, R.B., Eger, E.I., Holmes, M.A., Yasuda, N., Johnson, B.H., Targ, A.G., Rampil, I.J. Cardiovascular actions of common anesthetic adjuvants during desflurane (I-653) and isoflurane anesthesia in swine, *Anesth Analg*, 71(2):144-148, 1990.

38. Ducey, J.P., Deppe, S.A., Foley, K.T. A comparison of the effects of suxamethonium, atracurium and vecuronium on intracranial haemodynamics in swine, *Anaesth Intens Care*, 17:448-455, 1989.

39.   Muir, A.W., Marshall, R.J. Comparative neuromuscular blocking effects of vecuronium, pancuronium, Org 6368 and suxamethonium in the anaesthetized domestic pig, *Br J Anaesth*, 59:622-629, 1987.

40.   Assem, E.S., Ezeamuzie, I.C. Suxamethonium-induced histamine release from the heart of naive and suxamethonium-sensitized guinea-pigs: evidence suggesting spontaneous sensitization in naive animals, and relevance to anaphylactoid reactions in man, *Agents Actions*, 27(1-2):146-149, 1989.

41.   Hackett, G.H., Jantzen, J.P., Earnshaw, G. Cardiovascular effects of vecuronium, atracurium, pancuronium, metocurine and RGH-4201 in dogs, *Acta Anaesthesiol Scand*, 33(4):298-303, 1989.

42.   Sugai, Y., Sugai, K., Hirata, T., Okuda, C., Miyazak, M. The interaction of pancuronium and vecuronium with cardiac muscarinic receptors, *Acta Anaesthesiol Scand*, 31:224-226, 1987.

43.   Wolfson, M.R., Shaffer, T.H. Differential effects of pancuronium bromide on cardiopulmonary function in the neonatal lamb, *Pediatric Pulmonology*, 8:233-239, 1990.

44.   Deam, R.K., Soni, N. Effects of pipecuronium and pancuronium on the isolated rabbit heart, *Br J Anaesth*, 62:287-289, 1989.

45.   Wali, F.A., Makinde, V. Effects of pancuronium and vecuronium on creatine phosphokinase in rat isolated heart, liver, kidney and diaphragm, *Gen Pharmacol*, 22(2):310-304, 1991.

46.   Chapple, D.J., Miller, A.A., Ward, J.B., Wheatly, P.L. Cardiovascular and neurological effects of laudanosine. Studies in mice and rats and in conscious anesthetized dogs, *Br J Anaesth*, 59(2):218-225, 1987.

47.   Giffen, J.P., Litwak, B., Cottrell, J.E., Hartung, J., Capuano, C. Intracranial pressure mean arterial pressure and heart rate after rapid paralysis with atracurium in cats, *Can Anaesth Soc J*, 32(6):618-621, 1985.

48.   Hildebrand, S.V., Howitt, G.A., Arpin, D. Neuromuscular and cardiovascular effects of atracurium in ponies anesthetized with halothane, *Am J Vet Res*, 47(5):1096-1000, 1986.

49.   Hildebrand, S.V., Arpin, D. Neuromuscular and cardiovascular effects of atracurium administered to healthy horses anesthetized with halothane, *Am J Vet Res*, 49(7):1066-1071, 1988.

50.   Bellis, D.J., Day, S., Barnes, P.K. The chronotropic effect of acetylcholine in the presence of vecuronium and atracurium, *Anaesthesia*, 45:118-119, 1990.

51.   Schmeling, W.T., Kampine, J.P., Warltier, D.C. Negative chronotropic actions of sufentanil and vecuronium in chronically instrumented dogs pretreated with propranolol and/or diltiazem, *Anesth Analg*, 69:4-14, 1989.

52.   Cason, B., Baker, D.G., Hickey, R.F., Miller, R.D., Agoston, S. Cardiovascular and neuromuscular effects of three steroidal neuromuscular blocking drugs in dogs (ORG 9616, ORG 9426, ORG 9991), *Anesth Analg*, 70:482-488, 1990.

53.   Giffen, J.P., Hartung, J., Cottrell, J.E., Capuano, C., Shwiry, B. Effect of vecuronium on intracranial pressure, mean arterial pressure and heart rate in cats, *Br J Anaesth*, 58:441-443, 1986.

54.   Muir, A.W., Houston, J., Marshall, R.J., Bowman, W.C., Marshall, I.G. A comparison of the neuromuscular blocking and autonomic effects of two new short-acting muscle relaxants with those of succinylcholine in the anesthetized cat and pig, *Anesthesiology*, 70:533-540, 1989.

55.   Muir, A.W., Houston, J., Green, K.L., Marshall, R.J., Bowman, W.C., Marshall, I.G. Effects of a new neuromuscular blocking agent (ORG 9426) in anesthetized cats and pigs and in isolated nerve-muscle preparations, *Br J Anaesth*, 63:400-410, 1989.

56.   Gibbs, N.M., Larach, D.R., Schuler, H.G. The effect of neuromuscular blockade with vecuronium on hemodynamic responses to noxious stimuli in the rat, *Anesthesiology*, 71:214-217, 1989.

57.   Stick, J.A., Arden, W.A., Chou, C.C., Parks, A.H., Wagner, M.A., Johnston, C.C. Effects of flunixin meglumine on jejunal blood flow, motility and oxygen consumption in ponies, *Am J Vet Res*, 49(7):1173-1178, 1988.

58.   Davenport, N., Goldstein, R.E., Capurro, N., Lipson, L.C., Bonow, R.O., Shulman, N.R., Epstein, S.E. Sulfinpyrazone and aspirin increase epicardial coronary collateral flow in dogs, *Am J Cardiol*, 47(4):848-854, 1981.

59.   Jackson, H.R., Johnson, S.L.M., Ng, K.H., Pye, W., Hall, R.C. The effect of acetylsalicylic acid on the response of the cardiovascular system to catecholamines, *Eur J Pharmacol*, 28(1):119-124, 1974.

60.   Lee, D.C., Lee, M.O., Clifford, D.H. Inhibition of the cardiovascular effects of lysine acetylsalicylate by propranol in dogs during halothane anesthesia, *Can Anaesth Soc J*, 29(4):349-354, 1982.

61.   Radegran, K. The effect of acetylsalicylic acid on the peripheral and pulmonary vascular responses to thrombin, *Acta Anaes Scan*, 16(3):140-146, 1972.

62. Moschos, C.B., Halder, B., de la Cruz, C. Jr., Lyons, M.M., Regan, T.J. Antiarrhythmic effects of aspirin during nonthrombin coronary occlusion, *Circ*, 57(4):681-684, 1978.

63. Sakanashi, M., Araki, H., Furukawa, T., Rokutanda, M., Yonemura, K. A study on constrictor response of dog coronary arteries to acetylsalicylic acid, *Arch Int Pharmacodyn Ther*, 252(1):86-96, 1981.

64. Toda, N., Okunishi, H., Taniyama, K., Miyazaki, M. Responses to adenine nucleotides and related compounds of isolated dog cerebral, coronary and mesenteric arteries, *Blood Vessels*, 19(5):226-236, 1982.

65. Miyajima, S., Aizawa, Y., Shibata, A. Attenuation of reactive hyperemia caused by aspirin in canine coronary artery, *Angiology*, 40(9):824-829, 1989.

66. Hofman, W.F., Ehrhart, I.C. Effects of cyclooxygenase inhibition on pulmonary vascular responses to serotonin, *J Appl Physiol*, 62(3):1192-1200, 1987.

67. Regan, T.J., Arena, J., Torres, R.B., Baktah, S. Electrophysiologic effects of aspirin on myocardium:interaction with catecholamine, *Trans Assoc Am Physicians*, 101:257-263, 1988.

68. Ogletree, M.L., Lefer, A.M. Influence of nonsteroidal anti-inflammatory agents on myocardial ischemia in the cat, *J Pharmacol Exp Ther*, 197(3):582-593, 1976.

69. Schaub, R.G., Gates, K.A., Roberts, R.E. Effect of aspirin on collateral blood flow after experimental thrombosis of the feline aorta, *Am J Vet Res*, 43(9):1647-1650, 1982.

70. Levy, J.V. Effect of choline magnesium trisalicylate on prostacyclin production by isolated vascular tissue of the rat, *Thromb Res*, 29(2):149-154, 1983.

71. Hashimoto, H., Ogawa, K. Effects of sulfinpyrazone, aspirin and propranolol on the isoproterenol-induced myocardial necrosis, *Jpn Heart J*, 22(4):643-652, 1981.

72. Vercesi, A.E., Pocesi, A. Jr. The effects of salicylate and aspirin on the activity of phosphorylase A in perfused hearts of rats, *Experientia*, 33(2):157-158, 1977.

73. Karmazyn, M., Beamish, R.E., Fliegel, L., Dhalla, N.S. Adrenochrome-induced coronary artery constriction in the rat heart, *J Pharmacol Exp Ther*, 219(1):225-230, 1981.

74. Cerletti, C., Gambino, M.C., Garattini, S., de Gaetano, G. Biochemical selectivity of oral versus intravenous aspirin in rats. Inhibition by oral aspirin of cyclooxygenase activity in platelets and presystemic but not systemic vessels, *J Clin Invest*, 78(1):323-326, 1986.

75. Taube, C., Martin, S., Kohler, A.H., Kohler, A.R., Mest, H.J. Influence of acetylsalicylic acid and BM 13177 on blood pressure and efficacy of antihypertensive drugs in spontaneously hypertensive rats, *Biomed Biochim Acta*, 47(10-11):S94-S99, 1988.

76. Kohler, A.H., Kohler, A.R., Taube, C., Mest, H.J. Decrease in arterial blood pressure in spontaneously hypertensive rats by the TXA2 receptor antagonist BM 13177 and by acetylsalicylic acid, *Biomed Biochim Acta*, 47(10-11):S269-S273, 1988.

77. Bomberger, R.A., DePalma, R.G., Ambrose, T.A., Manalo, P. Aspirin and dipyridamole inhibit endothelial healing, *Arch Surg*, 117(11):1459-1464, 1982.

78. de Kergommeaux, B.D., Ali, M., McDonald, J.W.D. Effects of ASA on thromboxane and prostacyclin synthesis by rabbit aorta and pulmonary artery, *Prostaglandins, Leukotrienes and Medicine*, 11:225-231, 1983.

79. Neto, F.R. Electrophysiological effects of the salicylates on isolated atrial muscle of the rabbit, *Br J Pharm*, 77:285-292, 1982.

80. Cottle, M.K., van Petten, G.R., van Muyden, P. Effects of phenylephrine and sodium salicylate on maternal and fetal cardiovascular indices and blood oxygenation in sheep, *Am J Obstet Gyn*, 143(2):170-176, 1982.

81. Heymann, M.A., Rudolph, A.M. Effects of acetylsalicylic acid on the ductus arteriosus and circulation in fetal lambs in utero, *Circ Res*, 38(5):418-422, 1976.

82. Cohen, I., Nobel, D., Ohba, M., Ojeda, C. The interaction of ouabain and salicylate on sheep cardiac muscle, *J Physiol*, 297:187-205, 1979.

83. Cohen, I., Nobel, D., Ohba, M., Ojeda, C. Action of salicylate ions on the electrical properties of sheep cardiac Purkinje fibers, *J Physiol*, 297:163-185, 1979.

84. Coates, G., OBrodovich, H., Jefferies, A.L. Pulmonary haemodynamics during exercise after low and high doses of acetylsalicylic acid in sheep, *Respiration*, 52(2):94-100, 1987.

85. Crutchley, D.J., Ryan, U.S., Ryan, J.W. Effects of aspirin and dipyridamole on the degradation of adenosine diphosphate by cultured cells derived from bovine pulmonary artery, *J Clin Invest*, 66(1):29-35, 1980.

86. Kanke, Y., Bashey, R.I., Mori, Y., Angrist AA; Effect of puromycin and salicylate on biosynthesis of mucopolysaccharides and glycoproteins in bovine heart valve, *Exp Mol Pathol*, 15(3):336-344, 1971.

87. Zambraski, E.J., Guidotti, S.M., Atkinson, D.C., Diamond, J. Salicylic acid causes a diuresis and natriuresis in normal and common bile-duct-ligated cirrhotic miniature swine, *J Pharmacol Exp Ther*, 247(3):983-988, 1988.

88. del Basso, P., Iacobacci, O., Carpi, A. Action of salicylate on failing heart lung preparations of guinea-pig perfused with red blood cells suspended in Tyrode-dextran, *Arch Int Pharmacodyn Ther*, 236(1):137-153, 1978.

89. Hollander, W., Kirkpatrick, B., Paddock, J., Colombo, M., Nagraj, S., Prusty, S. Studies on the progression and regression of coronary and peripheral atherosclerosis in the cynomolgus monkey. 1. Effects of dipyridamole and aspirin, *Exp Mol Path*, 30(1):55-73, 1979.

90. Humphrey, S.J., Zins, G.R. The effects of indomethacin on systemic hemodynamics and blood flow in the conscious dog, *Res Comm Chem Path Pharm*, 39(2):229-240, 1983.

91. Ezrailson, E.G., Hanley, H.G., Hartley, C.J., Lewis, R.L.M., Entman, M.L., Schwartz, A. Studies on the mechanism of an antibiotic ionophore, RO2-2985, in the conscious chronically instrumented dog: Involvement of the prostaglandin synthetic pathway, *Cardiovasc Res*, 16(11):670-674, 1982.

92. Uchida, Y., Murao, S. Effects of thromboxane synthetase inhibitors on cyclical reduction of coronary blood flow in dogs, *Jpn Heart J*, 22(6):971-975, 1981.

93. Gaffney, G.R., Williamson, H.E. Effect of indomethacin and meclofenamate on canine mesenteric and celiac blood flow, *Res Comm Chem Path Pharm*, 25(1):165-168, 1979.

94. Sakanashi, M., Araki, H., Yonemura, K.I. Indomethacin-induced contractions of dog coronary arteries, *J Cardiovasc Pharm*, 2(5):657-665, 1980.

95. Sakanashi, M., Takeo, S., Miyamoto, Y., Aniya, Y., Higuchi, M. Effects of 2-nicotinamidoethyl nitrate (SG-75, nicorandil) on indomethacin-induced contractions of isolated dog coronary arteries, *Jpn Heart J*, 24(2):289-295, 1983.

96. Goldberg, M.R., Joiner, P.D., Greenberg, S., Hyman, A.L., Kadowitz, P.J. Effects of indomethacin on veno-constrictor responses to bradykinin and norepinephrine, *Prostaglandins*, 9(3):385-390, 1975.

97. Bedard, M.P., Kotagal, U.R., Kleinman, L.I. Acute cardiovascular effects of indomethacin in anesthetized newborn dogs, *Dev Pharmacol Ther*, 6:179-186, 1983.

98. Nyhan, D.P., Chen, B.B., Fehr, D.M., Goll, H.M., Murray, P.A. Pentobarbital augments pulmonary vasoconstrictor response to cyclooxygenase inhibition, *Am J Physiol*, 257(4 pt 2):H1140-H1146, 1989.

99. Blaise, G., Iqbal, A., Vanhoutte, P.M. Inhibitors of cyclooxygenase augment serotonergic responsiveness in canine coronary arteries, *Am J Physiol*, 255(5 pt 2):H1032-H1035, 1988.

100. Lipton, H.L., Chapnick, B.M., Hyman, A.L., Glass, F.L., Kadowitz, P.J. the influence of indomethacin on vasodilator responses to bradykinin and nitroglycerin in the cat, *Peptides*, 2(2):165-169, 1981.

101. Posner, P., Peterson, C.V. Cardiac electrophysiologic effect of indomethacin, *Eur J Pharm*, 77(2-3):193-195, 1982.

102. Lipton, H.L., Armstead, W.M., Hyman, A.L., Kadowitz, P.J. Characterization of the vasoconstrictor activity of indomethacin in the mesenteric vascular bed of the cat, *Prostaglandins Leukot Med*, 27(1):81-91, 1987.

103. Manku, M.S., Horrobin, D.F. Indomethacin inhibits responses to all vasoconstrictors in the rat mesenteric vascular bed: restoration of responses by prostaglandin E_2, *Prostaglandins*, 12(3):369-376, 1976.

104. Kondo, K., Okuno, T., Suzuki, H., Handa, M., Saruta, T. Effects of captopril and prostaglandin I_2 on vasoconstrictor responses to norepinephrine and potassium ions in rat mesenteric artery, *Jpn Heart J*, 22(4):617-625, 1981.

105. Plotkine, M., El Bouchi, N., Allix, M., Capdeville, C., Bouchon, V., Boulu, R.G. Effect of indomethacin on the coupling of cerebral blood flow to brain metabolism, *J Pharmacol (Paris)*, 17(3):286-294, 1986.

106. Sakanashi, M., Takeo, S., Nakasone, J., Nagamine, F., Miyamoto, Y., Kato, T. An analysis of the depressant effect of indomethacin on contractions of isolated and perfused rat hearts, *Jpn J Pharmacol*, 43(4):465-468, 1987.

107. Brodowicz, G.R., Lamb, D.R. Exercise training, indomethacin, and isoproterenol-induced myocardial necrosis in the rat, *Basic Res Cardio*, 86(1):40-48, 1991.

108. Gardiner, S.M., Compton, A.M., Bennett, T. Effects of indomethacin on the regional haemodynamic responses to low doses of endothelins and sarafotoxin, *Br J Pharmacol*, 100(1):158-162, 1990.

109. Baur, T.S., Brodowicz, G.R., Lamb, D.R. Indomethacin suppresses the coronary flow response to hypoxia in exercise trained and sedentary rats, *Cardiovasc Res*, 24(9):733-736, 1990.

110. Hadhazy, P., Nador, T. Effects of indomethacin and PGE_1 on the vasoconstrictor responses of the rabbit ear artery to nerve stimulation, *Prostaglandins*, 11(2):241-250, 1976.

111. Bill, A. Effects of indomethacin on regional blood flow in conscious rabbits-a microsphere study, *Acta Physiol Scand*, 105:437-442, 1979.

112. Rowe, B.P. The influence of indomethacin on blood pressure during the infusion of vasopressors, *Hypertension*, 8(9):772-778, 1986.

113. Cornish, E.J., Goldie, R.G., Krstew, E.V., Miller, R.C. Effect of indomethacin on responses of sheep isolated coronary artery to arachidonic acid, *Clin Exp Pharm Phys*, 10(2):171-175, 1983.

114. Yabek, S.M., Avner, B.P. Effects of prostacyclin (PGI_2) and indomethacin on neonatal lamb mesenteric and renal artery responses to electrical stimulation and norepinephrine, *Prostaglandins*, 19(1):23-29, 1980.

115. Newton, S.G., McClure, D.E., Selna, L.A., Weidner, W.J. The effect of indomethacin on plasma and lung lymph angiotensin converting enzyme activity in sheep, *Prostaglandins Leukot Med*, 26(3):179-188, 1987.

116. Paulick, R.P., Meyers, R.L., Rudolph, C.D., Rudolph, A.M. Venous and hepatic vascular responses to indomethacin and prostaglandin E1 in the fetal lamb, *Am J Obstet Gynecol*, 163(4 Pt 1):1357-1363, 1990.

117. Lundell, B.P.W., Sonesson, S-E., Sundell, H. Cerebral blood flow following indomethacin administration, *Dev Pharmacol Ther*, 13:139-144, 1989.

118. Burvenich, C., Peeters, G. Effects of prostaglandin synthetase inhibitors on mammary blood flow during experimentally induced mastitis in lactating goats, *Arch Int de Pharm et de Thera*, 258(1):128-137, 1982.

119. Boyd, L.M., Ezra, D., Feuerstein, G., Goldstein, R.E. Effects of FPL-55712 or indomethacin on leukotriene-induced coronary constriction in the intact pig heart, *Eur J Pharm*, 89(3-4):307-311, 1983.

120. Mirro, R., Leffler, C.W., Armstead, W., Beasley, D.G., Busija, D.W. Indomethacin restricts cerebral blood flow during pressure ventilation of newborn pigs, *Pediatr Res*, 24(1):59-62, 1988.

121. Leffler, C.W., Busija, D.W., Fletcher, A.M., Beasley, D.G., Hessler, J.R., Green R.S. Effects of indomethacin upon cerebral hemodynamics of newborn pigs, *Pediatr Res*, 19(11):1160-1164, 1985.

122. Leffler, C.W., Busija, D.W., Beasley, D.G. Effect of therapeutic dose of indomethacin on the cerebral circulation of newborn pigs, *Pediatr Res*, 21(2):188-192, 1987.

123. Leffler, C.W., Busija, D.W., Beasley, D.G., Fletcher A.M., Green R.S. Effects of indomethacin on cardiac output distribution in normal and asphyxiated piglets, *Prostaglandins*, 31(2):183-190, 1986.

124. Chemtob, S., Laudignon, N., Beharry, K., Rex, J., Varma, D., Wolfe, L,, Aranda, J.V. Effects of prostaglandins and indomethacin on cerebral blood flow and cerebral oxygen consumption of conscious newborn piglets, *Dev Pharmacol Ther*, 14:1-14, 1990.

125. Schror, K., Krebs, R., Nookhwun, C. Increase in the coronary vascular resistance by indomethacin in the isolated guinea pig heart preparation in the absence of changes in mechanical performance and oxygen consumption, *Eur J Pharmacol*, 39:161-169, 1976.

126. D'Souza, S.J., Biggs, D.F. Tartrazine and indomethacin increase firing rates in the carotid sinus nerves of guinea pigs, *Proc West Pharmacol Soc*, 28:135-137, 1985.

127. Northover, A.M. The effects of indomethacin and verapamil on the shape changes of vascular endothelial cells resulting from exposure to various inflammatory agents, *Agents Actions*, 24(3-4):351-355, 1988.

128. Weiss, H.R., Winbury, M.M. Intracoronary nitroglycerin, pentaerythritol trinitrate and dipyridamole on intramyocardial oxygen tension, *Microvasc Res*, 4(3):273-284, 1972.

129. Rosenblum, W.I., El-Sabban, F. Effect of dipyridamole on platelet aggregation in cerebral microcirculation of the mouse, *Thromb Res*, 12(1):181-185, 1978.

130. Walker, B.R., Erickson, A.L., Arnold, P.E., Burke, T.J., Berl, T. Reduced osmotic and non-osmotic release of vasopressin after meclofenamate in the conscious dog, *Am J Physiol*, 250(6 Pt 2):R1028-RR1033, 1986.

131. Harrison, G.L., McMurtry, I.F., Moore, L.G. Meclofenamate potentiates vasoreactivity to alpha-adrenergic stimulation in chronically hypoxic guinea pigs, *Am J Physiol*, 251(3 Pt 2):H496-H501, 1986.

132. Stanton, B.J., Coupar, I.M., Burcher, E. The activity of non-steroidal anti-inflammatory drugs in the rat mesenteric vasculature, *J Pharm Pharmacol*, 38(9):674-678, 1986.
133. Meerdink, D.J., Okada, R.D., Leppo, J.A. The effect of dipyridamole on transmural blood flow gradients, *Chest*, 96(2):400-405, 1989.
134. Fujita, M., Mikuniya, A., McKown, D.P., McKown, M.D., Franklin, D. Effects of dipyridamole on collateral flow and regional myocardial function in conscious dogs with newly developed collaterals, *Basic Res Cardiol*, 85(2):142-152, 1990.
135. Li, Y.J., Zhang, G.L., Suzuki, H., Kuriyama, H. Actions of dipyridamole on endogenous and exogenous noradrenaline in the dog mesenteric vein, *Br J Pharmacol*, 102(1):51-56, 1991.
136. Chilian, W.M., Layne, S.M., Klausner, E.C., Eastham, C.L., Marcus, M.L. Redistribution of coronary microvascular resistance produced by dipyridamole, *Am J Physiol*, 256(2 Pt 2):H383-390, 1989.
137. Mall, G., Schikora, I., Mattfeldt, T., Bodle, R. Dipyridamole-induced neoformation of capillaries in the rat heart, *Lab Invest*, 57(1):86-93, 1987.
138. Puiroud, S., Pinard, E., Seylaz, J. Dynamic cerebral and systemic circulatory effects of adenosine, theophylline and dipyridamole, *Brain Res*, 453(1-2):287-298, 1988.
139. Boeynaems, J.M., Van Coevorden, A., Demolle, D. Dipyridamole and vascular prostacyclin production, *Biochem Pharmacol*, 35(17):2897-2902, 1986.
140. Bult, H., Fret, H.R., Jordaens, F.H., Herman, A.G. Dipyridamole potentiates the anti-aggregating and vasodilator activity of nitric oxide, *Eur J Pharmacol*, 199(1):1-8, 1991.
141. Laughlin, M.H., Klabunde, R.E., Delp, M.D., Armstrong, R.B. Effects of dipyridamole on muscle blood flow in exercising miniature swine, *Am J Physiol*, 257(5 Pt 2):H1507-H1515, 1989.
142. Raeder, E.A., Verrier, R.L., Lown, B. Effects of sulfinpyrazone on ventricular vulnerability in the normal and the ischemic heart, *Am J Cardiol*, 50(2):271-275, 1982.
143. Thomas, M., Gabe, I.T., Mills, C.J. Vasodilator effects of sulfinpyrazone in dogs, *J Cardiovasc Pharm*, 2(6):7710776, 1980.
144. Banditt, D.G., Grant, A.O., Hutchinson, A.B.S., Strauss, H.C. Electrophysiological effects of sulfinpyrazone on canine cardiac Purkinje fibers, *Can J Physiol Pharmacol*, 58:738-742, 1979.
145. Cairncross, K.D., Bassett, J.R., Martin, C. the effect of sulfinpyrazone on morphological changes in the coronary vasculature induced by prolonged unpredictable stress in the rat, *Pharm Biochem Behav*, 10(2):285-291, 1979.
146. Kristiansen, O., Refsum, H., Hotuedt, R. Electrophysiological and mechanical effects of sulphinpyrazone on isolated rat atria, *Clin Physiol*, 2:299-306, 1982.
147. Marissak, K. Effects of butorphanol, flunixin, levorphanol, morphine, pentazocine and xylazine in horses, *Dissertation Abstracts Int*, 43(3):646-647, 1982.
148. Chay, S., Woods, W.E., Nugent, T., Blake, J.W., Tobin, T. The pharmacology of nonsteroidal anti-inflammatory drugs in the horse: flunixin meglumine (Banamine), *Equine Prac*, 4(10):16-23, 1982.
149. Bottoms, G.D., Fessler, J.F., Roesel, O.F., Moore, A.B. Endotoxin-induced hemodynamic changes in ponies: effects of flunixin meglumine, *Am J Vet Res*, 42(9):1514-1518, 1981.
150. Wong, S., Gardocki, J.F., Pruss, T.P. Pharmacologic evaluation of tolectin (tolmetin, MCN-2559) and MCN-2891, two anti-inflammatory agents, *J Pharm Exp Ther*, 185(1):127-138, 1973.
151. Apstein, C.S., Vogel, W.M. Coronary arterial vasodilator effect of ibuprofen, *J Pharm Exp Ther*, 220(1):167-171, 1982.
152. Adams, H.R. Acute adverse effects of antibiotics, *J Am Vet Med Assoc*, 166:983-984, 1975.
153. Adams, H.R. Antibiotic-induced alterations of cardiovascular reactivity, *Fed Proc*, 35(5):1148-1150, 1976.
154. Cohen, L.S., Wechsler, A.S., Mitchell, J.H., Gick, G. Depression of cardiac function by streptomycin and other antimicrobial agents, *Am J Cardiol*, 26:505-511, 1970.
155. Gross, D.R., Dodd, K.T., Williams, J.D., Adams, H.R. Adverse cardiovascular effects of oxytetracycline preparations and vehicles in intact, awake calves, *Am J Vet Res*, 42(8):1371-1377, 1981.
156. Adams, H.R. Cardiovascular depressant effects of the neomycin-streptomycin group of antibiotics, *Am J Vet Res*, 36:103-108, 1975.
157. Adams, H.R., Goodman, F.R. Differential inhibitory effects of neomycin on contractile responses of various canine arteries, *J Pharm Exp Ther*, 193:393-402, 1975.
158. Goodman, F.R., Weiss, G.B., Adams, H.R. Alterations by neomycin of ^{45}Ca movements and contractile responses in vascular smooth muscle, *J Pharm Exp Ther*, 188:472-480, 1974.

159. Adams, H.R. Cardiovascular depressant effects of neomycin and gentamicin in rhesus monkeys, *Br J Pharm*, 54:453-462, 1975.

160. Swain, H.H., Kiplinger, G.F., Brady, T.M. Actions of certain antibiotics on the isolated dog heart, *J Pharm Exp Ther*, 117:151-159, 1956.

161. Hashimoto, H., Yanagisawa, T., Taira, N. Differential antagonism of the negative inotropic effect of gentamicin by calcium ions, Bay K 8644 and isoprenaline in canine ventricular muscle: comparison with cobalt ions, *Br J Pharmacol*, 96(4):906-912, 1989.

162. Gotanda, K., Yanagisawa, T., Satoh, K., Taira, N. Are the cardiovascular effects of gentamicin similar to those of calcium antagonists?, *Jpn J Pharmacol*, 47(3):217-227, 1988.

163. Adams, H.R. Direct myocardial depressant effects of gentamicin, *Eur J Pharm*, 30:272-279, 1975.

164. De la Chapelle-Groz, B., Athias, P. Gentamicin causes the fast depression of action potential and contraction in cultured cardiocytes, *Eur J Pharmacol*, 152(1-2):111-120, 1988.

165. Lullman, H., Schwarz, B. Effects of aminoglycoside antibiotics on bound calcium and contraction in guinea-pig atria, *Br J Pharmacol*, 86(4):799-803, 1985.

166. Hubbell, J.A.W., Muir, W.W., Robertson, J.T., Sams, R.A. Cardiovascular effects of intravenous sodium penicillin, sodium cefazolin and sodium citrate in awake and anesthetized horses, *Vet Surg*, 16(3):245-250, 1987.

167. Daubeck, J.L., Daughety, M.J., Petty, C. Lincomycin-induced cardiac arrest: a case report and experimental investigation, *Anesth Analg*, 53:5630567, 1974.

168. Nattel, S., Ranger, S., Talajic, M., Lemery, R., Roy, D. Erythromycin-induced long QT syndrome: concordance with quinidine and underlying cellular electrophysiologic mechanism, *Am J Med*, 89(2):235-238, 1990.

169. Teske, R.H., Carter, G.G. Effect of chloramphenicol on pentobarbital-induced anesthesia in dogs, *J AVMA*, 159:777-780, 1971.

170. Adams, H.R., Dixit, B.N. Prolongation of pentobarbital anesthesia by chloramphenicol in dogs and cats, *J AVMA*, 156:902-905, 1970.

171. Gross, D.R., Kitzman, J.V., Adams, H.R. Cardiovascular effects of intravenous administration of propylene glycol and of oxytetracycline in propylene glycol in calves, *Am J Vet Res*, 40(6):783-791, 1979.

172. Sangiah, S., Burrows, G.E. Hypotension produced by rapid intravenous administration of chloramphenicol in anaesthetized dogs, *Res Vet Sci*, 46:62-67, 1989.

173. Rion, J.L., Duckett, W.M., Riviere, J.E., Jernigan, A.D. Spurlock SL; Concerned about intravenous use od doxycycline in horses, *J AVMA*, 195(7):846-848, 1989.

174. Blood, B.E. The action of salicylate on sheep cardiac Purkinje fibre contractility, *J Physiol (Lond)*, 269(1):85P-86P, 1977.

175. Fessler, J.F., Bottoms, G.D., Roesel, O.F., Moore, A.B. Frauenfelder HC, Boon GD; Endotoxin-induced change in hemograms, plasma enzymes and blood chemical values in anesthetized ponies: effects of flunixin meglumine, *Am J Vet Res*, 43(1):140-144, 1982.

176. Colbert, W.E., Turk, J.A., Williams, P.D., Buening, M.K. Cardiovascular and autonomic pharmacology of the macrolide antibiotic LY281389 in anesthetized beagles and in isolated smooth and cardiac muscles, *Antimicrob Agents Chemother*, 35(7):1365-1369, 1991.

177. Murray, B.M., Paller, M.S., Ferris, T.F. Effect of cyclosporine administration on renal hemodynamics in conscious rats, *Kidney Int*, 28(5):767-774, 1985.

178. Nicholson, A., Ilkiw, J.E. Neuromuscular and cardiovascular effects of atracurium in isoflurane-anesthetized chickens, *Am J Vet Res*, 53:2337-2342, 1992

5.   General anesthesia

In 1978 Pratila and Pratilas published an extensive review of the effects of anesthetic agents on the electromechanical activity of the heart.[20] They reviewed data obtained from microelectrode studies of single cardiac cells, isolated hearts and intact animals. Pentobarbital, injected into the sinus node artery produces a dose-dependent negative chronotropy, SA nodal block and AV nodal rhythms, at high doses. Barbiturates, in general, prolong AV junctional conduction times, reset baroreceptor control with higher heart rates for a given blood pressure. All of these effects are produced by a type of vagolytic activity.

Although many investigators have shown increases in heart rate following ketamine injection in intact animals these effects are not seen in isolated heart experiments.[20] Ketamine-induced tachycardia can be blocked by synaptic blockade (hexamethonium) or by combined vagal and α-adrenergic blockade. There seems to be strong evidence of central sympathetic stimulation and parasympathetic inhibition by ketamine. Ketamine also increases tolerance to digitalis.[20]

Halothane has been shown to have dose-dependent effects on SA nodal fibers resulting from a reduction in the rate of slow diastolic depolarization and an increase in threshold potential.[20] There is also a concentration-dependent depression of AV nodal conduction, a depression of intraventricular conduction, a depression of ventricular automaticity, and a significant reduction in digitalis-induced cardiotoxicity. All of the above points to an antidysrhythmic action of halothane. There is also considerable experimental work which indicates halothane-catecholamine-induced dysrhythmia is a serious problem.[20]

Methoxyflurane also demonstrates dose-dependent depression of the AV conduction system, apparently independent of vagal control. There is a direct depression of SA nodal activity and, when circulating epinephrine levels are increased, the combination with methoxyflurane can result in severe dysrhythmias. There is also a decrease in the level of the threshold potentials and increased re-entry phenomena.[20]

Other halogenated inhalant anesthetics have been shown to have the same type of chronotropic and dysrhythmic potential. The differences seem to be related to sensitivity relative to the effective anesthetic dose required.

The intravenous administration of most anesthetics, in sufficient dosage to result in a surgical plane of anesthesia, is known to induce peripheral vasodilation and hypotension in mammals. There is increasing evidence that, especially in the microcirculation, these dosages can exert direct depressant and vasodilator effects on vascular smooth muscle. Anesthetic agents appear to be able to; 1) directly inhibit vascular smooth muscle vasomotion, and 2) nonspecifically depress the vascular smooth muscle contractile response to a variety of neurohumoral substances and certain ions. This depressant activity seems to be related to the movement and/or translocation of Ca^{2+} across the vascular membranes and intracellularly. There is some evidence that venous smooth muscle cells are more sensitive to these agents than are arterial smooth muscle cells.[1] Smaller (20 μm diameter) arterioles tend to be more profoundly affected than larger arterioles. Influences on the microvascular beds tend to be both dose-dependent and tissue-specific.[2]

Anesthetic agents also affect the formed elements of the blood and macrophages of the reticuloendothelial system. Many of these cells participate in phagocytosis, cell locomotion and diapedesis. Contractility in these cells is affected by Ca^{2+}-dependent depression of smooth muscle fiber. The production of bone marrow granulocytes has been shown to be depressed by anesthetic agents as has *in vitro* lymphocyte transformation. Erythrocyte cell membranes are made more resistant to rupture following exposure to many anesthetic agents.[3] Various anesthetic agents can affect other peripheral systems in a selective manner. These effects could be very relevant to the experimental design.[4]

All general anesthetic agents studied, thus far, cause myocardial depression at all concentrations that are clinically or experimentally useful. This result is apparently produced both by decreasing Ca^{2+} influx across the plasma membrane and by reducing the calcium ion concentrations in the sarcoplasmic reticulum.[5] We have been warned repeatedly about the pitfalls involved in accepting, without question, data collected from animals under various forms of anesthesia.[6-17] Despite these warnings, the current literature is replete with many examples of conclusions made on the effect of some perturbation, pharmacological, physiological or physical, on the cardiovascular system of an acute preparation in an anesthetized animal. These conclusions are usually based on an interpretation of results using the assumption that the general anesthesia and the surgical trauma involved do not exert a major effect on the cardiovascular parameter(s) being monitored or, at least, do not change the normal response to the perturbation. We do, however, know that complex interactions, particularly between drugs, frequently occur.

Anesthetic agents have a profound effect on cardiac control mechanisms. The Frank-Starling mechanism seems to play a small role in conscious, reclining dogs, since the left ventricle operates near the inflection of its diastolic pressure-dimension curve. A large increase in left ventricular end-diastolic pressure is associated with a negligible increase in left ventricular end-diastolic diameter. These responses are dramatically altered by anesthesia. The Anrep effect, obtained using afterload manipulation, also appears to be a phenomenon of general anesthesia. It is difficult to document and of minimal, if any, significance in the conscious animal. The treppe or Bowditch phenomenon (i.e. positive inotropy induced by increased frequency of contraction) has been well documented in isolated cardiac muscle and in anesthetized preparations but does not appear to be significant in conscious animals over the normal physiological range of heart rates.[18]

The mechanisms involved in the baroreceptor response to acute hypertension differs in the conscious and anesthetized state. In the conscious animal, with high basal parasympathetic tone, baroreceptor responses are predominantly mediated by increases in vagal tone. Several studies in anesthetized subjects indicate that the bradycardia resulted primarily from a withdrawal of sympathetic tone.[18]

Since autonomic reflexes are mediated by supramedullary areas of the central nervous system it is not surprising that general anesthetic agents modify reflex circulatory control mechanisms. This has been shown to be true in the coronary, renal, mesenteric and hindlimb circulatory systems.[18] There have been qualitative and quantitative differences noted in the response to digitalis glycosides, catecholamines, morphine and other pharmacologic agents between anesthetized and conscious animals.[18] These differences are probably due to the influence of the general anesthetics on the various control mechanisms as well as their direct depressant activity.

General anesthetics can be divided on the basis of their ability to sensitize the heart to the arrhythmogenic effects of the catecholamines, and to their ability to stimulate sympathetic nervous system activity. Some agents tend to abolish the baroreceptor reflexes, while stimulating the sympathetic system. Others reset the baroreceptors to favor a reduced level of arterial pressure, while reducing efferent sympathetic activity to the heart.[5]

Recently considerable work has been reported on the role of a variety of neuropeptide vasoactive substances on the normal control of the circulation.[21] Some of these agents are found in sensory afferent nerve fibers that supply the adventitial-media junction of muscular arteries in almost all circulatory beds that have been investigated thus far. Of particular interest are the sensory nerve terminals that store and release potent vasodilator neuropeptides including substance P, calcitonin gene-related peptide (CGRP) and neurokinin A.[22] Von Euler and Gaddum[23] isolated a peptide subsequently called substance P (SP) from extracts of brain and intestine and demonstrated its strong peripheral vasodilatory effects. This agent is now included in a long list of endogenously released substances (at least 38) that have been shown to cause endothelium-dependent vasodilation.[21] The half-life of SP, when injected intravenously in conscious dogs, is approximately 30 seconds,[24] so it is possible that it functions as a circulating hormone. SP has been shown to enter the bloodstream, at least from its intestinal site of origin.[25] It can, apparently, cross the lung without being inactivated[26] and is a potent vasodilator.[27] Immunohistochemical techniques have been used to demonstrate that SP is co-localized with calcitonin gene-related peptide (CGRP) in a distinct pattern of distribution particularly at sensory nerve terminals supplying the adventitial-medial border of most muscular arteries.[22,27]

Sensory nerve fibers which store and release CGRP, SP and neurokinin A innervate pial blood vessels ranging in size from approximately 60-160 μm in diameter in the cat.[28,29] Capsaicin, the pungent volatile oil responsible for the "hotness" of chili peppers, causes neuropeptide release from perivascular pial fibers, as well as from fibers from other muscular arteries, and sufficiently high dose treatment will deplete neuropeptide stores.[30] CGRP was isolated after two messenger RNA's were described in the rat and its existence was predicted.[31] The local release of CGRP and SP around blood vessels is thought to be a major component of the "Triple Response of Lewis" and of neurogenic inflammation.[32] More recently evidence has been presented which seems to suggest that the cerebral arteriolar vasodilator responses to nitroprusside and nitroglycerin are dependent upon the local release of CGRP.[33] This new information substantiates the contention that the neuropeptide vasodilators play an important physiological role in the control of local blood flow.

Since SP and CGRP are co-released at sensory afferent nerve terminals there is good reason to believe that these agents, working together on vascular endothelial and smooth muscle cells, play a major role in maintaining normal vascular tone and, perhaps more importantly, in response to a wide variety of noxious stimuli. Nicotine, at a high concentration has been shown to stimulate release of CGRP and, presumably SP, from cardiac nerves in isolated, perfused, guinea pig hearts.[40] Ischemia can also stimulate release of CGRP from cardiac nerves in the same preparation, suggesting that there is a potentially important physiological function of CGRP and SP in coronary vasodilation during ischemia.[40] Ischemia-induced release of these neuropeptides may be the neural component of the well-recognized anoxia-induced vasodilation of coronary blood vessels, which is thought to involve the release of adenosine and other local factors. These responses may be either depleted or their receptors down-regulated as a result of exposure to anesthetic agents.

If noxious exposure to noxious stimuli can trigger the release of SP, this may explain the transient hypotensive response observed following administration of nicotine in chloralose-anesthetized cats.[41] Vagal afferent nerves in the lung are known to contain both SP and CGRP and to release these neuropeptides after stimulation of nicotinic, cholinergic receptors.[41] This could come about because of inadequate release of neuropeptides, decreases in receptor affinity or numbers, reduced release or depletion of endothelial-dependent relaxant factor(s) [EDRF(s)] or endothelium-dependent hyperpolarizing factors [EDHF(s)], or changes in the guanylate cyclase, cyclic GMP, cyclic AMP, cyclic GMP-kinase and/or Ca^{2+} utilization mechanisms or any combination of these or other, as yet undefined, factors. There is evidence for defective release of CGRP from perivascular nerves in the spontaneously hypertensive rat (SHR) model of hypertension and in human patients with essential hypertension.[42]

The distribution pattern of Neuropeptide Y (NPY)-immunoreactive nerves in the arterial system is co-localized with the noradrenergic innervation.[34] Well-developed nerve fibers containing this neuropeptide are localized in the adventitia and along the adventitia-media border in the thoracic aorta, carotid, mesenteric and cerebral arteries and the Circle of Willis, with greater density in the muscular, smaller, arteries.[25] NPY is a potent vasoconstrictor both *in vivo* and *in vitro*.[35] The main physiological action of NPY in the circulation seems to be to potentiate the vasoconstrictor effects of other agents, particularly norepinephrine and histamine.[36] Low levels of sympathetic nerve stimulation results in release of norepinephrine and the resulting vasoconstriction can be blocked by α-adrenergic blocking agents. Higher levels of stimulation release both norepinephrine and NPY and the vasoconstriction is not blocked by α-blockers.[38-40]

There is considerable evidence that normal vascular tone is maintained via a basal level of constant stimulation of both vasodilator and vasoconstrictor mechanisms. This is easily shown by administration of a nitric oxide synthase inhibitor(s) or capsaicin in conscious animals and the resulting hypertension, i.e. withdrawal of vasodilator tone. Control of tissue blood flow, under normal circumstances, is thus regulated by increasing or decreasing any or all of the dilator or constrictor pathways in an almost infinite variety of combinations. This scenario provides for an extremely sensitive level of control with considerable reserve capability. If the sensory neuropeptides do play an important role in these mechanisms, and there is considerable evidence that they do, anesthetic agents which have any effect on sensory nerve responses must interfere with these mechanisms. Very recent work indicates that anesthetic agents (in the case of these studies, volatile anesthetics) modify the compensatory responses to hypoxemia that occur in awake animals (i.e. vasodilatory responses). The end result is decreased blood flow to the brain and heart.[43]

Since the first edition of this text an excellent 2 volume series edited by

Altura and Haleny has been published which deals with the cardiovascular actions of anesthetic agents. This multi-author text covers this subject with more detail than can be included in this chapter and interested readers are advised to refer to that source.[19]

The purpose of the next three chapters in this text is to tabulate some of what has been substantiated about the cardiovascular effects of the more commonly used anesthetic regimens and to cite the conditions under which these results were obtained.

References

1. Altura, B.M., Altura, B.T., Carella, A., Turlapty, D.D.M.V., Weinberg, J. Vascular smooth muscle and general anesthetics, *Fed Proc*, 39:1584-1592, 1980.
2. Longnecker, D.E., Harris, P.D. Microcirculatory actions of general anesthetics, *Fed Proc*, 39:1580-1583, 1980.
3. Bruce, D.L. Anesthesia formed elements of the blood and macrophages, *Fed Proc*, 39:1588-1594, 1980.
4. Roth, S.H. Membrane and cellular actions of anesthetic agents, *Fed Proc*, 39:1595-1599, 1980.
5. Price, H.L., Ohnishi, S.T. Effects of anesthetics on the heart, *Fed Proc*, 39:1575-1579, 1980.
6. Smith, H.W. The kidney: structure and function in health and disease, Oxford University Press, New York, 1951.
7. Manders, W.T., Vatner, S.F. Effects of sodium pentobarbital anesthesia on left ventricular function and distribution of cardiac output in dogs, with particular reference to the mechanism for tachycardia, *Circ Res*, 39:512-517, 1976.
8. Priano, L.L., Traber, D.L., Wilson, R.D. Barbiturate anesthesia: an abnormal physiologic situation, *J Pharmacol Exp Ther*, 165:126-135, 1969.
9. Vatner, S.F., Smith, N.T. Effects of halothane on left ventricular function and distribution of regional blood flow in dogs and primates, *Circ Res*, 34:155-167, 1974.
10. Forsyth, R.P., Hoffbrand, B.I. Redistribution of cardiac output after sodium pentobarbital anesthesia in the monkey, *Am J Physiol*, 218:214-217, 1970.
11. Westermark, L., Wahlin, A. Blood circulation in the kidney of the cat under halothane anesthesia, *Acta Anaesthesiol Scand*, 13:185-208, 1969.
12. Westermark, L. Blood circulation in the skeletal muscles and the skin of the cat under halothane anesthesia, *Acta Anaesthesiol Scand*, 13:209-227, 1969.
13. Vatner, S.F., Franklin, D., Braunwald, E. Effects of anesthesia and sleep on circulatory response to carotid sinus nerve stimulation, *Am J Physiol*, 200:1249-1255, 1971.
14. Vatner, S.F., Higgins, C.B., Franklin, D. *et al.* Extent of carotid sinus regulation of the myocardial contractile state in conscious dogs, *J Clin Invest*, 51:995-1008, 1972.
15. Higgins, C.B., Vatner, S.F., Franklin, D. *et al.* Extent of regulation of the heart's contractile state in the conscious dog by alteration in the frequency of contraction, *J Clin Invest*, 52:1187-1194, 1973.
16. Vatner, S.F., Higgins, C.B., Franklin, D. *et al.* Effects of a digitalis glycoside on coronary and systemic dynamics in conscious dogs, *Circ Res*, 28:470-479, 1971.
17. Vatner, S.F., Higgins, C.B., Patrick, T. *et al.* Effects of cardiac depression and of anesthesia on the myocardial action of a cardiac glycoside, *J Clin Invest*, 50:2585-2595, 1971.
18. Vatner, S.F. Effects of anesthesia on cardiovascular control mechanisms, *Environ Health Perspect*, 26:193-206, 1978.
19. Altura, B.M., Haleny, S. (editors); Cardiovascular actions of anesthetics and drugs used in anesthesia, Vol 1; Basic Aspects, Vol 2; Regional blood flow and clinical considerations, Multi-author text, Karger, ISBN# 3-8055-4159-7, 1986.
20. Pratila, M.G., Pratilas, V. Anesthetic agents and cardiac electromechanical activity, *Anesthesiology*, 49:338-360, 1978.
21. Fiscus, R.R. Molecular mechanisms of endothelium-mediated vasodilation, *Seminars in Thrombosis and Hemostasis - Suppl.*, Thieme Med Publish Inc, NY, 14:12-22, 1988.

22. Reinecke, M., Forssmann, W.G. Peptidergic innervation of the coronary vessels, Chp 4 in *Nonadrenergic Innervation of Blood Vessels*, Vol II: Region, eds. Burnstock G, Griffith SG, CRC Press, Boca Raton, 1988.

23. Von Euler, U.S., Gaddum, J.H. An unidentified depressor substance in certain tissue extracts, *J Physiol (London)*, 72:74-82, 1931.

24. Yeo, C.J., Jaffe, B.M., Zinner, M.J. The effects of intravenous Substance P infusion on hemodynamics and regional blood flow in conscious dogs, *Surgery*, 95:175-182, 1984.

25. Gamse, R., Mroz, E., Leeman, S., Lembeck, F. The intestine as a source of immunoreactive substance P in plasma of the cat, *Arch Pharmacol*, 305:17-22, 1978.

26. Lembeck, F., Holzer, P., Schweditsch, M., Gamse, R. Elimination of substance P from the circulation of the rat and its inhibition by bacitracin, *Arch Pharmacol*, 305:9-15, 1978.

27. Owman, C. role of neural substance P and coexisting calcitonin-gene related peptide (CGRP) in cardiovascular function, Chp 5 in *Nonadrenergic Innervation of Blood Vessels, Vol I: Putative Neurotransmitters*, eds. Burnstock G, Griffith SG, CRC Press, Inc., Boca Raton, 1988.

28. Mayberg, M.R., Zervas, N.T., Moskowitz, M.A. Trigeminal projections to supratentorial pial and dural blood vessels in cats demonstrated by horseradish peroxidase histochemistry, *J Comp Neurol*, 223:46-56, 1984.

29. Mayberg, M.R., Langer, J.R.S., Zervas, N.T., Moskowitz, M.A. Perivascular meningeal projections from cat trigeminal ganglia: Possible pathway for vascular headaches in man, *Science*, 213:228-230, 1981.

30. Moskowitz, M.A., Brody, M., Liu-Chen, L.-Y. *In vitro* release of immunoreactive substance P from putative afferent nerve endings in bovine pial arachnoid, *Neuroscience*, 9:809-814, 1983.

31. Rosenfeld, M.G., Mermod, J.J., Amara, S.G., Swanson, L.W., Sawchenko, P.E., Rivier, J., Vale, W.W., Evans, R.M. Production of a novel neuropeptide encoded by the calcitonin gene via tissue specific RNA processing, *Nature*, 304:129-135, 1983.

32. Barnes, P.J., Belvisi, M.G., Rogers, D.F. Modulation of neurogenic inflammation: Novel approaches to inflammatory disease, *TIPS*, 11:185-189, 1990.

33. Wei, E.P., Moskowitz, M.A., Boccalini, P., Kontos, H.A. Calcitonin gene-related peptide mediates nitroglycerin and sodium nitroprusside-induced vasodilation in feline cerebral arterioles, *Circ Res*, 70:1313-1319, 1992.

34. Polak, J.M., Bloom, S.R. Atrial natriuretic peptide (ANP), neuropeptide Y (NPY), and calcitonin gene-related peptide (CGRP) in the cardiovascular system of man and animals, Chp 7, *Nonadrenergic innervation of blood vessels*, Burnstock G, Griffith SG (eds), CRC Press, Boca Raton, 1988.

35. Lundberg, J.M., Tatemoto, K. Pancreatic polypeptide family (APP, BPP, NPY and PYY) in relation to sympathetic vasoconstriction resistance to adrenoceptor blockade, *Acta Physiol Scand*, 116:393-401, 1982.

36. Edvinsson, L., Emson, P., McCulloch, J., Tatemoto, K., Uddman, R. Neuropeptide Y: cerebrovascular innervation and vasomotor effects in the cat, *Neurosci Lett*, 43:79-84, 1983.

37. Edvinsson, L., Emson, P., McCulloch, J., Tatemoto, K., Uddman, R. Neuropeptide Y: immunocytochemical localization to and the effect upon feline pial arteries and vein *in vitro* and *in situ*, *Acta Physiol Scand*, 122:155-159, 1984.

38. Edvinsson, L. Functional role of perivascular peptides in the control of cerebral circulation, *TINS*, 8:126-131, 1985.

39. Dahlof, C., Dahlof, P., Lundberg, J. Neuropeptide Y (NPY): Enhancement of blood pressure increase upon adrenoceptor activation and direct pressor effects in pithed rats, *Eur J Pharmacol*, 109:289-295, 1985.

40. Franco-Cereceda, A., Saria, A., Lundberg, J.M. Ischaemia and changes in contractility induce release of calcitonin gene-related peptide but not neuropeptide Y from the isolated perfused guinea-pig heart, *Acta Physiol Scand*, 131:319-320, 1987.

41. Armitage, A.K., Hall, G.H. Mode of action of intravenous nicotine in causing a fall of blood pressure in the cat, *Eur J Pharmacol*, 7:23-30, 1969.

42. Xu, D., Wang, X., Wang, J.P., Yuan, Q.X., Fiscus, R.R., Chang, J.K., Tang, J. Calcitonin gene-related peptide (CGRP) in normotensive and spontaneously hypertensive rats, *Peptides*, 10:309-312, 1989.

43. Durieux, M.E., Sperry, R.J., Longnecker, D.E. Effects of hypoxemia on regional blood flows during anesthesia with halothane, enflurane, or isoflurane, *Anesthesiology*, 76:402-408, 1992.

6. Cardiovascular effects of intravenous anesthetic agents

The most commonly used anesthetic agents of this kind are the barbiturates. The duration of action of these agents is tied to their fat solubility. Since the thiobarbiturates are more fat soluble (classified as ultra-short acting), they provide a surgical plane of anesthesia for less time than the short acting agents such as pentobarbital sodium. Most of these drugs are, however, metabolized at about the same rate. If the ultra-short acting barbiturates are used and additional drug is given to achieve a longer duration of anesthesia, the pool of unmetabolized drug is expanded and the recovery period can be very prolonged.

As a class of drugs, the barbiturates interfere with Ca^{2+} transport in cardiac tissue and with uptake into the sarcoplasmic reticulum. They may also interfere with Ca^{2+}-mediated events in the excitation-contraction-coupling mechanism. They generally tend to result in an increase in preload, a decrease in the various indices of contractility, decreases in afterload and increases in heart rate.[1] There is an apparent decrease in plasma K^+. This may be due to an increase in extracellular fluid volume which would act to dilute the extracellular potassium.

Two agents, α-chloralose and urethane, have been promoted for use in cardiovascular studies because of their purported lack of cardiovascular effects. Some cardiovascular effects will be documented in this chapter for these agents. Perhaps more to the point, it is all but impossible to have animals recover full normal function following anesthesia with these drugs. Renal damage is particularly evident. With such severe sequelae, it is difficult to believe that physiological preparations can be maintained during this form of anesthesia.

Another important observation is that not all cardiovascular effects caused by the anesthetic agents are gone when the animal regains consciousness. Persistent sinus tachycardia following apparent recovery from the anesthetic has been reported following the use of pentobarbital, for example.[2]

There has been considerable controversy about the effects of intravenous anesthetic agents on the reflex control of arterial blood pressure. Vatner and Braunwald feel that pentobarbital has almost the same effect as sinoaortic denervation with regard to baroreflex responses.[64] This view is supported by Cox and Bagshaw[65] and another group of workers from Vatner's laboratory.[66] Workers associated with Sagawa, on the other hand, found that baroreceptor responses were not significantly impaired in rabbits[63,67,68] and others have reported no substantial impairment of overall blood pressure control in dogs.[69-72] For the researcher interested in blood pressure responses it seems obvious that it will be necessary to confirm that any anesthetic agents being used have either no response, or a well described response in the particular model being used.

Recently a new class of nonbarbiturate, intravenously administered anesthetic agents have become available. These include both steroid anesthetic agents and another novel agent called propofol. Some discussion of the cardiovascular effects of these agents will be included in this chapter.

Table 6.1: Cardiovascular effects of pentobarbital sodium

Conditions of the experiment	Dose	Cardiovascular Effects	Reference
6.1:1 Pentobarbital-Dogs			
Intact, awake, previously instrumented, effects of an abrupt, sustained increase in left ventricular pressure for periods of 7 and 65 seconds	30 mg/kg, IV	The Anrep effect could be observed in conscious dogs with slow heart rates but it was much more pronounced at faster rates and even more obvious after anesthesia	3,4
Intact, awake, previously instrumented, controlled ventilation with blood gas values held constant	30 mg/kg, IV	There was an initial, transient, peripheral vasodilation. Steady state effects were measured 15-30 min post-injection. There was a slight decrease in mesenteric flow and cardiac output. Mesenteric and systemic resistances increased but there were no changes in iliac and renal resistances. When the HR increased the end-systolic diameter increased, coronary arterial resistance decreased along with LV end-diastolic diameter, LV dP/dt/P and LV shortening velocity. With the HR held constant, the end-systolic diameter increased, shortening velocity and dP/dt/P decreased but LV end-diastolic diameter increased. There was no change in coronary artery resistance but a marked depression of the myocardium. The tachycardia which resulted was not only due to vagolytic effects, it seems to be mediated through baroreceptor reflexes.	5
Intact, awake, previously instrumented, Treppe or Bowditch effect tested	30 mg/kg, IV	Increases in contractility indices associated with increases in HR can be demonstrated in isolated cardiac muscle and in anesthetized preparations but this phenomenon appears to have little, if any, role in conscious dogs	4

Conditions	Dose	Cardiovascular effects	Reference
Intact, awake, previously instrumented	30 mg/kg, IV	In the conscious dog basal parasympathetic tone is relatively high. This aspect of autonomic control is more potent than it is in the pentobarbital anesthetized animal where parasympathetic tone decreases	4
Same as above with volume loading to test the Frank-Starling mechanism	Same	In the intact conscious dog increasing the preload increased the LV end-diastolic diameter slightly (i.e. no Frank-Starling effect). In the pentobarbital anesthetized, open chest dog, increases in preload resulted in significant decreases in LV end-diastolic diameter	4
Intact, awake, previously instrumented	Same	There were minor effects on cardiac output, mean aortic pressure and systemic vascular resistance but significant decreases in stroke volume and contractility	4
Same as above	22 mg/kg, IV	HR increased, systolic duration decreased by 25%, diastolic interval decreased, pronounced sinus tachycardia which often persisted for several days after recovery of consciousness. Systemic blood pressure decreased during induction but usually recovered rapidly and then stayed only slightly below control values. There was a decrease in peak LV dP/dt, no change in cardiac output, except for the early transient. Stroke volume decreased with increases in HR. There were also decreases in peak ejection velocity into the aorta, decreases in stroke work and LV peak power	2
Intact, awake, previously instrumented and tested for positive inotropic response to ouabain with and without anesthesia	30 mg/kg, IV	In conscious dogs with non-failing hearts, there were minor inotropic effects but much more striking inotropic responses after pentobarbital	6

Conditions	Dose	Cardiovascular effects	Reference
Previously instrumented, intact, awake, ventilation held constant, response to carotid chemoreceptor stimulation with intracarotid injection of nicotine	25 mg/kg, IV	Marked cardiac depression, intense decrease in HR, increase in initial cardiac cycle length and iliac vascular resistance in the awake state. After anesthesia these responses were depressed	7
Intact, vagotomized and trimethadinium pretreated. Compared response to saline infusion at 0.76 ml/min versus ouabain at equal volume and rate (36 µg/kg/hr)	44 mg/kg, IV	The functional refractory period of the A-V nodal system is less affected by pentobarbital than by halothane or methoxyflurane. Ouabain infusion produced a marked increase in the A-V functional refractory period. Did not interfere with the positive inotropic effect of ouabain	8
Previously instrumented with left atrial catheter, injection of radio-opaque media and cineangiography	27 mg/kg, IV	Depressed ejection fraction, segmental circumferential fiber shortening velocity and end-diastolic volume	9
Intact, awake, previously instrumented, evaluated effects of atropine and isoprenaline	25 mg/kg, IV	Increased HR, usually caused the "Wenckebach Point" (1 or 2 systole block at end expiration) to disappear. Reduced effects of atropine but did not modify effects of isoprenaline	10
Morphine sulfate (0.4 mg/kg, IM), acute, isolated and perfused carotid sinus preparation, instrumentation of thorax and abdomen, thorax then closed	25 mg/kg, IV	Mean arterial pressures and peripheral resistance depressed moderately, less depressed than with halothane and more than with α-chloralose. Carotid sinus reflexes significantly depressed	11
Right heart by-pass, 0.2% V/V, end-expiratory halothane, N_2O 70%, steady state control, left anterior descending coronary artery ligation	40 mg/kg, IV	ATP depleted 43.5%, decreased myocardial oxygen consumption, no change in blood pressure or HR	12

Conditions	Dose	Cardiovascular effects	Reference
Cardiopulmonary by-pass using the sagittal sinus outflow technique, anesthetized with thiopental (13-25 mg/kg, IV), gallamine (2-8 mg/kg), mechanical ventilation, maintained anesthesia with halothane (1-1.5% with 20-25% O_2), cardioplegia with 1 M KCl after aortic cross-clamping	40 mg/kg, IV	Cardiopulmonary by-pass circulation held constant at 100 ml/kg/min flow, mean aortic pressure held at 50-100 mmHg with occasional injection of 0.5-1 mg methoxamine or 1-2 mg chlor-promazine. Pentobarbital had no inhibitory effect on cerebral metabolism in the absence of synaptic activity	13
Anesthetized with pentobarbital (25 mg/kg, IV), positive pressure ventilation	1-2 mg/kg every 30 min, additional doses per 8 hours of anesthesia	No changes in monophasic action potential recordings, conduction velocity, refractoriness or peak LV dP/dt. Immediately after catheterization, during anesthesia, the HR decreased slightly, decreased conduction velocity and increased functional refractory period of the A-V node. After 15-30 min no further changes occurred.	14
Tested tolerance to ouabain sufficient to produce ventricular tachycardia and death. Positive pressure ventilation with 100% O_2, $PaCO_2$ maintained at 35 mmHg	35 mg/kg, IV + maintenance as needed	Increased the dose of ouabain required to cause both ventricular tachycardia and the LD_{50}. Was less protective than either Innovar or ketamine	15
Phencyclidine (2 mg/kg, IM), α-chloralose IV until first sign of pupillary constriction (60-80 mg/kg), bilateral cervical vagotomy, positive pressure ventilation	5 mg/kg, IV	Depressed cardiovascular responses to stimulation of the medulla, hypothalamus, and sciatic nerve, but not to stimulation of the stellate ganglia. Cardiovascular responses to hypothalamic stimulation were depressed more than those elicited by stimulation of the dorsal medullary reticular formation	16

Conditions	Dose	Cardiovascular effects	Reference
In situ, constant pressure perfusion of the sinus node artery at 10 mmHg. Dogs were anesthetized with pentobarbital (30 mg/kg, IV), positive pressure ventilation	30 µg to 10 mg infusions into the SA nodal artery	Doses greater than 100 µg decreased HR. Doses greater than 3 mg resulted in SA nodal block followed by A-V nodal rhythm. This direct depression of the SA nodal pacemaker activity could be partially antagonized by infusion of norepinephrine	17
Perfused hindlimb preparation using constant flow, heparin (3 mg/kg + 0.5 mg/kg/hr), aortic sinus nerve stimulation	30 mg/kg, IV	Stimulation of the carotid sinus nerve augmented the vasoconstrictor effects of the pressor reflex. Pentobarbital seems to enhance the aortic nerve pressor reflex	18
Intact, awake, previously instrumented	30 mg/kg, IV	In combination with 10 mg/kg hemorrhage there was a significant decrease in the renal autoregulatory limits. Not seen with hemorrhage or pentobarbital alone. The lower limit of renal autoregulation is significantly changed by even minor hemorrhage in the pentobarbital anesthetized dog	73
Anesthetized with pentobarbital (25 mg/kg, IV), volume ventilation, maintained for 8 hours with supplemental doses, closed chest, 15 ml saline + 15 ml 5.5% glucose/hr, IV	25 mg/kg + 1-2 mg/kg every 30 min as required	Immediately after catheterization there was a slight decrease in HR, decreased conduction velocity, increased functional refractory period of A-V node. 15-30 min post catheterization there was no change in cardiac electro-physiology for 8 hours. Decreased LV dP/dt towards end of 8 hours of anesthesia	74
Conscious, previously instrumented	30 mg/kg, IV	Prolonged PR and QT intervals, ventricular tachycardia inducible in 6 or 10 dogs with no change in cycle length or number of extra stimuli required	75
Evaluated vagal tone in intact, awake animals using time-series analysis of R-R intervals	25 mg/kg, IV	No consistent change in vagal tone using this analysis	76

Conditions	Dose	Cardiovascular effects	Reference
Previously instrumented, intact, awake vs 1 hr after pentobarbital, IV	Dosed IV sufficient to achieve serum conc. approx. 25 mg/l	Measured ejection fraction and end-systolic pressure-volume relationships. No decrease in contractility with anesthesia	77
Right trabecular *in vitro* preparation	1 hr after exposure to same dose as above	Only a minimal decrease in isometric tension	77
Awake vs anesthetized, compared pulmonary pressure/flow relationships	30 mg/kg, IV	No effect on baseline pressure/flow relationship. α-adrenergic receptor block (prazosin) leads to vasodilation in awake, vasoconstriction in anesthetized. β-adrenergic receptor block (propranolol) causes constriction in awake and anesthetized states but the pentobarbital attenuated the response. Cholinergic receptor blockade (atropine) caused vasodilation in awake dogs, vasoconstriction in anesthetized state	78
Awake vs anesthetized, renal response to IV infusion of human atrial natriuretic peptide (25 ng/kg/min for 60 min, IV)	25 mg/kg, IV	Increased sodium excretion significantly after pentobarbital, response attenuated by renal denervation	79
Ketamine (10 mg/kg), exsanguinated, isolated helical strips of cerebral and mesenteric arteries	10^{-5} to 10^{-3} mol/L, dose-response	Dose-related vasodilation associated, in part, with inhibition of transmembrane influx of Ca^{2+}	80

Conditions	Dose	Cardiovascular effects	Reference
Compared to conscious controls, inhibition of cyclooxygenase pathway with indomethacin (5 mg/kg, IV), or meclofenamate (2.5 mg/kg, IV), measured pulmonary artery pressure/flow relationship	30 mg/kg, IV	Magnitude of the pulmonary vasoconstrictor response to indomethacin was increased over a broad range of flow. Pulmonary vasoconstrictor response to meclofenamate was increased over the entire range of flows tested. Pentobarbital alters regulation of baseline pulmonary vascular pressure/flow relationships by endogenous metabolites or cyclooxygenase pathway	**81**
Anesthetized with pentobarbital (25 mg/kg, IV), pancuronium (0.1 mg/kg + 1-2 mg/hr + approx. 1 mg/hr in control group	Treatment group received 4 mg/kg/hr after loading dose	After 30 min decreased mean aortic pressure, systemic oxygen consumption and oxygen extraction ratio, increased oxygen delivery	**82**
Intact, awake, previously instrumented	30 mg/kg, IV	No change in mean aortic pressure, mean pulmonary arterial pressure, pulmonary arterial wedge pressure, renal arterial pressure, pulmonary arterial flow, heart rate, arterial pH, or blood gases. Angiotensin II caused pulmonary arterial vasoconstriction both before and after pentobarbital. Vasodilation of ACE inhibitor was reduced after pentobarbital	**83**
6.1:2 Pentobarbital- Cats			
Isolated mesenteric vessels for direct microvascular observation	not given	Completely abolished mesenteric vessel vasomotion	**19**

Conditions	Dose	Cardiovascular effects	Reference
Induced with face mask with halothane, gallamine (1 mg/kg), positive pressure ventilation, maintained anesthesia with 69.2% N_2O, 0.8% halothane, occlusion og middle cerebral artery	50 mg/kg, slow IV infusion	Decreased local cortical blood flow and metabolism in the well perfused cortex so that oxygen availability remains constant while increasing local cortical blood flow in the poorly perfused areas, this tends to increase oxygen availability	20
Isolated atrial preparation	$1\text{-}5 \times 10^{-4}$ M in the bath	Dose-dependent weakening of the negative inotropic effects of vagal stimulation. Inhibition of acetylcholine evoked an overflow from the postganglionic parasympathetic neurones of the heart	21
Anesthetized with pentobarbital (35 mg/kg), exsanguinated, femoral arteries and arteries of the circle of Willis used in isolated vascular ring experiments	$10^{-4}\text{-}10^{-3}$ M	Antagonized the release of norepinephrine from the tissues, probably by interfering with Ca^{2+} entry into the adrenergic nerve endings	22
Isolated middle cerebral arteries, isometric contraction recordings	3×10^{-4} M	Maximum contractions to K^+, norepinephrine and $PGF_{2\alpha}$ were all reduced	23
Catheters in veins and the aorta, stimulation of the carotid sinus, aortic and vagus nerves	35-40 mg/kg, IP	Selective blockade of baroreceptor reflexes, possible γ-aminobutyric acid mimetic at the ventral vasomotor synapses	24
Isolated femoral artery preparation. 5-HT-induced dose-dependent contractions. Anesthetized with pentobarbital (35 mg/kg, IP), killed by bleeding	10^{-5} to 10^{-3} M	5-HT-induced contraction was essentially due to direct interaction with 5-HT receptors. Pentobarbital relaxed arteries previously contracted with 5-HT, probably by interfering with Ca^{2+} entry into the cells	84

Conditions	Dose	Cardiovascular effects	Reference
Acute instrumentation, anesthetized with pentobarbital (35 mg/kg, IP)	Dose response greater than 35 mg/kg, (i.e. added doses to initial dose required for instrumenta-tion	Diaphragmatic excitation-contraction coupling not affected. Contribution of the diaphragm to the breathing movements did not change with increased depth of anesthesia. Increased doses decreased the rate of rise of the integrated phrenic activity, decreased transdiaphragmatic pressure and lung volume, but no effect on the mechanical properties of the respiratory system. There was a decrease in ventilation not proportional to the drop in central inspiratory activity	**25**
Intact awake, previously instrumented	25-30 mg/kg, IV	Initial decrease then increase in renal sympathetic nerve activity, aortic pressure and heart rate	**85**
Isolated middle cerebral arteries	Dose-response 10^{-4} M 10^{-3} M	Concentration-dependent vasodilation Inhibited contractions induced by 10^{-5} M 5-HT or 75 mM K^+ Reduced concentration-dependent contractions induced by Ca^{2+}	**86**
6.1:3 Pentobarbital- Rats			
Evaluation of the duration of anesthesia	40 mg/kg, IP	Sleep time 130.4 ± 3.6 min	**26**
Previously instrumented, intact, awake, cannulae in aorta and peritoneal cavity, aortic samples of blood used	35 mg/kg, IP + 5 mg/kg/hr	Sustained a 2-3 fold increase in plasma renin concentrations with 10-15 mmHg decrease in mean aortic pressure. Levels of circulating epinephrine and norepinephrine were unchanged	**27**

Conditions	Dose	Cardiovascular effects	Reference
Langendorff type isolated heart preparation, anesthetized with pentobarbital to remove heart, compared to decapitation without anesthesia	5 mg/100 g body wt, prior to decapitation	Left ventricular mechanical performance and O_2 consumption not changed by pentobarbital, but caused a significant decrease in coronary resistance and increased spontaneous heart rates. During pacing from 240-480/min there was no change in mechanical performance. Pentobarbital treated hearts were completely insensitive to X 3 increases of Ca^{2+} in the perfusate	28
Aortic strips and portal veins, isolated vascular strip preparations	1×10^{-4} M	In portal vein prep, decreased total Ca^{2+} exchange and also decreased intracellular $[Ca^{2+}]$	29
	$5\text{-}20 \times 10^{-4}$ M	Decreased Ca^{2+} exchange (portal vein prep)	
	5×10^{-4} M	Decreased intracellular $[Ca^{2+}]$ (aortic strip prep)	
	2×10^{-3} M	Decreased intracellular $[Ca^{2+}]$ (aortic strip prep)	
Evaluation of the effects of hemorrhage, against a predetermined pressure, on relative O_2 tension in the kidney. Ether anesthesia, placement of O_2 electrode in the kidney 24 hr prior to the experiment, also aortic catheter	50 mg/kg, IP	Two conditions evaluated; bleeding and held 30 min at 40 mmHg and 60 min at 50 mmHg. Pentobarbital reduced the fall in relative O_2 tension, protected against kidney lesions	30
Previously instrumented with an aortic cannula	6.2 - 50 mg/kg, IP	Marked protection against mortality and kidney lesions following bleeding to 30-50 mmHg for 60 min	31
Previously instrumented with aortic cannulae, decapitation at various intervals for plasma renin activity assays	35 mg/kg, IP	Slight increase in plasma renin activity, not as marked as that seen with ether or urethane, marked initial drop in aortic pressure followed by a gradual return to baseline	32

Conditions	Dose	Cardiovascular effects	Reference
Anesthetized with halothane in O_2, cannulae in femoral artery, vein and trachea, tubocurarine (1.5 mg/kg, IV), ventilated with 30 % O_2, measured movement of phenylalanine	50 mg/kg, IV	Decreased phenylalanine influx to brain little, if any, effect on neutral amino acid transport process	33
Decerebrated at mid-collicular level under halothane anesthesia at least 90 min prior to study	12.5 mg/kg, IV	Decreased HR, blood pressure and respiratory rate, decreased occlusion, tilt and sodium cyanide chemoreceptor responses	34
Previously instrumented, intact, awake	35 mg/kg, IP + 5 mg/kg/hr	Sustained 2-3 fold increase in plasma renin concentrations with 10-15 mmHg decrease in mean aortic pressure, circulating epinephrine and norepinephrine levels unchanged	27
Isolated, perfused heart (Langendorff) prep	5 mg/100 g body wt, prior to decapitation	LV mechanical performance and oxygen consumption no changed by pentobarbital, but caused significant decrease in coronary resistance and increased spontaneous HR. During pacing from 240-480 b/min there was no change in mechanical performance. Pentobarbital treated hearts were completely insensitive to a 3-fold increase of Ca^{2+} in the perfusate	28
Previously instrumented with aortic cannula	6.2-50 mg/kg, IP, Dose-response	Marked protection against mortality and kidney lesions following bleeding to 30-50 mmHg for 60 min	35
Previously cannulated aorta for blood pressure, decapitation at various intervals for plasma renin activity	35 mg/kg, IV	Slight increase in plasma renin activity, not as marked as with ether or urethane. Marked initial drop in blood pressure followed by a gradual return to baseline	32

Conditions	Dose	Cardiovascular Effects	Ref
Compared to intact, awake, previously instrumented group	50 mg/kg, IP + 500 µg/kg/min, IV	Cardiac output and regional blood flows reduced, lactate/pyruvate ratio increased	87
Pressor response to nitric oxide synthase inhibitor, L-NNA	65 mg/kg, IP + 0.06-0.12 mg/kg/min, IV	Pressor response the same as in conscious rats	88
Cremaster muscle preparation, Serotonin response curves	To effect, general anesthesia	Small arterioles maintain a large dilator capacity. Good dilator response to serotonin with constriction of large arterioles	89
Urethane anesthesia (1.1-1.3 g/kg, IP), pentobarbital applied directly to the ventral medullary surface of the brain	16 or 32 mg/ml (1-4 µl), directly applied using small pieces of gelfoam	Decreased baseline mean aortic pressure and ventilation, attenuated the baro-pressure reflex but not the baro-ventilatory reflex	90
Previously instrumented compared to conscious	8 mg/kg/hr, IV	Decreased respiratory rate, increased mean aortic pressure, no change in heart rate, decreased cardiac output	91
Compared isolated hearts (Langendorff) from pentobarbital anesthetized vs decapitated	60 mg/kg, IP	At lower Ca^{2+} concentrations of 0.5 and 1.0 mM inotropic activity was greater in hearts from anesthetized than from the non-anesthetized rats. At higher $[Ca^{2+}]$ heart from non-anesthetized rats showed greater inotropic responses. No differences in HR between groups. The effects of T_3 (thyroid) was much greater in the unanesthetized hearts	92

Conditions	Dose	Cardiovascular Effects	Ref
Capsaicin-denervated vs controls	50 mg/kg, IP	Both groups showed the same aortic pressure prior to anesthesia. After pentobarbital the mean aortic pressure decreased to 6 min. In controls there was a slow compensatory increase in BP to higher than baseline, maintained for 1 hr. No compensation in capsaicin-denervated animals. Capsaicin-denervated rats seem to have increased dependence on angiotensin II-mediated blood pressure regulation. Blood pressure regulation during pentobarbital anesthesia seems to depend on signals conveyed to the CNS via capsaicin-sensitive afferent neurons which activate efferent adrenergic mechanisms	93
Comparison of responses in conscious rats vs pentobarbital anesthesia to L-NMMA (N^G-monomethyl-L-arginine; 0.1-10 mg/kg, IV)	65 mg/kg, IP	No change in blood pressure, increase in heart rate. Dose-response to L-NMMA increased blood pressure more in the anesthetized than in the conscious rats. Pressor response to phenylephrine not different between the two groups	94
Intact, awake, previously instrumented, cisterna magna cannulae and arterial cannulae	50 mg/kg, IV	Decreased norepinephrine concentrations in cisternal cerebrospinal fluid and plasma and decreased epinephrine concentrations in plasma. Data suggest both central and peripheral suppression of noradrenergic activity	95
Conscious vs pentobarbital anesthetized, previously instrumented	55 mg/kg, IP	Reflex bradycardia significantly decreased, parasympathetic blockade with methyl-atropine produced relatively less inhibition of baroreflex gain in the anesthetized group. Results suggest pentobarbital anesthesia lowers the baroreflex gain by inhibiting vagally mediated reflex bradycardia	96

Conditions	Dose	Cardiovascular Effects	Ref
Isolated intracerebral arterioles and venules (diameter 30-90 μM), pH 7.3	10^{-6} to 10^{-2} mol/L	No significant changes in diameter of venules but dilated arterioles in a dose-dependent manner at pH 7.3, maximum dilation of approx. 130% of control diameter at 10^{-3} mol/L	**97**
	10^{-3} mol/L	Significantly inhibited arteriolar constriction by KCl (120 m mol/L) but did not alter venular constriction	
IV bolus response to L-NNA (32 mg/kg)	65 mg/kg, IP + 0.06-0.12 mg/kg/min continuous IV infusion	Increased mean aortic pressure; anesthetized increased 61 ± 10 mmHg, conscious increased 51.3 mmHg	**88**
Measured local cerebral blood flow 5, 10, 25 & 60 min after pentobarbital	50 mg/kg, IP	More strongly decreased local cerebral blood flow (LCBF) in the forebrain than in the hindbrain and produces different patterns of changes in LCBF than in local cerebral glucose utilization	**98**
Measured cerebral plasma volume	50 mg/kg, IV over 8 min	Cerebral plasma volume = 2.1 ± 0.26 ml/100 g brain tissue. Significantly less than CPV with halothane or isoflurane.	**99**
Coronary artery ligation	60 mg/kg, IP	High incidence to V-tach and fibrillation	**100**
Compared urethane (1.6 g/kg) to pentobarbital (30 mg/kg) anesthetized animals with measurement of renal vascular resistance. Comparisons were made following area postrema stimulation	1.6 g/kg and 30 mg/kg	Pentobarbital decreased renal flow and increased renal resistance, response blocked by ganglionic blockade	**101**

6.1:4 Pentobarbital-Rabbits, Conditions of the experiment	Dose	Cardiovascular Effects	Reference
Isolated left atrial preparation, electrically stimulated, measured contractile force and effective refractory period	0.1 to >200 µg/ml added to bath	Dose-dependent decrease in contractile force and increase in effective refractory period	36
Intact, awake, femoral artery and vein cannulation with local anesthesia and physical restraint	10 mg/kg, IV, 3 cumulative doses at 15 min intervals	Each dose produced transient decreases in blood pressure, not modified by prior muscarinic receptor blockade, β-receptor blockade or combined blockade. Pentobarbital produced total loss of resting vagal tone without impairment of reflex vagal activation	37
Isolated lung preparation	Dose-response	Partially blocked lipid peroxide tertiary butyl hydroperoxide-induced pulmonary vasoconstriction, possibly by inhibiting calcium entry	102
Previously instrumented, intact, awake	40 mg/kg, IV	Decreased aortic pressure, hypercapnia and respiratory acidosis	103
6.1:5 Pentobarbital- Pigs			
Surgical preparation enabling stepwise decrease in hepatic blood flow without hepatic hypoperfusion	30 mg/kg, IV + 1-2 mg/kg/hr	Decreased hepatic oxygen delivery and decreased hepatic lactate uptake at lowered hepatic blood flows	104
Preanesthesia with ketamine (20 mg/kg), Xylazine (2 mg/kg), skin, myocutaneous and fasciocutaneous flaps, blood flow measured with microspheres	30 mg/kg, IV + additional doses as required	No change in aortic blood pressure or HR, decreased cardiac output, stroke volume, LV work, systemic resistance increased compared to awake animals, increased blood flow in all viable portions of arterial and random skin flaps	105

6.1:6 Pentobarbital- Sheep, Conditions of the experiment	Dose	Cardiovascular Effects	Reference
Intact, awake, previously instrumented lambs	4.0 mg/kg, IV	No change in cardiac output, mean aortic blood pressure, heart rate, cerebral blood flow, oxygen transport or consumption, kidney blood flow or GI blood flow	**106**
6.1:7 Pentobarbital- Cattle			
Cultured adrenal chromaffin cells in presence of ouabain	Dose-response	Potentiated effects of GABA on catecholamine release and phosphoinositide metabolism	**107**
6.1:8 Pentobarbital- Gerbils			

Carotid ligation, bilateral, combined pentobarbital, ether or sham injection (50 mg/kg, IP pentobarbital)	Additional 30 mg/kg 4 hr after ligation	Brain edema as evaluated by swelling percentage:
		    ether 6.374 ± 0.89
		(SEM)
		    sham 0.491 ± 0.15
		    pentobarbital 3.359 ± 0.68
		Neurologic deficit decreased by 56-79% in pentobarbital versus ether anesthesia. Mortality at 8 hr decreased by 75% in pentobarbital versus ether anesthesia
			38

6.1:9 Pentobarbital- Chickens			
Isolated heart preparation (Langendorff)	1×10^{-7} to 1×10^{-2} M in perfusate	Dose-dependent decrease in evoked overflow of acetylcholine	**21**
Isolated atria	$1\text{-}5 \times 10^{-4}$ M	Weakened negative inotropic effects of vagal stimulation, probably due to a reduction of the Ca^{2+} inward current into the nerve terminals	**21**

6.1:10 Pentobarbital-Primates, Conditions of the experiment	Dose	Cardiovascular Effects	Reference
Baboons anesthetized with α-chloralose (60 mg/kg, IV), immobilized with gallamine (repeated doses), positive pressure ventilation with 100% oxygen, measured brain blood flow	Dose not given	If flow after occlusion of the middle cerebral artery was greater than 25 ml/100 g/min the pentobarbital decreased the flow further	**39**
Previously instrumented, intact, awake	30 mg/kg, IV	Decreased aortic pressure, systemic resistance, cardiac output, LV end-diastolic pressure and arterial pH. Increased percentage of cardiac output delivered to the kidneys, skin, bronchial circulation and bone, decreased % of cardiac output to brain, skeletal muscle, adrenals and chest wall	**40**

Table 6.2: Cardiovascular effects of thiopental sodium and sodium pentothal

Conditions of the experiment	Dose	Cardiovascular Effects	Reference
6.2:1 Thiopental-Dogs			
Intact, awake, previously instrumented	20 mg/kg, IV	Initial increase then a decrease in aortic pressure; renal blood flow was preserved	**41**
Intact, awake, previously instrumented	24 mg/kg, IV	Immediate and persistent increase in HR, decrease in aortic pressure, decrease in systemic vascular resistance, decrease in LV dP/dt max and decrease in stroke volume. At 5 min post-induction the aortic pressure and systemic resistance decreased less than after minaxolone. There was a rebound in aortic pressure, systemic resistance and LV dP/dt max 1-2 min after induction	**42**

Conditions	Dose	Cardiovascular effects	Reference
Intact, awake, previously instrumented, measurements taken 30, 60 and 90 min following injection	15-25 mg/kg, IV, to effect (surgical plane of anesthesia)	At 30-60 min there was a decrease in cardiac output, decreased LV work and decreased blood flow to lungs, kidney and liver. At 60-90 min, no change in the measured parameters except for a decrease in coeliac artery and total liver blood flow	43
Anesthetized with halothane (1.09% end-tidal) or the same preceded by thiopental, positive pressure ventilation	20 mg/kg, IV	Potentiates ventricular, but not supraventricular sensitization to epinephrine during halothane anesthesia	44
Anesthetized with α-chloralose (50 mg/kg) and urethane (500 mg/kg), 70% nitrous oxide and 30% oxygen, morphine sulfate (1 mg/kg, as needed), pancuronium bromide (0.1 mg/kg/dose), positive pressure ventilation	Sufficient thiopental to produce 30 sec burst suppression of EEG	Resulted in a significant decrease in spinal cord blood flow in both the cervical and thoracic segments	45
Anesthetized with ketamine (10 mg/kg, IV), gallamine (5-8 mg/kg, IV, repeated every 30 min), Halothane (1-1.5%) in 50% nitrous oxide/oxygen, cardiopulmonary bypass, off halothane, ketamine (2 mg/kg, IV, every 30 min), produced complete global ischemia by stopping the pump	40 mg/kg, IV	No effect on potassium efflux during ischemia	46

Conditions	Dose	Cardiovascular effects	Reference
Anesthetized with α-chloralose (50 mg/kg, IV), urethane (500 mg/kg, IV), nitrous oxide (70%), morphine (2.5-5 mg/kg) and pancuronium (0.1-0.3 mg/kg), hyperventilation	High doses sufficient to produce 30-60 sec burst suppression of EEG	After thiopental no significant difference in cerebral blood flow or cerebral vascular resistance with $PaCO_2$ held between 30-40 mmHg. when $PaCO_2$ increased to >40 mmHg, cerebral blood flow increased and cerebral vascular resistance decreased	47
Anesthetized with α-chloralose (50 mg/kg), urethane (500 mg/kg), IV, maintained with 70%/30% nitrous oxide:oxygen + morphine (1 mg/kg/dose) + pancuronium bromide (0.1 mg/kg/dose)	Dose-response according to duration of EEG burst suppression	Beyond 30 sec of burst suppression doe-dependent decrease in mean aortic pressure and cardiac index, increased HR, decreased hematocrit, $PaCO_2$, PaO_2 and pH unchanged, decreased spinal cord blood flow	45
Halothane anesthetized at 1 MAC + 50% nitrous oxide:oxygen, succinylcholine (2 mg/kg, IV) immediately following induction dose of thiopentone	25-30 mg/kg, IV	More sensitive than midazolam, induced dogs to arrhythmogenic effects of epinephrine-aminophylline dose-response	108
Intact, awake, previously instrumented	19.4 mg/kg, IV	At 15 & 30 sec post-injection: decreased stroke volume; HR, left atrial pressure & mean pulmonary arterial pressure increased; cardiac index, contractility, systemic resistance and pulmonary resistance unchanged; mean aortic pressure was unchanged at 15 sec but increased at 30 sec to 2 min; by 7.5 min all values returned to baseline except HR, pO_2, pH decreased and pCO_2 increased	109
Ketamine (10 mg/kg), exsanguinated, isolated helical strips of cerebral & mesenteric arteries	10^{-5} to 10^{-3} mol/L, dose-response	In lower concentrations constriction; at higher concentrations profound relaxation; contractions greater in mesenteric than in cerebral arteries	80

Conditions	Dose	Cardiovascular effects	Reference
Evaluated vagal tone in intact animals using time-series analysis of R-R intervals	25 mg/kg, IV	Decreased vagal tone	76
6.2:2 Thiopental-Cats			
Intact, previously instrumented control vs thiopental treated 6,24,48 & 72 hrs after occlusion of the middle cerebral artery	10 mg/kg	Decreased aortic blood pressure and heart rate, PaO_2 increased, no change in $PaCO_2$, size and distribution of the infarct significantly decreased, SGOT and LDH activity in serum and cerebrospinal fluid of thiopental treated groups was decreased	48
Pretreated with combination of acepromazine (0.02 mg/kg), meperidine (4.0 mg/kg) & atropine (0.05 mg/kg) all IM	10 mg/kg thiopental with incremental doses until a surgical plane of anesthesia was achieved	Decreased cardiac output, cardiac index, stroke volume; no change in HR, aortic pressure or peripheral resistance	110
6.2:3 Thiopental-Rats			
Isolated atria and isolated portal vein preparations	Dose-response, 2.5-160 µg/ml perfusate	Depression of atrial rate, Ca^{2+} dependent and depression of amplitude of myogenic activity, also Ca^{2+} dependent	49
Langendorff isolated heart prep., standard perfusion with 95% oxygen, 5% CO_2, with glucose; hypoxic perfusion with 95% N_2, 5% CO_2 and mannitol (no glucose). Stabilized for 15 min, perfused for 40 min with hypoxic medium, then for 30 min with oxygen, thiopental added to the hypoxic medium	50 & 200 mg/L	50 mg/L decreased creatine kinase released during hypoxia and reoxygenation, 200 mg/L decreased creatine kinase even more during both hypoxia and reoxygenation	50

6.2:4 Thiopental-Rabbits	Dose	Cardiovascular effect	Reference
Isolated arterial perfused interventricular septum, heparinized and killed with a blow to the head or anesthetized with pentobarbital, electrically stimulated at 48-60 beats/min, thiopental added to perfusate	28 & 227 μmoles/L	Reduced developed tension by 50 & 80%, dose-dependent, effect was rapid, reversible and independent of heart rate; 227 μmoles/L inhibited K^+ influx and efflux, Ca^{2+} influx and efflux were also reduced but no displacement of Ca^{2+} from the myocardium; maximum rate of depolarization of the action potential and time to 50% repolarization decreased, resting membrane potential amplitude and time to 90% depolarization were unchanged. The negative inotropic effect was apparently due to reduced availability of Ca^{2+} to the myofibrils	51
Isolated lung preparation	Dose-response	Completely blocked lipid peroxide tertiary butyl hydroperoxide-induced pulmonary vasoconstriction, possibly by inhibition of Ca^{2+} entry	102
6.2:5 Thiopental-Pigs			
Anesthetized with Desflurane or Isoflurane, 1.2 MAC	2.5 & 5.0 mg/kg, IV	Decreased mean aortic pressure, cardiac output, stroke volume and peripheral resistance; no change in HR, left or right-sided cardiac filling pressures	111
6.2:6 Thiopental-Sheep			
70 min maintenance of anesthesia	750 mg, IV in 1 min + 25 mg/min for 30 min + 10 mg/min for 70 min	Doubled blood concentrations of cefoxitin over control, awake animals, renal extraction ratio decreased 50-60%	112
Intact, awake, previously instrumented; measurements made during the last 30 min of the anesthesia period	750 mg, IV bolus + 25 mg/min for 30 min + 10 mg/min for 70 min	Decreased total body oxygen consumption, increased HR and mean aortic pressure, cardiac output decreased, no change in hepatic blood flow, decreased renal blood flow	113

Conditions	Dose	Cardiovascular effects	Reference
Previously instrumented, comparisons made to awake state	750 mg, IV in 1 min + 25 mg/min + 10 mg/min for 70 min	Modest changes in hepatic and renal blood flows associated with doubling of arterial pethidine concentrations, and disturbed pethidine kinetics	62
6.2:7 Pentothal-Goats			
Intact, awake, previously instrumented	9 mg/kg, IV	Increased HR, decreased stroke volume, slight initial decrease in pulmonary artery flow which returned to baseline and an associated decrease then increase in pulmonary arterial flow acceleration	52
6.2:8 Pentothal-Primates			
Anesthetized with halothane (0.5-1%), nitrous oxide (66%) and oxygen (34%), pancuronium (0.05 mg/kg, IV), positive pressure ventilation, aortic pressure reduced to 50 mmHg with repeated injections of trimethophan (10 mg,IV), a neck tourniquet was inflated to 1,500 mmHg, maintained aortic pressure at approx. 50 mmHg for 16 min with 4-5% halothane in oxygen, norepinephrine infusion started approx. 4 min prior to end of ischemia to increase aortic pressure to approx. 80 mmHg	90 mg/kg, IV, 5 and 15 min after ischemia	Significant improvement in neurologic recovery	54
Same model as above	90 mg/kg, Iv over a variety of time intervals	No beneficial effects on neurologic outcome after global ischemia	54

Conditions	Dose	Cardiovascular Effects	Ref
Anesthetized with halothane (1%), nitrous oxide (66%), oxygen (34%), subjected to 16 min of global ischemia, post-ischemia treated with thiopental	90 mg/kg, IV, infused over 60 min	Total and regional cerebral blood flow increased in thiopental treated, improves distribution of brain blood flow and brain glucose uptake early post-ischemia and depresses cerebral metabolic rate of oxygen later post-ischemia	55
6.2:9 Thiopental-Harbor seals			
Awake, previously instrumented (24-48 hrs) with catheters in the pulmonary artery and aorta	10 mg/kg, IV + 1% halothane up to 9.5 hrs	Decreased cardiac output, decreased aortic pressure and PaO_2, increased HR and hypothermia during the first hour of anesthesia but hyperthermia during prolonged anesthesia	56

Table 6.3: Cardiovascular effects of Methohexital

Conditions of the experiment	Dose	Cardiovascular effects	Ref
6.3:1 Methohexital-Dogs			
Intact, awake, previously instrumented	12 mg/kg, IV	Marked increase in HR, decrease in aortic pressure, decreased systemic vascular resistance, decrease in LV dP/dt max, rebound recoveries 1-2 min after injection, cardiac output increased only during period of maximum increase in HR	42
Intact, awake, previously instrumented	9.7 mg/kg, IV	Mean aortic pressure decreased at 15 sec; stroke volume decreased, cardiac index increased at 30 sec, 1 & 2 min; contractility increased at 1,2 & 2.5 min, pO_2 & pH decreased, pCO_2 increased	109

6.3:2 Methohexital-Cats, Conditions of the experiment	Dose	Cardiovascular Effects	Ref
Catheters is precava and aorta, stimulation of carotid sinus, aortic and vagus nerves, pancuronium bromide (200 µg/kg + 75 µg/kg every 30 min), positive pressure ventilation	35-40 mg/kg, IP	Selective blockade of baroreceptor reflexes, possible gamma-aminobutyric acid mimetic at central vasomotor synapses	24
Halothane anesthesia with high concentrations for induction, then positive pressure ventilation and 0.7% halothane with nitrous oxide (70%), selective perfusion of the 4th cerebral ventricle	20, 40, 80, 160 and 320 µg/ml (0.15 ml/min)	Dose-dependent decrease in aortic pressure and heart rate, no effect with same infusions into the lateral ventricles and 3rd ventricle	57
6.3:3 Methohexital-Primates			
Baboons, anesthetized with α-chloralose (60 mg/kg, IV), repeated doses of gallamine triethiodide (1 mg/kg, IV, as needed), positive pressure ventilation with 100% O_2	25, 50 & 100 mg/kg/hr at 24, 68 & 120 min after middle cerebral artery occlusion, infusions topped approx. 142 min after occlusion, 7 animals preloaded with 25 mg/kg/hr, 12 mg/kg/hr or 6 mg/kg/hr 46 min prior to occlusion	If flow after occlusion was greater than 25 ml/100 g/min methohexital reduced flow, but if flow was less than 20 ml/100 g/min a significant increase in flow was achieved	58

Table 6.4: Cardiovascular effects of secobarbital

Conditions of the experiment	Dose	Cardiovascular effects	Reference
6.4:1 Secobarbital-Dogs			
Acute, open chest preparation, coronary occlusion, SA node region crushed, 15 min wait after drug administration before any recordings were made	30 mg/kg, IV	Reduction in regional myocardial blood flow resulted in changes in the degree of bipolar ECG recordings that were greater than those changes seen with α-chloralose	59

Table 6.5: Cardiovascular effects of thiamylal

Conditions of the experiment	Dose	Cardiovascular effects	Reference
6.4:1 Thiamylal-Dogs			
Ketamine (10 mg/kg), exsanguinated, isolated helical strips of cerebral & mesenteric arteries	10^{-5} to 10^{-3} mol/L, Dose-response	In lower concentrations constriction, at 10^{-3} mol/L profound relaxation, contractions greater in mesenteric than in cerebral arteries	80
Intact, awake, previously instrumented	18.4 mg/kg, IV	Increased systemic resistance at 1 min post-injection, increased pulmonary arterial resistance at 1 & 2 min, pO_2 & pH decreased, pCO_2 increased	109

Table 6.6: Cardiovascular effects of α-chloralose

Conditions of the experiment	Dose	Cardiovascular Effects	Reference
6.6:1 α-chloralose-Dogs			
Intact, awake, previously instrumented	80 mg/kg, IV	No significant change in HR, no effect on atrioventricular conduction, significantly decreased effect of atropine on heart rate and A-V conduction, no effect on isoprenaline response	10

Conditions	Dose	Cardiovascular Effects	Reference
Intact, awake, previously instrumented	60 mg/kg, IV	Transient changes during induction in rates, flows and pressures, marked sinus arrhythmia in normal resting animals converted to regular sinus rhythm, no change in LV pressure waveforms or values, cardiac output decreased transiently but then returned to baseline within 5 min. Transient changes included an increase in flow acceleration and increases work and power of the heart, stroke work increased slightly	2
Previously instrumented, intact, awake, ventilation held constant, response to carotid chemoreceptor stimulation with intracarotid injection of nicotine	100 mg/kg, IV	Striking depression of carotid chemoreceptor stimulation response, less than that of pentobarbital or halothane but still a marked depression of this response	7
Acute open chest preparation, coronary occlusion, 15 min wait after drug administration before recordings, SA node region crushed, morphine (2.25 mg/kg, SQ)	50-100 mg/kg, IV, repeated as necessary	Reductions in regional myocardial blood flow resulted in changes in the degree of bipolar ECG recordings but changes were less than those seen with secobarbital	59
Hindlimb perfusion at constant flow rate, heparin (3 mg/kg, SQ), aortic and carotid sinus nerve stimulation	100 mg/kg, IV + 25 mg/hr	Carotid sinus nerve stimulation augmented the vasoconstrictor effects of the pressor reflex (i.e. enhanced the aortic nerve pressor reflex)	18
Morphine sulfate (0.4 mg/kg, IM), acute, isolated and perfused carotid sinus preparation with instrumentation of the abdomen, thorax then closed, positive pressure ventilation	80 mg/kg, IV	Mean arterial pressure and peripheral resistance were high compared to values obtained with pentobarbital or halothane. The carotid sinus reflexes are sensitive and well maintained	11

6.6:2 α-chloralose-Cats, Conditions of the experiment	Dose	Cardiovascular Effects	Reference
Induced with halothane, catheters in vein and aorta, stimulation of carotid sinus, aortic and vagus nerves	50-60 mg/kg, IV	Selective blockade of baroreceptor reflexes, possible gamma-aminobutyric acid mimetic at central vasomotor synapses	**24**
Measured renal sympathetic nerve activity, arterial blood pressure and HR	40-50 mg/kg, IV at 2 ml/min (10-19 ml total vol)	Sustained increase in renal sympathetic nerve activity, no effect on aortic pressure or heart rate	**85**
6.6:3 α-chloralose-Rats			
Decerebrated at mid-collicular level under halothane anesthesia at least 90 min prior to the study	60 mg/kg, IV	Decreased HR, blood pressure and respiratory rate, decreased responses to carotid vasomotor synapses	**24**
IV bolus response to L-NNA (32 mg/kg) (nitric oxide synthase inhibitor), compared anesthetized to conscious	90 mg/kg, IP + 15 mg/kg/30 min, IV	Increased mean aortic pressure more in the anesthetized than in the conscious rats	**88**
Pressor response to nitric oxide synthase inhibitor	90 mg/kg, IP + 15 mg/kg/30 min, IV	Pressor response same in anesthetized and conscious rats	**88**

6.6:4 α-chloralose-Rabbits, Conditions of the experiment	Dose	Cardiovascular Effects	Reference
Anesthetized with pentobarbital (30 mg/kg), urethane (800 mg/kg), α-chloralose-urethane combination, open-loop characteristic of carotid sinus reflex	80 mg/kg, IV	The response range and the slope parameters under α-chloralose anesthesia were significantly smaller than those obtained from the other regimens. The solvent propylene glycol, used for the chloralose, did not affect this parameter. Concluded that α-chloralose weakens the reflex control of arterial pressure in the rabbit even though it is supposed to maintain same in dogs	63
6.6:5 α-chloralose-Sheep			
Intact, awake, previously instrumented lambs	30, 60 or 90 mg/kg, IV	Significant decrease in baroreflex activity in all doses tested, mean aortic pressure and HR increased at 30 and 60 mg/kg doses; at 90 mg/kg mean aortic pressure decreased but no change in HR	114
6.6:6 α-chloralose-Bats			
Conscious	80 mg/kg, IV	Dilates arterioles in wing	60

Table 6.7: Cardiovascular effects of urethane

Conditions of the experiment	Dose	Cardiovascular effects	Reference
6.7:1 Urethane-Dogs			
Hindlimb perfusion with constant flow rate, heparin (3 mg/kg + 0.5 mg/kg/hr), aortic nerve and carotid sinus nerve stimulation	750 mg/kg, IP	Failed to demonstrate any interaction between the aortic nerve and carotid sinus nerve pressor reflexes	18

6.7:2 Urethane-Cats	Dose	Cardiovascular effects	Reference
Catheters in vein and aorta, stimulation of carotid sinus, aortic and vagus nerves	1250 mg/kg, IP	No selective blockade of baroreceptor reflexes	24
Measured renal sympathetic nerve activity, arterial pressure and heart rate	0.5-1.0 g/kg, IV ethyl carbamate in a 20% solution dissolved in 0.9% saline total vol = 4-10 ml	Animals usually vomited immediately after injection, some suffered cardiac arrest, also depressed ventilation, transient decrease in renal sympathetic nerve activity, no effect on aortic pressure or HR	84
6.7:3 Urethane-Rats			
Decerebrated at mid-collicular level under halothane anesthesia at least 90 min prior to study	750 mg/kg, IV	Decreased HR, blood pressure and respiratory rate, decreased responses to carotid occlusion, tilt and sodium cyanide chemoreceptor responses	34
Previously cannulated aorta, decapitation at various intervals after urethane administration for plasma renin activity	1250 mg/kg, IP	No significant change in blood pressure, increased plasma renin activity, sustained and marked plasma renin activity response, inhibited by propranolol	32
Previously instrumented with aortic cannulae	1000 mg/kg, IP	Little or no protection against mortality and kidney lesions following bleeding to 30-50 mmHg for 60 min	35

Conditions	Dose	Cardiovascular Effects	Reference
Effect of bleeding against various pre-determined pressures on relative oxygen tension in the kidney, oxygen electrode was placed in the kidney under ether anesthesia 24 hrs prior to the experiment, heparinized at the time of the experiment	1000 mg/kg, IV	Did not reduce the fall in relative oxygen tension following bleeding against 40 mmHg for 30 min or against 50 mmHg for 60 min, also did not protect against kidney lesions	30
Aortic strips and portal vein segments after decapitation, male rats only	10^{-3} to 10^{-4} in bath	Inhibited development of spontaneous mechanical activity, even at concentrations equivalent to 10% of anesthetic levels (i.e. 10^{-3} M). Dose-dependent attenuation of contractility induced by adrenaline, angiotensin and KCl, as well as Ca^{2+}, induced contractions of K^+-depolarized preparations, found that plasma concentrations of urethane at anesthetic levels can directly induce vascular smooth muscle relaxation	61
Compared urethane to pentobarbital anesthesia, response of renal vasculature to Area Postrema stimulation	1.6 g/kg	Increased renal flow and mean aortic pressure but no change in renal vascular resistance	101
Coronary artery ligation	1.25 g/kg, IP	High incidence of ventricular tachycardia and fibrillation	100
IV bolus response to nitric oxide synthase inhibitor (L-NNA, 32 mg/kg)	1 g/kg, IP	Increased mean aortic pressure the same as in conscious rats	88
Pressor response to nitric oxide synthase inhibitor (L-NNA)	1 g/kg, IP	Very modest effect on pressor response	88
6.7:4 Urethane-Bats			
Conscious, bat wing preparation	800 mg/kg	Dilutes arterioles in the bat wing	60

Table 6.8: Cardiovascular effects of α-chloralose and urethane combinations

Conditions of the experiment	Dose	Cardiovascular effects	Reference
6.8:1 α-chloralose-urethane- Dogs			
Hindlimb perfusion with constant flow rate, heparin (3 mg/kg + 0.5 mg/kg/hr), stimulation of aortic and carotid sinus nerves	α-chloralose (50 mg/kg), urethane (500 mg/kg), IV	Carotid sinus nerve stimulation (i.e. stimulation of depressor reflexes) augmented the vasoconstrictor effects of the pressor reflex (i.e. enhanced the aortic nerve pressor reflex)	**18**
6.8:2 α-chloralose-urethane- Cats			
Induced with halothane, catheters in vein and aorta, stimulation of carotid sinus, aortic and vagus nerves, pancuronium bromide (200 μg/kg + 75 μg/kg/30 min), positive pressure ventilation	α-chloralose (40 mg/kg), urethane (250 mg/kg), IV	Selective blockade of baroreceptor reflexes, perhaps related to enhancement or imitation of the action of gamma-aminobutyric acid at central vasomotor synapses	**24**
6.8:3 α-chloralose-urethane- Rats			
Decerebration, a complete midcollicular transection, cremaster muscle preparation for direct microvascular observation, allowed to recover from α-chloralose (57 mg/kg, IP) and urethane (760 mg/kg, IP), pancuronium (800 mg/ml) added to cremaster bath	α-chloralose (22.8 mg/kg), urethane (304 mg/kg) IP (40% of original dose)	Anesthesia inhibited vasomotion and increased arteriolar diameters by 16-36%, during decerebrate recovery from the anesthesia phase the 8-50 μm diameter arterioles exhibited amplitude changes of diameters of approximately 35% with a mean frequency of 31 cycles/min	**62**

Conditions	Dose	Cardiovascular Effects	Reference
Two hours allowed for recovery, observed for 1 1/2 hrs after reanesthesia	same as above	Reanesthesia decreased heart rate and mean aortic pressure, average diameter for 2nd, 3rd, 4th and 5th order arterioles increased by anesthesia, decreased spontaneous vasomotion activity to zero	62
Compared to intact, awake, previously instrumented group	α-chloralose (60 mg/kg), urethane (800 mg/kg),IP + 10% of initial doses as required	Cardiac output and regional blood flows to cerebrum, cerebellum, heart, kidney, stomach, small bowel, GI tract, spleen, liver, skin, diaphragm, cremaster muscle, rectus abdominous muscle, gastrocnemius muscle all decreased; lactate/pyruvate ratio increased	87
Comparison of responses in conscious rats vs chloralose/urethane anesthetize rats to L-NMMA (nitric oxide synthase inhibitor-0.1-10 mg/kg, IV)	α-chloralose (100 mg/kg), urethane (500 mg/kg), IP	Decreased blood pressure, increased heart rate, dose-response increase in mean aortic pressure greater in anesthetized than in conscious rats; pressor response to phenylephrine not different between groups	94
Cremaster muscle preparation in decerebrated rats anesthetized with chloralose/urethane and allowed to recover following decerebration	α-chloralose (57 mg/kg), urethane (760 mg/kg), IP	Decreased respiratory rate, heart rate and mean aortic pressure, decreased vasomotion in 8-50 μm diameter arterioles and resulted in 16-36 % dilation of these vessels	62
6.8:4 α-chloralose-urethane- Mice			
Intact, awake	α-chloralose (80 mg/kg), urethane (800 mg/kg), IV	Dilates cutaneous arterioles	2

Propofol is a new, nonbarbiturate, intravenously administered anesthetic agent that has been recommended as a safe agent for induction and maintenance of anesthesia.

Table 6.9 Cardiovascular effects of Propofol

Conditions of the experiment	Dose	Cardiovascular effects	Reference
6.9:1 Propofol-Dogs			
Intact, awake, hemorrhaged to 60 mmHg mean aortic pressure and held at this level for 60 min, then propofol administered	6 mg/kg, IV	Three min after propofol mean pulmonary arterial pressure, pulmonary arterial resistance, O_2 utilization ratio, venous admixture of $PaCO_2$ and $PvCO_2$ all increased; mean aortic pressure, PaO_2, PvO_2, arterial and venous pH all decreased; after 15 min $PvCO_2$ still increased, all other parameters back to pre-propofol levels; after 30 min all parameters back to pre-propofol levels	**116**
Isotope dilution technique to measure norepinephrine kinetics compared to awake dogs	6 mg/kg + 0.8 mg/kg/min, IV	Decreased aortic pressure, decreased sympathetic tone, less effect than 2.0 MAC halothane on norepinephrine clearance	**117**
Chronically instrumented conscious vs anesthetized with autonomic nervous system blocked	Dose-response, 25, 50 & 100 mg/kg/hr, IV	No change in isovolumetric relaxation or regional chamber stiffness, i.e. no change in diastolic function. No change in diastolic compliance of the left ventricle	**118**
Intact, awake, effects on propranolol distribution and metabolism	6 mg/kg + 0.8 mg/kg/min, IV	Decreased intrinsic clearance but no significant difference in systemic clearance or hepatic plasma flow; marked changes in volume of distribution; modest inhibitor of drug metabolism, major effects on propranolol distribution	**119**
Intact, awake, previously instrumented	3.2 ± 0.1 mg/kg, IV + 0.4 mg/kg/min for 60 min, + 100% oxygen	No change in aortic pressure, heart rate, respiratory rate; increased $PaCO_2$, no change in packed cell volume or total plasma proteins	**120**

Conditions	Dose	Cardiovascular Effects	Reference
Same above except done in greyhound dogs	Same as above	Same as above, mild respiratory acidosis	**120**
Intact, awake, chronically instrumented dogs	5 mg/kg bolus IV, and 15 min infusions of 15, 30, 60 and 120 mg/kg/hr	Dose-dependent decrease in preload recruitable stroke work and other measures of contractility (dP/dtmax and % segment shortening); Decreased systemic vascular resistance	**123**
Anesthetized with thiopental (15 mg/kg, IV), fentanyl (12 μg/kg/hr) and midazolam (0.6 mg/kg/hr), IV. In some animals additional bolus doses of fentanyl were required to maintain heart rate constant	150, 300, 600 & 1200 μg/min infused directly into the LAD coronary artery	At 150 & 300 μg/min infusion rates (clinical range), no negative inotropic effects; Higher doses increased coronary venous oxygen tensions and decreases in contractility (% segmental shortening)	**124**
6.9:2 Propofol-Rats			
Isolated superfused neonatal rat spinal cord	0.5 to 10 μM, Dose-response curves	Depressed the response evoked by direct application of Substance P; No anti-analgesic or hyperalgesic effect observed	**125**
Anesthetized with urethane	2.5-40 mg/kg, IV	Transient decrease in mean aortic pressure followed by transient increase in aortic pressure above baseline at most doses, increased heart rate accompanied drops in pressure; except at high doses cardiovascular changes returned to baseline values by 8 min; no changes in arterial blood gases	**121**

Conditions	Dose	Cardiovascular effects	Reference
SHR rats anesthetized with halothane for surgical preparation, then decreased to 0.5 to 0.7% in half animals and propofol given to other half (n=14 in each group), ligation of middle cerebral artery for 2 hr at normothermia	1% IV infusion in dose sufficient to suppress EEG bursts	No difference between propofol and halothane anesthesia groups for neurologic deficits and infarct volumes	122
6.9:3 Propofol-Sheep			
Conscious, previously instrumented	250-300 mg IV bolus + 20-25 mg/min, IV	Decreased total body O_2 consumption, heart rate and mean aortic pressure increased, cardiac output unchanged, hepatic blood flow decreased, renal blood flow decreased	113
70 min maintenance of anesthesia	250-300 mg, IV induction (1 min) + 20-25 mg/min, IV	Doubled blood concentrations of cefoxitin over control awake animals, renal extraction ratio decreased 50-60%	112
Previously instrumented, comparisons made to awake animals	250-300 mg, IV over 1 min + 20-25 mg/min, IV	Doubled arterial pethidine concentrations, hepatic extraction ratio of pethidine unchanged, flux increased 20% & clearance decreased 10%; modest changes in hepatic and renal blood flow with disturbed pethidine kinetics for several hours	115

References

1.   Parker, J.L., Adams, H.R. The influence of chemical restraining agents on cardiovascular function: A review, *Lab Anim Sci*, 28:575-583, 1978.
2.   Van Critters, R.L., Franklin, D.L., Rushmer, R.F. Left ventricular dynamics in dog during anesthesia with α-chloralose and sodium pentobarbital, *Am J Cardiol*, 13:349-354, 1964.
3.   Vatner, S.F., Monroe, R.G., McRitchie, R.J. Effect of anesthesia, tachycardia and autonomic blockade on the Anrep effect in intact dogs, *Am J Physiol*, 226:1450-1456, 1974.
4.   Vatner, S.F. Effects of anesthesia on cardiovascular control mechanisms, *Environ Health Perspect*, 26:193-206, 1978.
5.   Manders, W.T., Vatner, S.F. Effects of sodium pentobarbital anesthesia on left ventricular function and distribution of cardiac output in dogs, with particular reference to the mechanism for tachycardia, *Circ Res*, 39:512-517, 1976.

6. Vatner, S.F., Higgins, C.B., Patrick, T. Effects of cardiac depression and of anesthesia on the myocardial action of a cardiac glycoside, *J Clin Invest*, 50-2585-2595, 1971.

7. Zimpfer, M., Sit, S.P., Vatner, S.F. Effects of anesthesia on the canine carotid chemoreceptor reflex, *Circ Res*, 48:400-406, 1981.

8. Morrow, D.H., Haley, J.V., Logic, J.R. Anesthesia and digitalis, VII. The effect of pentobarbital, halothane, and methoxyflurane on AV node conduction and inotropic responses to ouabain, *Anesth Analg*, 51:430-438, 1972.

9. Laks, M.M., Greenless, L., Garner, D. Comparison of ejection fraction and segmental circumferential fiber shortening velocity in the anesthetized and conscious canine, *Jpn Heart J*, 20:359-365, 1979.

10. Duchene-Marullaz, P., Fabry-Delaigue, R., Gueorguiev, G., Kantelip, J.P. Influence of chloralose and pentobarbitone sodium on atrioventricular conduction in dogs, *Br J Pharmacol*, 77:309-317, 1982.

11. Cox, R.H., Bagshaw, R.J. Effects of anesthesia on carotid sinus reflex control of arterial hemodynamics in the dog, *Am J Physiol*, 239:H681-H691, 1980.

12. Tinker, J.H., Harrison, C.E. Protection from myocardial ischemia role of anesthetics, *Anesthe*, 51(3 suppl.):S58, 1979.

13. Astrup, J., Sorensen, P.M., Sorensen, H.R. Inhibition of cerebral oxygen and glucose consumption in the dog by hypothermia pentobarbital and lidocaine, *Anesthe*, 55:263-268, 1981.

14. Amlie, J.P., Owren, T. The effect of prolonged pentobarbital anaesthesia on cardiac electrophysiology and inotropy of the dog heart *in situ*, *Acta Pharmacol Toxicol* (Copenhagen), 44:264-271, 1979.

15. Ivankovich, A.D., El-Etr, A.A., Janeczko, G.F. The effects of ketamine and of Innovar anesthesia on digitalis tolerance in dogs, *Anesth Analg* (Cleveland), 54:106-111, 1975.

16. Peiss, C.N., Manning, J.W. Effects of sodium pentobarbital on electrical and reflex activation of the cardiovascular system, *Circ Res*, 14:228-235, 1964.

17. Chiba, S., Nakajima, T. Effect of sodium pentobarbital on the SA nodal activity of the dog heart *in vivo*, *Tohoku J Exp Med*, 106:381-385, 1972.

18. Kendrick, J.E., Matson, G.L. Effect of anesthetics on the interaction between pressor and depressor reflexes in dogs, *Proc Soc Exp Biol Med*, 165:100-106, 1980.

19. Chambers, R., Zweifach, B.W. Topography and function of the mesenteric capillary circulation, *Am J Anat*, 75:173-205, 1944.

20. Feustel, P.J., Ingvar, M.C., Severinghaus, J.W. Cerebral oxygen availability and blood flow during middle cerebral artery occlusion, effects of pentobarbital, *Stroke*, 12:858-863, 1981.

21. Weide, W., Loffelholz, K. Aminopyridine antagonizes the inhibitory effect of pentobarbital on acetylcholine release in the heart, *Naunyn Schmiedebergs Arch Pharmacol*, 312:7-13, 1980.

22. Marin, J., Recio, L. Effect of pentobarbital on the noradrenaline release induced by drugs and field electrical stimulation from cerebral and femoral arteries of the cat, *Biochem Pharmacol*, 31:1567-1571, 1982.

23. Edvinsson, L., McCulloch, J. Effects of pentobarbital on contractile responses of feline cerebral arteries, *J Cereb Blood Flow Metab*, 1:437-440, 1981.

24. Lalley, P.M. Inhibition of depressor cardiovascular reflexes by a derivative of gamma amino butyric-acid and by general anesthetics with suspected gamma amino butyric-acid mimetic effects, *J Pharmacol Exp Ther*, 215:418-425, 1980.

25. Siafakas, N.M., Bonora, M., Duron, B., Gautier, H., Milic-Emili, J. Dose effect of pentobarbital sodium on control of breathing in cats, *J Appl Physiol*, 55:1582-1592, 1983.

26. Sanchez, E., Tampier, L., Dolz, H., Mardones, J. The effects of methohexital in untreated and nalorphine-pretreated rats, *Anesthe*, 37:40-46, 1972.

27. Carvalho, J.S., Cherkes, J.K. Renin release by pentobarbital anesthesia in the rat: a role for vascular mechanisms, *Life Sci*, 30:887-897, 1982.

28. Rubanyi, G., Kovach, A.G. Effect of pentobarbital anesthesia on contractile performance and oxygen-consumption of perfused rat heart, *Circ Shock*, 7:121-127, 1980.

29. Altura, B.T., Turlapaty, P.D., Altura, B.M. Pentobarbital sodium inhibits calcium uptake in vascular smooth muscle, *Biochem Biophys Acta*, 595:309-312, 1980.

30. van der Meer, C., Valkenburg, P.W. Effect of pentobarbital and urethane on the oxygen tension in the kidney of hypotensive rats, *Arch Int Pharmacodyn Ther*, 238:154-164, 1979.

31. Bell, F.P., Hubert, E.V. Membrane active agents effect of various anesthetics and chlorpromazine on arterial lipid metabolism, *Atherosclerosis*, 39:517-526, 1981.

32.   Leenen, F.H.H., Provoost, A.P. Maintenance of blood pressure by β-adrenoceptor mediated renin release during different forms of anesthesia in rats, *Can J Physiol Pharmacol*, 59:364-370, 1981.

33.   Hawkins, R.A., Mans, A.M., Biebuyck, J.F. Amino-acid supply to individual cerebral structures in awake and anesthetized rats, *Am J Physiol*, 242:E1-E11, 1982.

34.   Sapru, H.N., Krieger, A.J. Cardiovascular and respiratory effects of some anesthetics in the decerebrate rat, *Eur J Pharmacol*, 53:151-158, 1979.

35.   Peters, J.M., van der Meer, C., Czanky, J.C., Spierdijk, J. Effect of anesthetics on mortality and kidney lesions caused by hypotension, *Arch Int Pharmacodyn Ther*, 238:134-153, 1979.

36.   Plizga, A., Holl, J.E. Myocardial depression associated with effective refractory period prolongation after pentobarbital and procainamide but not after dantrolene, *Res Commun Chem Pathol Pharmacol*, 28:13-26, 1980.

37.   Murthy, V.S., Zagar, M.E., Vollmer, R.R., Schmidt, D.H. Pentobarbital-induced changes in vagal tone and reflex vagal activity in rabbits, *Eur J Pharmacol*, 84:41-50, 1982.

38.   Lawner, P., Laurent, J., Simeone, F., Fink, E., Rubin, E. Attenuation of ischemic brain edema by pentobarbital after carotid ligation in the gerbil, *Stroke*, 10:644-647, 1979.

39.   Branston, N.M., Hope, D.T., Symon, L. Barbiturates in focal ischemia of primate cortex, effects on blood flow distribution, evoked potential and extracellular potassium, *Stroke*, 10:647-653, 1979.

40.   Forsyth, R.P., Hoffbrand, B.I. Redistribution of cardiac output after sodium pentobarbital anesthesia in the monkey, *Am J Physiol*, 218:214-217, 1970.

41.   Priano, L.L. Comparative renal vascular effects of thiopental, diazepam, ketamine and halothane, *Anesthesiol*, 57:A34, 1982.

42.   Twissell, D.J., Dodds, M.G. The systemic hemodynamic effects of minaxolone, a comparison with other anesthetics in the dog, *Br J Anaesth*, 51:995P-996P, 1979.

43.   Ahlgren, I., Aronsen, D.F., Bjorkman, I., Wetterlin, S. Hemodynamics during superficial thiopental anesthesia in the dog, *Acta Anaes Scand*, 22:76-78, 1978.

44.   Atlee, J.L., Malkinson, C.E. Thiopental potentiation of epinephrine sensitization with halothane, *Anesthe*, 53:S133, 1980.

45.   Hitchon, P.W., Kassell, N.F., Hill, T.R., Gerk, M.K., Sokoll, M.D. The response of spinal cord blood flow to high-dose barbiturates, *Spine*, 7:4-45, 1982.

46.   Astrup, J., Skovsted, P., Gjerris, F., Sorensen, H.R. Increase in extracellular potassium in the brain during circulatory arrest, effects of hypothermia, lidocaine and thiopental, *Anesthe*, 55:256-262, 1981.

47.   Kassell, N.F., Hitchon, P.W., Gerk, M.K., Sokoll, M.D., Hill, T.R. Influence of changes in arterial carbon dioxide partial pressure on cerebral blood flow and metabolism during high dose barbiturate therapy in dogs, *J Neurosurg*, 54:615-619, 1981.

48.   Kim, D.S. Effect of thiopental in acute focal cerebral infarction assessed by enzyme activities in serum and cerebrospinal fluid, *J Catho Med Coll*, 34:493-506, 1981.

49.   Hall, P.J., Pleuvry, B.J. An *in vitro* study of the effects of calcium on the cardiovascular actions of thiopentone, althesin and ketamine in the rat, *J Pharm Pharmacol*, 31:460-465, 1979.

50.   Sinclair, D.M., deMoss, D., Boink, A.B., Ruigrok, T.J. A protective effect of thiopentone on hypoxic heart muscle, *J Mol Cell Cardiol*, 12:225-227, 1980.

51.   Frankel, W.L., Poole-Wilson, P.A. Effects of thiopental on tension development, action potential and exchange of calcium and potassium in rabbit ventricular myocardium, *J Cardiovas Pharmacol*, 3:554-564, 1981.

52.   Foex, P., Prys-Roberts, C. Pulmonary haemodynamics and myocardial effects of Althesin (CT 1341) in the goat, *Postgrad Med I (June Suppl.)*, 48:24-31, 1972.

53.   Bleyaert, A.L., Nemoto, E.M., Safar, P., Stezoski, S.W., Mickell, J.J., Moosby, J., Rao, G.R. Thiopental amelioration of brain damage after global ischemia in monkeys, *Anesthe*, 49:390-398, 1978.

54.   Gisvold, S.E., Safar, P., Hendrickx, H.H.L., Alexander, H. Thiopental treatment after global brain ischemia in monkeys, *Anesthe, 55 (Suppl 3)*:A97, 1981.

55.   Kofke, W.A., Nemoto, E.M., Hossmann, K.A., Taylor, F., Kessler, P.D., Stezoski, S.W. Brain blood flow and metabolism after global ischemia and post insult thiopental therapy in rhesus monkeys, *Stroke*, 10:554-560, 1979.

56.   Sinnett, E.E., Wahrenbrock, E.A., Kooyman, G.L. Cardiovascular depression and thermoregulatory disruption caused by pentothal/halothane anesthesia in the harbor seal, *Phoca vitulina*, *J Wildl Dis*, 17:121-130, 1981.

57.   Freye, E., Gupta, B.N. Cardiovascular effects on selective perfusion of the 4th cerebral ventricle in cats with fentanyl naloxone and methohexital, *Indian J Exp Biol*, 18:29-31, 1980.

58.   Branston, N.M., Hope, D.T., Symon, L. Barbiturates in focal ischemia of primate cortex: effects on blood flow distribution, evoked potential and extracellular potassium, *Stroke*, 10:647-653, 1979.

59.   Ruffy, R., Lovelace, D.E., Knoebel, S.B., Zipes, D.P. Influence of secobarbital and α-chloralose and of vagal and sympathetic interruption, on left ventricular activation after acute coronary artery occlusion in the dog, *Circ Res*, 48:884-894, 1981.

60.   Harris, P.D., Hodoval, L.F., Longnecker, D.E. Quantitative analysis of microvascular responses to carotid occlusion after pentobarbital, urethane and α-chloralose, *Microvasc Res*, 4:325, 1972.

61.   Altura, B.M., Weinberg, J. Urethane and contraction of vascular smooth muscle, *Br J Pharmacol*, 67:255-263, 1979.

62.   Faber, J.E., Harris, P.D., Wiegman, D.L. Anesthetic depression of microcirculation, central hemodynamics and respiration in decerebrate rats, *Am J Physiol*, 243:H837-H843, 1982.

63.   Ishikawa, N., Kallman, C.H., Sagawa, K. Rabbit carotid sinus reflex under pentobarbital, urethan, and chloralose anesthesia, *Am J Physiol*, 246:H696-H701, 1984.

64.   Vatner, S.F., Braunwald, E. Cardiovascular control mechanism in the conscious state, *N Engl J Med*, 293:970-976, 1975.

65.   Cox, R.H., Bagshaw, R.J. Influence of anesthesia on the response to carotid hypotension in dogs, *Am J Physiol*, 237:H424-H432, 1979.

66.   Zimplfer, M., Manders, W.H., Barger, A.C., Vatner, S.F. Pentobarbital alters compensatory neural and humoral mechanism in response to hemorrhage, *Am J Physiol*, 243:H713-H724, 1982.

67.   Ishikawa, N., Sagawa, K. Nonlinear summation of depressor effect of carotid sinus pressure changes and aortic nerve stimulation in the rabbit, *Circ Res*, 52:401-410, 1983.

68.   Yamazaki, T., Sagawa, K. Effect of thiamylal on the response to carotid occlusion and mild hemorrhage in rabbits, *Am J Physiol*, 246:H806-H810, 1984.

69.   Johnson, M.D., Malvin, R.L. Plasma renin activity during pentobarbital anesthesia and graded hemorrhage in dogs, *Am J Physiol*, 229:1098-1101, 1975.

70.   Walgenbach, S.C., Donald, D.E., Mecher, A. Inhibition of carotid pressor response by left aortic depressor nerve in dogs, *Am J Physiol*, 240:H555-H560, 1981.

71.   Kirckheim, H., Gross, R. Hemodynamics of the carotid sinus reflex elicited by bilateral carotid occlusion in the conscious dog, *Pfluegers Arch*, 327:203-224, 1971.

72.   Stephenson, R.B., Donald, D.E. Reflex from isolated carotid sinuses of intact and vagotomized conscious dogs, *Am J Physiol*, 238:H815-H822, 1980.

73.   Kremser, P.C., Gewertz, B.L. Effect of pentobarbital and hemorrhage on renal autoregulation, *Am J Physiol*, 249:F356-F360, 1985.

74.   Amlie, J.P., Owen, T. The effect of prolonged pentobarbital anaesthesia on cardiac electrophysiology and inotropy of the dog heart *in situ*, *Acta Pharmacol et Toxicol*, 44:264-271, 1979.

75.   Hunt, G.B., Ross, D.L. Comparison of effects of three anesthetic agents on induction of ventricular tachycardia in a canine model of myocardial infarction, *Circ*, 78:221-226, 1988.

76.   Halliwill, J.R., Billman, G.E. Effect of general anesthesia on cardiac vagal tone, *Am J Physiol*, 262:H1719-H1724, 1992.

77.   Unruh, H.W., Wang, R., Bose, D., Mink, S.N. Does pentobarbital anesthesia depress left ventricular contractility in dogs?, *Am J Physiol*, 261:H700-H706, 1991.

78.   Nyhan, D.P., Goll, H.M., Chen, B.B., Fehr, D.M. *et al.* Pentobarbital anesthesia alters pulmonary vascular response to neural antagonists, *Am J Physiol*, 256:H1384-H1392, 1989.

79.   Madwed, J.B., Wang, B.C. Pentobarbital anesthesia alters renal actions of alpha-hANP in dogs, *Am J Physiol*, 258:R616-R623, 1990.

80.   Moriyama, S., Nakamura, K., Hatano, Y., Harioka, T., Mori, K. Responses to barbiturates of isolated dog cerebral and mesenteric arteries contracted with KCl and prostaglandin F2 alpha, *Acta Anaesthesiol Scand*, 34:523-529, 1990.

81.   Nyhan, D.P., Chen, B.B., Fehr, D.M., Goll, H.M., Murray, P.A. Pentobarbital augments pulmonary vasoconstrictor response to cyclooxygenase inhibition, *Am J Physiol*, 257:H1140-H1146, 1989.

82.   Van der Linden, P., Gilbart, E., Engelman, E., Schmartz, D., Vincent, J.L. Effects of anesthetic agents on systemic critical O_2 delivery, *J Appl Physiol*, 71:83-93, 1991.

83.   Nyhan, D.P., Chen, B.B., Fehr, D.M., Rock, P., Murray, P.A. Anesthesia alters pulmonary vasoregulation by angiotensin II and captopril, *J Appl Physiol*, 72:636-642, 1992.

84. Marin, J., Gonzalez, J.C., Salaices, M., Sanchez, C.F., Rico, M.L. Contractile responses and noradrenaline release evoked by serotonin in cat femoral artery: influence of pentobarbital, *Gen Pharmacol*, 13:117-123, 1982.

85. Matsukawa, K., Ninomiya, I. Anesthetic effects on tonic and reflex renal sympathetic nerve activity in awake cats, *Am J Physiol*, 256:R371-R378, 1989.

86. Marin, J., Martinez-Aldma, J., Salaices, M. Interference of pentobarbital and verapamil with the reactivity of middle cerebral artery of cat exposed to experimental subarachnoid hemorrhage, *Gen Pharmacol*, 20:243-248, 1989.

87. Seyde, W.C., McGowan, L., Lund, N., Duling, B., Longnecker, D.E. Effects of anesthetics on regional hemodynamics in normovolemic and hemorrhaged rats, *Am J Physiol*, 249:H164-H173, 1985.

88. Wang, Y.X., Zhou, T., Chua, T.C., Pang, C.C. Effects of inhalation and intravenous anesthetic agents on pressor response to NG-nitro-L-arginine, *Eur J Pharmacol*, 198:183-188, 1991.

89. Asher, E.F., Alsip, N.L., Zhang, P.Y., Harris, P.D. Prostaglandin-related microvascular dilation in pentobarbital- and etomidate-anesthetized rats, *Anesthesiology*, 76:271-278, 1992.

90. Jung, R., Bruce, E.N., Katona, P.G. Tonic and baroreflex effects on arterial pressure and ventilation of pentobarbital and nicotine on the rat ventral medullary surface, *Brain Res*, 485:399-402, 1989.

91. Schaefer, C.F., Brackett, D.J., Biber, B., Lerner, M.R. *et al.* Respiratory and cardiovascular effects of thyrotropin-releasing hormone as modified by isoflurane, enflurance, pentobarbital and ketamine, *Regul Pept*, 24:269-282, 1989.

92. Segal, J., Schwalb, H., Shmorak, V., Uretzky, G. Effect of anesthesia on cardiac function and response in the perfused rat heart, *J Mol Cell Cardiol*, 22:1317-1324, 1990.

93. Bramhall, T., Decrinis, M., Donnerer, J., Lembeck, F. Capsaicin-sensitive afferents and blood pressure regulation during pentobarbital anaesthesia in the rat, *Naunyn Schmiedebergs Arch Pharmacol*, 339:584-589, 1989.

94. Aisaka, K., Mitani, A., Kitajima, Y., Ohno, T., Ishihara, T. Difference in pressor responses to NG-monomethyl-L-arginine between conscious and anesthetized rats, *Jpn J Pharmacol*, 56:245-248, 1991.

95. Takemoto, Y. decreases in catecholamine concentrations of cisternal cerebrospinal fluid and plasma in rats caused by pentobarbital anesthesia, *Jpn J Physiol*, 42:141-145, 1992.

96. Watkins, L., Maixner, W. The effect of pentobarbital anesthesia on the autonomic nervous system control of heart rate during baroreceptor activation, *J Auton Nerv Syst*, 36:107-114, 1991.

97. Ogura, K., Takayasu, M., Dacey, R.G. Jr. Differential effects of pentobarbital on intracerebral arterioles and venules of rats *in vitro*, *Neurosurgery*, 28:537-541, 1991.

98. Otsuka, T., Wei, L., Acuff, V.R., Shimizu, A. *et al.* Variation in local cerebral blood flow response to high-dose pentobarbital sodium in the rat, *Am J Physiol*, 261:H110-H120, 1991.

99. Weeks, J.B., Todd, M.M., Warner, D.S., Katz, J. The influence of halothane, isoflurane, and pentobarbital on cerebral plasma volume in hypocapnic and normocapnic rats, *Anesthesiology*, 73:461-466, 1990.

100. Dai, S. Anaesthetic-related occurrence of early ventricular arrhythmias during acute myocardial ischaemia in rats, *Arch Int Physiol Biochim*, 97:341-346, 1989.

101. Hartle, D.K., Soliman, A.S. Area postrema stimulation induces differential renal hemodynamics with two anesthetics, *Am J Physiol*, 262:R289-R294, 1992.

102. McShane, A.J., Crowley, K., Shayevitz, J.R., Michael, J.R. *et al.* Barbiturate anesthetics inhibit thromboxane-, potassium-, but not angiotensin-induced pulmonary vasoconstriction, *Anesthesiology*, 70:775-779, 1989.

103. Borkowski, G.L., Danneman, P.J., Russell, G.B., Lang, C.M. An evaluation of three intravenous anesthetic regimens in New Zealand rabbits, *Lab Anim Care*, 40:270-276, 1990.

104. Nagano, K., Gelman, S., Parks, D.A., Bradley, E.L. Jr. Hepatic oxygen supply-uptake relationship and metabolism during anesthesia in miniature pigs, *Anesthesiology*, 72:902-910, 1990.

105. Thomson, J.G., Kerrigan, C.L., Abrahamowicz, M. Effects of sodium pentobarbital anesthesia on blood flow in skin, myocutaneous, and fasciocutaneous flaps in swine, *Plast Reconstr Surg*, 88:269-274, 1991.

106. Yaster, M., Koehler, R.C., Traystman, R.J. Interaction of fentanyl and pentobarbital on peripheral and cerebral hemodynamics in newborn lambs, *Anesthesiology*, 70:461-469, 1989.

107. Negishi, M., Ito, S. Involvement of phosphoinositide metabolism in GABA-induced catecholamine release from cultured bovine adrenal chromaffin cells, *Biochem Pharmacol*, 40:2719-2725, 1990.

108. Lina, A.A., Dauchot, P.J., Anton, A.H. Epinephrine-aminophylline-induced arrhythmias after midazolam or thiopentone in halothane-anesthetized dogs, *Can J Anaesth*, 38:1037-1042, 1991.
109. Turner, D.M., Ilkiw, J.E. Cardiovascular and respiratory effects of three rapidly acting barbiturates in dogs, *Am J Vet Res*, 51:598-604, 1990.
110. Dyson, D.H., Allen, D.G., Ingwersen, W., Pascoe, P.J. Evaluation of Acepromazine/Meperidine/Atropine premedication followed by thiopental anesthesia in the cat, *Can J Vet Res*, 52:419-422, 1988.
111. Weiskopf, R.B., Eger, E.I., Holmes, M.A., Yasuda, N., Johnson, B.H., Targ, A.G., Rampil, I.J. Cardiovascular actions of common anesthetic adjuvants during desflurane (I-653) and isoflurane anesthesia in swine, *Anesth Analg*, 71:144-149, 1990.
112. Selby, D.G., Mather, L.E., Runciman, W.B. Effects of propofol and of thiopentone anaesthesia on the renal clearance of cefoxitin in the sheep, *Br J Anaesth*, 65:360-364, 1990.
113. Runciman, W.B., Mather, L.E., Selby, D.G. Cardiovascular effects of propofol and of thiopentone anaesthesia in the sheep, *Br J Anaesth*, 65:353-359, 1990.
114. Konduri, G.G., Fewell, J.E. Influence of α-chloralose on reflex control of the cardiovascular system in lambs, *J Develop Physiol*, 13:87-91, 1990.
115. Mather, L.E., Selby, D.G., Runciman, W.B. Effects of propofol and of thiopentone anaesthesia on the regional kinetics of pethidine in the sheep, *Br J Anaesth*, 65:365-372, 1990.
116. Ilkiw, J.E., Pascoe, P.J., Haskins, S.C., Patz, J.D. Cardiovascular and respiratory effects of propofol administration in hypovolemic dogs, *Am J Vet Res*, 53:2323-2327, 1992.
117. Deegan, R., He, H.B., Wood, A.J., Wood, M. Effects of anesthesia on norepinephrine kinetics. Comparison of propofol and halothane anesthesia in dogs, *Anesthesiology*, 75:481-488, 1991.
118. Pagel, P.S., Schmeling, W.T., Kampine, J.P., Warltier, D.C. Alteration of canine left ventricular diastolic function by intravenous anesthetics *in vivo, Anesthesiology*, 76:419-425, 1992.
119. Perry, S.M., Whelan, E., Shay, S., Wood, A.J., Wood, M. Effect of i.v. anaesthesia with propofol on drug distribution and metabolism in the dog, *Br J Anaesth*, 66:66-72, 1991.
120. Robertson, S.A., Johnston, S., Beemsterboer, J. Cardiopulmonary, anesthetic, and postanesthetic effects of intravenous infusions of propofol in greyhounds and non-greyhounds, *Am J Vet Res*, 53:1027-1032, 1992.
121. Albertson, T.E., Tseng, C.C., Joy, R.M. Propofol modification of evoked hippocampal dentate inhibition in urethane-anesthetized rats, *Anesthesiology*, 75:82-90, 1991.
122. Ridenour, T.R., Warner, D.S., Todd, M.M., Gionet, T.X. Comparative effects of propofol and halothane on outcome from temporary middle cerebral artery occlusion in the rat, *Anesthesiology*, 76:807-812, 1992.
123. Pagel, P.S., Warltier, D.C. Negative inotropic effects of propofol as evaluated by the regional preload recruitable stroke work relationship in chronically instrumented dogs, *Anesthesiology*, 78:100-108, 1993.
124. Ismail, E.F., Song-Jung, K., Salem, R., Crystal, G.J. Direct effects of propofol on myocardial contractility in *in situ* canine hearts, *Anesthesiology*, 77:964-972, 1992.
125. Jewett, B.A., Gibbs, L.M., Tarasiuk, A., Kendig, J.J. Propofol and barbiturate depression of spinal nociceptive neurotransmission, *Anesthesiology*, 77:1148-1154, 1992.

7. Cardiovascular effects of inhalant anesthetic agents

Halothane and methoxyflurane have been the most commonly used halogenated inhalation anesthetic agents for general anesthesia in veterinary medicine. The use of other agents such as isoflurane, enflurane and desflurane are becoming more common. Methoxyflurane is used extensively in veterinary practice, primarily for cost considerations, while it is used very infrequently in research settings. The effects of these agents on the cardiovascular system are very commonly dose-dependent. They tend to increase the central venous pressure, i.e. right ventricular preload. Contractility, aortic pressure and cardiac output tend to decrease with a compensatory increase in heart rate. There is a direct depression of both the myocardium and vascular smooth muscle. These direct muscle cell effects seem to be associated with a disruption of Ca^{2+}-dependent contractile events. There is also a decrease in efferent sympathetic nervous activity and a decrease in reflex vasoconstriction. These agents also sensitize the heart to the arrhythmogenic activity of catecholamines.[1] Because of their effect on vascular smooth muscle, the halogenated agents produce marked changes in the peripheral circulation of some vascular beds, these effects are both concentration- and time-dependent.

At 1% end-tidal concentrations, halothane has been shown to result in marked renal vascular dilation, with somewhat less dilation of the iliac vascular beds. There was no change in the coronary circulation in these experiments, but a significant constriction of the mesenteric bed. After the anesthesia was prolonged for one hour there was a significant increase in resistance of the vascular beds with no change in regional flows. These changes were found concurrently with a constant cardiac output maintained by a slight increase in stroke volume in the presence of a decrease in heart rate, or vice versa.[2] The same laboratory studied the effects of halothane on intact, awake, previously instrumented dogs at 2% end-tidal concentrations. They noted a more marked myocardial depression, indicated by a 65% decrease in left ventricular dP/dt and a 63% decrease in the velocity of myocardial fiber shortening. The renal vascular bed exhibited the most intense dilation with the iliac circulation also dilating, but to a lesser extent. The coronary bed remained unchanged in these experiments while the mesenteric vascular bed constricted. When the anesthesia at this level was prolonged for 1 hour there was a progressive increase in aortic pressure and flow to all four regional beds being measured but no changes in vascular resistance in those beds.[2] More recent studies using isoflurane indicate significantly less negative inotropic effects and changes in renal vascular resistance.[116]

The halogenated agents seem to cause alterations in myofibrillar Ca^{2+} responsiveness but this effect is relatively insignificant compared to the anesthetic-induced decrease in availability of intracellular Ca^{2+} within the myocardium.[117] The volatile anesthetics may suppress autonomic reflexes to varying degrees and have many indirect actions that are mediated through an intact autonomic nervous system.[118] This always poses a problem in interpreting studies done in intact, awake, previously instrumented animals since the normal homeostatic response is for the body to compensate for whatever direct effects are caused by the anesthetic agent and to return the controlled variables to their set point levels.

As mentioned previously inhalation anesthetics can also sensitize the heart to the arrhythmogenic actions of catecholamines. There appears to be two mechanisms by which this occurs. The first is related to a reduction in supraventricular driving rate, caused both by direct depression from the anesthetic agent and by reflex response to the pressor effects of exogenous or endogenous catecholamines. The second mechanism, which predisposes to ventricular fibrillation, is caused by direct depression of the intraventricular conduction system. Halothane seems to have the most pronounced cardiac sensitization activity of all of the commonly used inhalation anesthetic agents.[3]

The cardiovascular effects of the most commonly used inhalant anesthetic agents are summarized in Tables 7.1-7.9. Halothane has been the most thoroughly studied of these agents but the effects typically seen with this drug may also be caused by the other agents.

Table 7.1: The cardiovascular effects of halothane

Conditions of the experiment	Dose	Cardiovascular Effects	Reference
7.1:1 Halothane-Dogs			
Intact, awake, previously instrumented for catheter electrocardiography	Dose-dependent	Depression of AV conduction, most marked proximal to the bundle of HIS. These effects are probably due to a prolongation of the refractory period	4
Isolated papillary muscle preparation	Anesthetic concentrations	Increased automaticity (i.e. re-entry), this seems to be responsible for the halothane-catecholamine-induced dysrhythmias	4
Intact, awake, previously instrumented with the ventilation held constant. Studied the response to carotid chemoreceptor stimulation (CCRS) with intra-carotid injections of nicotine	1 & 2 vol %	In unanesthetized dogs CCRS produced an intense decrease in heart rate, a very large increase in initial cardiac cycle length and mean iliac vascular resistance. Following anesthesia with 1% CCRS resulted in much smaller increases in cardiac cycle length and iliac resistance. After anesthesia with 2% halothane the response to CCRS was abolished	5

Conditions	Dose	Cardiovascular effects	Reference
Intact, awake, previously instrumented, compared results after anesthesia with the chest closed and the chest open	0.9% inhaled	**Chest closed:** There was no change in heart rate (HR), myocardial oxygen consumption (MVO_2), myocardial blood flow (MBF), endocardial to epicardial myocardial blood flow ratio (Endo/Epi), or peak to resting blood flow velocity ratio reserve (P/RV). Aortic pressure decreased significantly. **Chest open:** There was no change in HR, Endo/Epi or P/RV but aortic pressures, MVO_2 and MBF all decreased significantly	6
Intact, awake, following anesthesia with 1% end-tidal halothane in oxygen. Dogs were intubated, positive pressure ventilation, cannulation of the left coronary ostium, pacing electrode in the right atrium, single plane coronary cineangiograms, 5 ml injections of meglumine diatrizoate for contrast	1, 2 & 3 MAC	Results indicated that asynergy of contraction contributes little, if anything, to the halothane-induced impairment of myocardial performance	7
Intact, awake, previously instrumented, trained, morphine sulfate (0.2 mg/kg, IM), atropine (0.01 mg/kg, IM), otherwise awake. Measurements were made then given thiamylal (5 mg/kg, IV), masked with halothane, tracheal intubation with suxamethonium (2 mg/kg, IV), positive pressure ventilation	$0.75 \pm 0.1\%$, $0.94 \pm 0.02\%$, $1.13 \pm 0.02\%$, end-tidal concentrations	Brachiocephalic artery occlusion resulted in typical baroreceptor responses. There was a good linear correlation between the pressor response to brachiocephalic artery occlusion as a percentage of the response in "awake" animals and end-tidal halothane concentrations. This indicates a sensitive dose-response modification of the hemodynamic response to iatrogenically lowered pressures. At lower end-tidal concentrations (0.7-0.8%) the average pressor response to the occlusion was not significantly different than in "awake" dogs	8

Conditions	Dose	Cardiovascular effects	Reference
Intact, awake, previously instrumented. Compared pressor responses in awake, thiopental (25 mg/kg, IV) and N_2O (50%) treated dogs at various concentrations of halothane	0.0, 0.75, 1.5, inhaled	All anesthetic combinations attenuated reflex changes in heart rate produced by iatrogenic pressure changes, compared to the responses of the conscious dogs. There was a probable ganglionic blocking effect observed. Halothane was determined to have multiple sites of action, leading to its depression of the baroreflex	**9**
Previously instrumented, intact, awake, control vs aortic banded, LV hypertrophy	0.85, 1.3, 1.6 & 1.9%, end-tidal	Halothane anesthesia decreased the mean aortic pressure, cardiac output, stroke volume and LV dP/dt. There were no significant differences between the control and LV hypertrophy groups in these responses	**10**
Intact, awake, previously instrumented, breathing 100% oxygen	1 & 2%, inspired air	There was a concentration-dependent decrease in myocardial contractility, left ventricular end-diastolic diameter increased. At 1% conc. renal vascular resistance decreased and mesenteric resistance increased. At 2% regional blood flows increased with time	**11**
Intact, awake, previously instrumented	1.5 % in 2:1 N_2O	Decreased aortic pressure, preserved renal blood flow but renal vascular resistance was said to decrease	**12**
Intact, awake, previously instrumented	1.0, 1.5, & 2.0%, end-tidal	Increased HIS-Purkinje specialized conduction (not dose-dependent), no effect on spontaneous cycle length, A-V nodal or ventricular specialized conduction	**13**
Intact, awake, previously instrumented	1 & 2 %, end-tidal	There was a concentration-dependent decrease in LV dP/dt, LV end-diastolic diameter increased. At 1% there was a decrease in renal vascular resistance. With 1% concentrations regional vascular resistances tended to increase with time, with a 2% regional blood flows increased in time	**14**

Conditions	Dose	Cardiovascular effects	Reference
Compared response to saline infusion at 0.76 ml/min vs ouabain at equal volume and rate (36 μg/kg/hr) in intact, vagotomized and Trimethadinium pretreated dogs	1 & 2%, end-tidal	There was a dose-dependent increase in functional refractory period of the AV system, digitalization further increased this parameter along with an increase in the time of ouabain infusion required to produce ventricular arrhythmias	15
Anesthetized with thiopentone (up to 300 mg) with atropine (0.6 mg), intubation, alcuronium (2.5 mg), positive pressure ventilation	0.6 to 1.6%, end-tidal (0.7 to 1.8 MAC)	There was a dose-dependent myocardial depression; decreased cardiac index, decreased aortic pressure, no change in central venous pressure, a decrease in urine production and no change in effective renal plasma flow	16
Anesthetized with thiopentone (20 mg/kg, IV), suxamethonium (50-100 mg, IV), intubation, positive pressure ventilation with O_2, open chest, acute instrumentation	1% V/V	There was a decrease in aortic pressure, coronary artery flow, cardiac output, myocardial oxygen consumption and total body oxygen consumption with an increase in coronary vascular resistance. This dose of halothane did not influence the large increase in coronary artery flow produced by a $PaO_2 < 5.3$ kPa	17
Three groups of dogs compared; untreated, pretreated with Pargyline (100 mg/day), pretreated with Imipramine (25 mg/day), anesthetized with thiopental (15-20 mg/kg, IV), positive pressure ventilation, evaluated arterial pressure response to exogenous dose of epinephrine	1%, end-tidal	The no pretreatment group increased aortic pressure from 95 ± 23 to 147 ± 32 mmHg in response to the standard dose of epinephrine. The pretreatment with Pargyline (MAO inhibitor) group increased from 113 ± 21 to 143 ± 29 mmHg and the Imipramine (tricyclic antidepressant) group increased from 102 ± 25 to 180 ± 20 mmHg. Halothane offered the least amount of protection against epinephrine induced ventricular dysrhythmias compared to enflurane and methoxyflurane	18

Conditions	Dose	Cardiovascular effects	Reference
Anesthetized with thiopental (17.6 ± 0.5 mg/kg, IV), instrumented, positive pressure ventilation, arrhythmogenic dose of epinephrine, tested with Verapamil (0.2 mg/kg)	1% serum level (1.2 MAC)	Verapamil significantly and cumulatively increased the arrhythmogenic dose of epinephrine. Also were able to terminate ongoing epinephrine arrhythmias and convert ventricular tachycardia to sinus rhythm despite continuing epinephrine infusion	19
Anesthetized with thiopental (17.6 ± 0.5 mg/kg, IV), positive pressure ventilation	1.1 MAC	Verapamil increased the dose of epinephrine required to elicit a ventricular arrhythmia during halothane anesthesia	20
Anesthetized with thiopental (30 mg/kg, IV), 1-5% halothane in O_2 during the surgical prep., vagotomy, tracheal cannulation and positive pressure ventilation, open thorax, acute instrumentation, epinephrine infusion of 1 μg/kg/min	1%, end-tidal (1.2 MAC)	A constantly coupled bigeminal arrhythmia developed which was localized to the interventricular septum; simultaneously recorded echo-cardiograms showed early movement of the septum	21
Anesthetized with thiopental (25 mg/kg + 5 mg/kg/hr, IV), positive pressure ventilation with O_2, acute instrumentation, isolated, denervated carotid sinus preparation, localized administration of halothane with an isolated perfusion system	0.75 & 1.5 %	There was a dose-dependent sensitization of baroreceptors, a greater increase in carotid sinus afferent nerve activity for a given increase in sinus pressure; the changes observed could have been due to changes in sinus wall tension	22

Conditions	Dose	Cardiovascular effects	Reference
Induced with thiopental (15-20 mg/kg, IV), intubation, continued anesthesia with 0.5% halothane and 70% N_2O in O_2, intermittent positive pressure ventilation, acute, open thorax instrumentation, coronary sinus shunt	Increased concentrations until mean aortic pressure dropped to about 45 mmHg	Decrease in blood pressure, heart rate, cardiac output, stroke volume, maximum aortic dQ/dt and peak aortic flow; left ventricular end-diastolic pressure increased and LV dP/dt max decreased; there was a small decrease in systemic resistance and a decrease in coronary blood flow and myocardial oxygen consumption; the coronary artery sinus O_2 content was unchanged as were the arterial and coronary sinus levels of pyruvate; arterial and coronary sinus levels of lactate increased and there was a small but significant decrease in lactate consumption; coronary sinus levels of free fatty acids decreased	23
Acute instrumentation, thiopental (10 mg/kg, IV), morphine sulfate in 10 mg incremental doses to 4 mg/kg + 0.1 mg/kg/30 min, IV, succinylcholine (2 mg/ml) constant IV infusion at a rate just sufficient to prevent spontaneous breathing, positive pressure ventilation with 100% O_2	1.5%, end-tidal	Decreased myocardial O_2 consumption; the major portion of this change could be accounted for by decreases in aortic systolic pressure and heart rate	24
Induced with thiopental (17 mg/kg, IV), intubation, positive pressure ventilation with O_2; controls received incremental injections of thiopental (116 mg/kg, IV over the 6-10 hrs of the experiments)	1.5 to 2.4 % end-tidal	Increased epicardial activation times, ventricular functional refractory periods decreased; there was no change in effective refractory period of the ventricular conduction system; epicardial conduction delays at the effective refractory period decreased; increased concentrations of halothane decreased ventricular conduction and shortened the duration of the refractory periods in the ventricular conduction system	25

Conditions	Dose	Cardiovascular effects	Reference
Anesthetized with thiopental, intubated, positive pressure ventilation, maintained with halothane, acute instrumentation	1%	Sodium nitroprusside caused a decrease in directly measured myocardial O_2 consumption; this correlates well with a simultaneously observed decrease in the tension-related indirect indices of myocardial O_2 consumption	26
Thiopental (25 mg/kg, IV), pancuronium bromide (0.1 mg/ kg/hr), intubated, positive pressure ventilation; compared halothane treatment with N_2O (75-80%)	0.8 %	Decreased heart rate, aortic pressure, left ventricular pressure, LV dP/dt max and LV blood flow; the endocardial/ epicardial flow ratios were not significantly different; there was more coronary vascular bed reserve with halothane	27
Induced with thiopental (15 mg/kg, IV), premedicated with morphine sulfate (0.3 mg/kg, IM), open thorax, positive pressure ventilation, left anterior descending coronary artery (LAD) occlusion	0.5, 1, 1.5 & 2.0 %, inhaled	Regional ventricular function remained normal in the ischemic zone from LAD constriction; at higher concentrations, in the presence of LAD constriction, the area supplied by the LAD showed ischemic changes in function while the normally perfused regions maintained normal function	28
Previous implantation of a left atrial catheter; anesthetized with thiopental, place catheters in aorta and posterior vena cava; allowed to recover from 60 min then anesthetized with halothane	1.5% for 30 and 120 min	Decreased cardiac output, heart rate, left ventricular work, aortic pressure, left atrial mean pressure and coronary flow; flow to the lungs, kidneys and brain was well preserved; flow to the liver was unchanged in the 30 min group but markedly decreased in the 120 min group	29
Same preparation as above; studied normovolemic, moderately hypovolemic (withdrawal of 25 ml blood/kg) and hypovolemic hemorrhage to 60 mmHg mean aortic pressure	normovolemi c 1.5%, hypovolemic 0.5-1%	**Normovolemic**; decreased heart rate, cardiac output, blood pressure, left ventricular work and coronary flow **Moderate hypovolemia**; decreased blood pressure and coronary flow **Hemorrhagic hypovolemia**; increased blood pressure, coronary blood flow unchanged, decreased heart rate and increased stroke volume	30

Conditions	Dose	Cardiovascular effects	Reference
Thiopental (4 mg/kg, IV), morphine sulfate (1 mg/kg) & succinylcholine (0.5 mg/min) infusion, cardiac instrumentation	0.5, 1.0 & 2.0%, inhaled	Halothane depressed the slope of the relationship between blood pressure and heart rate; the reflex response range was only depressed at high halothane concentrations and the curve was displaced in the direction of lower heart rates at any given systemic pressure	31
Anesthesia induced with thiopental (20 mg/kg, IV), tracheal cannulation, positive pressure ventilation, bilateral vagotomy and carotid artery cannulation, open thorax, electrodes on the right atrium for pacing	0.8 %, inhaled	Found that changes in paced heart rate seemed to alter the electro-physiology of the halothane-sensitized myocardium to promote bigeminal arrhythmias by a re-entry mechanism	32
Anesthetized with pentobarbital (30 mg/kg, IV), 3 mg atropine, isoproterenol (0.1 μg/kg/min), propranolol (10 μg/kg, IV)	1 % in O_2	There was no change in heart rate, LV dP/dt, cardiac index, stroke volume, systemic resistance, pulmonary artery wedge pressures or mean aortic pressures; the isoproterenol infusion caused a decrease in HR, LV dP/dt, cardiac index and mean aortic pressures; Propranolol blocked all the responses to the isoproterenol infusion except for the decrease in mean aortic pressure; at 400 μg/kg, IV propranolol blocked all effects of isoproterenol; indicates that under these circumstances propranolol is additive not potentiated	33
Anesthesia with pentobarbital (30 mg/kg, IV + 3 mg/kg/hr, IV), positive pressure ventilation with 100% oxygen, decamethonium bromide (0.25-0.5 mg/kg, IV)	Interaction of halothane and hypocapnia tested	Both halothane and hypocapnia prolonged AV nodal conduction, halothane effects were more pronounced; halothane prolonged the atrial function, atrial effective and AV nodal functional refractory periods; these effects were linked to an increased incidence of repetitive atrial firing	34

Conditions	Dose	Cardiovascular effects	Reference
Anesthetized with pentobarbital (20-30 mg/kg, IV), acute instrumentation, positive pressure ventilation	1-2% in O_2	Decreased ventricular escape pacemaker activity during the supramaximal right vagal stimulation; suppressed ectopic pacemaker activity and markedly decreased ventricular automaticity in dogs given a toxic dose of ouabain; suggests differences between membrane activities of halothane in control versus ouabain treated dogs	35
Pentobarbital (30 mg/kg + 2 mg/kg as needed, IV), treatment group given Verapamil (0.2 mg/kg over a 10 min period)	1%, end-tidal	Single IV doses of Verapamil produce persistent hemodynamic interactions in dogs anesthetized with pentobarbital; under these circumstances halothane reduces systemic resistance, preserves cardiac output and decreases contractility	36
Digitalized for 7 days prior to the study with low doses (22 μg/kg/day) digoxin; anesthetized with pentobarbital (30 mg/kg + 3 mg/kg/ hr); positive pressure ventilation; decamethonium bromide (0.25-0.5 mg/kg,IV) to effect, acute instrumentation	1 % end-tidal	No protection against stimulated arrhythmias in hypocapnic or eucapnic, nontoxic, digitalized dogs	37
Pentobarbital (30 mg/ kg,IV), heart removed, crude membrane prep. from ventricular myocardial tissue	Dose-response, 3-5 vol%	No effect on either the affinity of canine myocardial β-adrenergic receptors for 3H-dihydroaloprenolol or 1-isoproterenol, nor does it alter the number of available receptors at binding equilibrium	38

Conditions	Dose	Cardiovascular Effects	Reference
Pentobarbital (30 mg/ kg,IV), positive pressure ventilation, heart removed, ventricular sarcoplasmic reticulum (SR) prep.	Dose-response	SR found to be an unlikely site of halothane-induced myocardial depression in the normal heart when substrate concentration and pH are maintained within normal limits. In the ischemic heart, in which the pH and substrate concentration have decreased, the interaction of halothane with the SR might contribute to a decrease in Ca^{2+} for contraction	39
Pentobarbital (30 mg/ kg,IV), pancuronium (0.06 mg/kg), positive pressure ventilation, closed chest, acute instrumentation	1.5% inspired	Pulmonary vascular response to alveolar hypoxia was manifested as an increased pulmonary arterial pressure and resistance, halothane increased the slope of the pulmonary resistance vs O_2 saturation curve because the reduction in cardiac output caused by halothane exceeded the decrease in pulmonary arterial pressure	40
Pentobarbital (30 mg/ kg, IV), ouabain (100-200 μg every 10 min until ventricular arrhythmias appeared), Lidocaine given as a bolus in increasing doses to 3 groups	>0.75% end-tidal	Halothane increased the elimination rate constants and the biological t/2 of lidocaine but not the volume of distribution; this indicates that the rate of lidocaine infusion should be decreased 4X to avoid toxic plasma levels during halothane anesthesia	41
Pentobarbital (30 mg/ kg,IV), suxamethonium (100 mg,IV), positive pressure ventilation, acute instrumentation, open thorax, occluded left main coronary	1% inspired	Approximate 40% decrease in blood flow to both ischemic and normal myocardium, 20% decrease in collateral perfusion pressure and 40% decrease in mean arterial pressure; ratio of oxygen availability/ consumption, in response to halothane, indicated improved oxygenation in acute ischemic vs nonischemic myocardium	42

Conditions	Dose	Cardiovascular Effects	Reference
Thiamylal (25 mg/kg,IV), succinylcholine (40 mg,IM), morphine (10 mg,IM),positive pressure ventilation, open thorax, left coronary artery perfusion	1,2 & 3%, inhaled	Without halothane left coronary flow was maintained constant, independent of perfusion pressure greater than 50 mmHg; 1 & 2% halothane decreased left coronary blood flow and perfusion pressure in a dose-dependent manner; there was also a shift in critical perfusion pressure; 3% halothane decreased left coronary flow with a decrease in perfusion pressure and a decrease in endocardial/epicardial blood flow ratio; there were also dose-dependent decreases in aortic pressure, left ventricular pressure, LV dP/dtmax and HR	**43**
Hexobarbital (no dose given), heparin (300 mg/kg), bled to cardiac arrest, isolated heart-lung preparation, perfused and ventilated	2.5-3%	No effects during normotonic perfusion or during enhanced pulmonary flow; decreased pulmonary vascular resistance during microembolism, i.e. induced pulmonary hypertension	**44**
Right heart by-pass, 0.2% V/V end-expired halothane with 70% N_2O for steady state, left anterior descending coronary artery ligation	0.9% V/V, end-expired	31% ATP depletion, decreased myocardial O_2 consumption, decreased mean arterial pressure, no change in HR	**45**
Closed chest catheterized prep.	1.6% compared to 3.2%, end-tidal	Increased left ventricular end-diastolic pressure, decreased aortic pressure, cardiac output, stroke volume, LV dP/dt, myocardial blood flow and myocardial oxygen consumption; no changes in systemic resistance, oxygen or lactate extraction by the heart	**46**
Halothane to effect, succinylcholine (20-30 mg + 5-10 mg,IV, as needed), 20 min allowed after succinylcholine before any measurements made, acute instrumentation using a multi-polar electrode catheter	1,1.5 & 2.0%, end-expired, steady state of 20 min prior to any recordings	Slowed conduction between the atria and the HIS bundle, also some ventricular slowing of conduction; work suggests that halothane-induced arrhythmias may be due, in part, to impaired conduction	**47**

Conditions	Dose	Cardiovascular Effects	Reference
Anesthetized with halothane, intubated and maintained with halothane during instrumentation then maintained on 70% N_2O, 30% O_2 + succinylcholine (1 mg/ min); some dogs received guanethidine (15 mg/kg 18 hrs prior to anesthesia + 5 mg/kg,IV after anesthesia), other dogs had guanethidine dosages switched; all animals given atropine (3.5 mg/kg,IV) just prior to each 1/2 of the experiment; some dogs received phenoxybenzamine	1.4 ± 0.1%	Decreased LV dP/dtmax, LV dP/dt/KPmax and Vmax; this depression of contractility was not reversed by autonomic blockade	48
Halothane and O_2 anesthesia, acute preparation, compared apneic and lethal concentrations in normal (39 ± 6) vs low (18 ± 6) hematocrit dogs	Dose-response	No significant differences between normal and anemic groups for mean alveolar concentrations, apneic or lethal concentrations; no differences in halothane dose-response curves for cardiac output, blood pressure, HR, LV end-diastolic pressure, arterial base excess; there was no redistribution of myocardial blood flow as a result of increased halothane doses	49
Halothane & O_2, positive pressure ventilation, acute instrumentation, mean arterial pressure reduced to 60% of control values for 1 hr with either pentolinium, trimethaphan or sodium nitroprusside	Mean alveolar concentrations determined during hypotension	Data indicate that anesthetic requirements decrease during deliberate hypotension using any of the three compounds	50

Conditions	Dose	Cardiovascular Effects	Reference
No premedication, induced with 4% halothane, positive pressure ventilation, acute instrumentation	1% inspired	No significant change in fraction of cardiac output perfusing A-V shunts, compared with awake control; no relationship between A-V shunts, as measured with a microsphere technique, and the physiological shunt fraction (Qs/Qt) using the oxygen technique and the standard shunt fraction equation. *This is an unusual result since Qs/Qt has been repeatedly shown to increase with general anesthesia*	51
Programmed stimulation of premature atrial beats	1,1.5 & 2.0 MAC	Lower concentrations increase the probability of spontaneous PVC's after programmed stimulation; the heart was more sensitive to this than it was with equal concentrations of Enflurane; increased concentrations prolonged the atrial effective refractory period and AV nodal functional refractory periods; also prolonged AV nodal internal-related conductivity; more frequent arrhythmias occurred than with Enflurane	52
Open chest, acute prep., masked to anesthesia, intubated, positive pressure ventilation, acute mid-left circumflex or left anterior descending coronary occlusion; compared to fentanyl anesthesia group	0.89 ± 0.2% end-tidal	Decreased regional blood flow within the infarcted region to approximately 3% of normal, decreased blood pressure, cardiac index, LV minute work index; increased HR, all compared to fentanyl group	53
Induced with mask, intubated, positive pressure ventilation, acute instrumentation	1% end-tidal (1.2 MAC)	Mediation of sensitization by halothane to epinephrine-induced arrhythmias, results indicated that this was, predominantly, due to an α-1-adrenergic receptor mechanism	54
Morphine (0.4 mg/ kg,IM), thiamylal (10 mg/kg, IV), positive pressure ventilation, acute instrumentation then thorax closed and air evacuated, isolated and perfused carotid sinus prep.	1%	Carotid sinus reflexes were sensitive and well maintained; resulted in lower mean arterial blood pressures than were seen with pentobarbital or α-chloralose in identical preparations	55

Conditions	Dose	Cardiovascular Effects	Reference
Morphine (4 mg/kg,IV + 0.1 mg/kg/hr,IV), induced with thiopentone (10 mg/kg,IV), succinylcholine (2 mg/ml continuous infusion to paralyzed respiration; afterload increased with phenylephrine	1.5%	Decreased aortic pressure, stroke volume and myocardial O_2 consumption; increasing afterload resulted in a further decrease in the 3 parameters; afterload increase also resulted in a 5% increase in LV end-diastolic diameter and a 32% increase in peak LV pressure	56
Morphine (0.2 mg/kg), atropine (0.01 mg/kg), after 1 hr thiamylal (5 mg/kg,IV), halothane by mask, intubation, positive pressure ventilation, isolated and perfused carotid sinus prep.	0.66 ± 0.02, 0.88 ± 0.02, 1.16 ± 0.03% end-tidal, with and without N_2O (67%)	Over a wide range of baroreceptor stimulation, pulmonary artery resistance and input resistance remained constant with end-tidal concentrations of approximately 0.9%, with or without N_2O; when halothane concentrations were significantly decreased or increased from the 0.9% level, reflex changes became significant, particularly pulmonary vascular resistance	57
Morphine sulfate (4 mg/kg + 0.1 mg/kg/hr,IV), intubation, positive pressure ventilation, succinylcholine (2 mg/ml) in a drip, open chest, acute instrumentation, phenylephrine (0.02 mg/ml/ infusion to 175 mmHg mean aortic pressure	1.5%, end-tidal	Decreased aortic pressure, stroke volume, myocardial oxygen consumption; when afterload was increased with phenylephrine there was a further decrease in stroke volume, cardiac output and myocardial oxygen consumption; left ventricular end-diastolic diameter and pressure were significantly increased by increases in afterload	58
Induced with fentanyl, anesthetized with 0.4% halothane, acute instrumentation	Conc. increased until aortic pressure decreased to approx. 50 mmHg	Cerebral blood flow unchanged, also no change in epidural pressure	59

Conditions	Dose	Cardiovascular Effects	Reference
Anesthetized with chloralose (100 mg/kg,IV), positive pressure ventilation with 100% O_2, Walton-Brodie strain gauge for contractility measurements	0.5 to 3%	Decreased HR, myocardial contractile force and systemic blood pressure	**60**
Induced with chloralose (90 mg/kg,IV) + urethane (900 mg/kg,IV), intubation, positive pressure ventilation, open chest, acute instrumentation, occlusion of LAD coronary	1.1%, end-tidal	Decreased aortic pressure, HR and LV dP/dt, LAD coronary occlusion did not change any of the hemodynamic parameters measured; a measurement of ischemia indicated that halothane was more protective than a nitroprusside-propranolol combination	**61**
Succinylcholine (3 mg/kg,IV), atropine (0.4 mg, IV), intubation, continuous succinylcholine infusion to maintain paralysis, positive pressure ventilation, naloxone (0.006 mg/kg, IV)	0.61 ± 0.03 to 0.73 ± 0.03%	Inconsistent arousal from anesthesia following naloxone indicated an opiate receptor independent action for halothane	**62**
In vitro Purkinje fiber prep.	Dose-response	Dose-dependent decrease in ventricular automaticity	**4**
In vitro Purkinje fiber prep., spontaneously active	2%	Slowing of spontaneous rate, increased threshold potential, decreased slope of phase 4 depolarization, also a steep increase in slope of phase 2, resulted in almost no plateau phase; action potential duration was decreased; sometimes saw no change in aortic pressure duration due to a decreased rate of phase 3; depressed intraventricular conduction	**4**
In vitro Purkinje fiber prep., quiescent	1%	No change in resting membrane potential, no effect on rate of slow diastolic depolarization	**4**

Conditions	Dose	Cardiovascular effects	Reference
Isotope dilution technique to measure norepi kinetics, compared to awake state	Dose-response 1., 1.5 & 2.0 MAC	Significant dose-dependent sympathetic inhibition, caused by decrease in norepi spillover and a decrease in norepi clearance, also decreased mean aortic pressure	**119**
Conscious, previously instrumented	Induction 4%, maintained at 2%, end-tidal	Prolonged PR interval & ventricular effective refractory period, abolished ability to induce ventricular tachycardia in 5 or 10 dogs, in inducible dogs cycle length of tachycardia was increased while number of extra-stimuli required was unchanged	**120**
Evaluated vagal tone in intact dogs using time-series analysis of R-R intervals	2%, inspired	Decreased respiratory sinus arrhythmias, i.e. decreased vagal tone	**121**
Anesthetized with pentobarbital (25 mg/kg,IV) + pancuronium (0.1 mg/kg + 1-2 mg/hr)	0.7 MAC	Decreased HR, mean aortic pressure, mean pulmonary artery pressure, cardiac index, stroke index, ventricular systolic stroke work index, oxygen diffusion and oxygen consumption; increased oxygen extraction ratio; no change in right atrial pressure, wedge pressure, systemic resistance, systolic oxygen consumption or lactate production	**122**
Same as above	1.0 MAC	Same as above but more depression, no change in right atrial pressure, wedge pressure, systemic resistance, all other parameters decreased	**122**
Intact awake, previously instrumented	1.2 %, end-tidal	No change in mean aortic pressure, mean pulmonary arterial pressure, pulmonary wedge pressure, right atrial pressure, pulmonary arterial flow, HR, pH, $PaCO_2$, PaO_2, oxygen saturation, $PvCO_2$, PvO_2 or venous oxygen saturations; Angiotensin II had reduced effect when animals under halothane; pulmonary vasodilator response to ACE inhibition is abolished	**123**
Compared to conscious & pentobarbital (30 mg/kg,IV) anesthetized dogs	Approx. 1.2 %, end-tidal	Active flow-independent pulmonary arterial constriction, decreased aortic pressure and aortic flow; effects not blocked by indomethacin, captopril or the combination of both	**124**

Conditions	Dose	Cardiovascular Effects	Reference
Same as above	Same as above	Active flow-independent pulmonary vasoconstriction at all levels of flow decreased both mean aortic pressure and flow; magnitude of response not significantly reduced by α-adrenergic blockade, angiotensin converting enzyme (ACE) inhibition, combined arginine vasopressin V1 + V2 receptor blockade or by cycloxygenase inhibition	**125**
Isolated cardiac sarcoplasmic reticulum vesicles	0.75 to 2.5%	Decreased net Ca^{2+} accumulation rate, increased ATP consumption, increased passive Ca^{2+} efflux, decreased Ca^{2+} retention	**126**
Thiopentone (500 mg,IV), positive pressure ventilation, maintained with pentobarbital as needed until preparation completed, succinylcholine (40 mg,IV), left lower lung lobe isolation	Dose-response; 0, 0.5, 1.0 & 2.0%	After cyclooxygenase blockade with indomethacin halothane inhibited hypoxic pulmonary artery vasoconstriction by acting on middle segment vessels	**127**
Intact, awake, previously instrumented	1.0 & 1.5 MAC	Dose-dependent prolongation of isovolumetric relaxation, decreased chamber stiffness during passive filling but no change in end-diastolic compliance by stress-strain relationships	**128**
Intact, awake, previously instrumented	1.0 MAC	Increased coronary blood flow secondary to increased HR, increased aortic pressure and pressure-work index; with autonomic blockade no change in coronary blood flow	**129**
Chronically instrumented, intact, awake	1.5 & 2.0 MAC	Decreased contractility in a dose-dependent manner	**130**

Conditions	Dose	Cardiovascular Effects	Reference
Compared to dogs anesthetized with fentanyl; LAD occlusion	0.75 & 1.5%	After 15 minutes of LAD occlusion cardiac output, mean aortic pressure & LV dP/dtmax were decreased in 1.5% but not in 0.75% or fentanyl groups; in all groups LAD occlusion resulted in decreased stroke volume, increased LV end-diastolic pressure and decreased anterior wall function; regional function in the non-ischemic wall improved with fentanyl, was maintained with 0.75% and decreased with 1.5% halothane	131
Anesthetized, measured contractile function of diaphragm, compared to pentobarbital anesthetized dogs	0, 1.0 & 2.0 MAC	Did not depress contractile function of either fresh or "fatigued" diaphragm *in vivo*	132
Intact, awake, slow progressive coronary occlusion of LAD with good collateral development; mean aortic pressure and HR adjusted to conscious levels following anesthesia by using phenylephrine and atrial pacing	1.5 & 2.5%	Dose-dependent decrease in global and regional indices of contractility & arterial pressure; decreased myocardial perfusion in both normal and collateral-dependent regions; decreased major determinants of myocardial oxygen consumption but did not unfavorably alter regional distribution of coronary blood flow in this model	133
Chronically instrumented, intact, awake, ganglionic cholinergic and β-adrenergic blockade + calcium channel stimulation	1.7%	Nonselective decrease of pressor response to both $\alpha 1$- & $\alpha 2$-adrenergic receptor stimulation, apparently not mediated by inhibition of transmembrane Ca^{2+} flux	134
Intact, awake, previously instrumented	Dose-response	Dose-dependent decrease in aortic pressure, LV dP/dt, stroke volume and other measures of myocardial function, increased HR; at 45 mmHg aortic pressure cardiac function was more depressed than it was with isoflurane but less depressed than with enflurane; coronary and renal flow were well maintained	135

Conditions	Dose	Cardiovascular Effects	Reference
Intact, awake, previously instrumented, studied effects of increases and decreases in [Ca^{2+}] in blood	1.2%, end-tidal	Depressed hemodynamic effects of increases and decreases in [Ca^{2+}]; less depressed than enflurane but more depressed than isoflurane; all responses depressed compared to awake dogs	**136**
Intact, awake, previously instrumented	1.25 & 1.75 MAC	Increased HR and systemic resistance; decreased mean aortic pressure and contractility	**118**
Intact, awake, previously instrumented	1.5 MAC	Infusions of CaCl$_2$ resulted in positive inotropic effects in both anesthetized and control states but CaCl$_2$ but did not alter diastolic function; reversed negative inotropic effects of halothane which suggested that the Ca^{2+} might have a diastolic as well as a systolic effect	**189**
7.1:2 Halothane-Cats			
In vitro SA nodal fibers	4%	Progressive decrease in maximum diastolic potential, overshoot and amplitude, with eventual fiber arrest	**4**
Same as above	1%	Moderate negative chronotropy, slightly reduced phase 4 rate and increased threshold potential	**4**
Same as above	2%	Negative chronotropy from reduced rate of phase 4 depolarization and increased threshold potential	**4**
Isolated papillary muscle preparation	Conc. equal to MAC for general anesth. for each individual	Depressed contractility	**63**
Isolated papillary muscle preparation	Dose-response	Dose-dependent decrease in contractility	**64**
Induced with 7% halothane; rapid IV admin. of guanethidine (dose-response)	1.5 to 3.5%, inspired	Severe and sustained ventricular arrhythmias in presence of halothane; more of this response evident in halothane vs urethane anesthetized cats	**65**

Conditions	Dose	Cardiovascular Effects	Reference
Pentobarbital (30 mg/kg,IP), hearts excised and homogenized tissue prep. of myocardium	Dose-response	Significantly decreased the stimulatory effect of catecholamines on myocardial adenylate cyclase without altering the basal or the sodium fluoride-induced adenylate cyclase activity	66
Isolated papillary muscle preparation	0.7 or 1.5%, in O_2 (95%) and CO_2 (5%)	Significantly decreased memory for potentiated state; this indicates that halothane may alter the filling of intracellular Ca^{2+} storage sites, which may be related to the negative inotropic action of halothane	67
Electrically driven and spontaneously beating isolated right ventricular papillary muscle preparations	Dose-response	Decrease in active tension, no change in spontaneous rate; decreased absolute active tension during staircase phenomenon and post-extrasystolic potentiation but this was probably due to a halothane increased percentage increase of developed tension during high voltage stimulation; when tyramine or norepinephrine was added to the bath, halothane decreased the preceding reactions; halothane also increased the threshold for electrical stimulation and lengthened the effective refractory period of the papillary muscle	68
Previously instrumented, microsphere measurements	0.5, 1.0 & 1.5 MAC	Retinal and cerebral blood flow were increased with 1.0 and 1.5 MAC, choroidal blood flow decreased at 1.0 & 1.5 MAC	137
7.1:3 Halothane-Rats			
Previously instrumented with an aortic cannula	2.5% induction, 0.8% maint.	Marked protection against mortality and kidney lesions following bleeding to 30-50 mmHg for 60 minutes	69
Anes. with halothane, cannulas in femoral artery and vein, intubation, tubocurarine (1.5 mg/kg,IV)	1% in 30% O_2	Decreased phenylalanine influx to brain, little, if any, effect on neutral amino acid transport processes	70

Conditions	Dose	Cardiovascular effects	Reference
Cremaster muscle preps., measured internal diameter of small arteries, response to hemorrhage to 30 mmHg aortic pressure	1.2 vol%, inspired	First order vessels; decreased approx. 10, 15 and 15% at 10, 20 & 30 min. respectively; 3rd order vessels, no change; 4th order vessels, decreased approx. 4, 10 & 10% at 10, 20 & 30 min respectively	71
Previously instrumented, measured distribution of blood flow using microsphere technique	1.3%	Flow increased to brain, decreased to heart, increased to kidneys, liver and large intestine, decreased to muscle; there was no change in flow to the lungs, skin, spleen, stomach or small intestine; cardiac output was decreased	72
Compared normal rats and rats with portal hypertension due to iatrogenic obstruction of the portal vein, performed 2 days earlier under ether anes.	Dosed to obtain a level of surgical anesth.	Decreased cardiac output, mean arterial pressure and portal venous pressure in both normal and portal hypertensive rats	73
Compared awake vs halothane anesth. after 1 hr of hemorrhagic shock (40 mmHg)	1.26 vol%	Plasma renin activity not altered by anesthesia, was altered by hemorrhage; results suggest that the influence of anesthesia on survival following severe hemorrhage does not result from anesthetic induced alterations of the renin-angiotensin system	74
Decapitation, isolated atrial prep.	Dose-response	Small, biphasic changes in HR, not mediated by either β-adrenergic or cholinergic mechanisms	75
Two pair of isolated lungs in series at constant pulmonary vascular flows; one of the preps was made atelectatic by airway occlusion, other by ventilation with 2% oxygen	Dose-response	The increase in pulmonary vascular resistance caused by atelectasis was decreased by halothane in a dose-dependent manner	76
Myocardial membrane prep.	5 vol%	No change in maximum response of adenylate cyclase activity to dobutamine and isoproterenol	77

Conditions	Dose	Cardiovascular effects	Reference
Blood flow measured using isotope techniques in awake vs anesth. groups previously instrumented with an aortic cannula	1 & 2 MAC	Decreased arterial pressure with no change in cerebral blood flow	78
Effects on global ischemia in isolated, perfused and pumping heart preps.	1.5%	Significant decrease in cardiac output and minute work, no change in HR or coronary flow; no change in ATP levels prior to ischemia; does not increase basal ATP stores prior to ischemia nor decrease ATP utilization during global ischemia; does not delay the onset of ischemic contracture	79
Decapitation, homogenized tissue preps. of myocardium	Dose-response	Significant decrease in stimulatory effect of catecholamines on myocardial adenylate cyclase without altering the basal or the sodium fluoride-induced adenylate cyclase activity	66
Isolated, cultured myocardial cells from 3-5 day old rats	Dose-response; 10, 20 & 30 mg% (substrate/anesth.	Potent metabolic depressant action on glucose metabolism and fatty acid metabolism	80
Microvascular mesocecum prep., direct observation of vessels after anesth. with pentobarbital (30 mg/kg,IP)	0.55, 1.10 & 1.65%, inspired	Increased vasodilation, venular flow maintained, capillary flow showed only small changes, increased vasomotion and increased sensitivity to norepi	81
Anesth. with diethyl ether, positive pressure ventilation, 100 IU heparin, isolated heart-lung prep.	Plasma conc. equal to those resulting in anesth., nebulized vs perfused	When given via airways halothane inhibits the pulmonary vasoconstrictor response to hypoxia; when given in the perfusate, it had no significant effect on the hypoxic response	82
Chronically instrumented, halothane admin. immediately after LAD occlusion	0. 0.5 or 1.0%	Was antiarrhythmic; decreased incidence of ventricular fibrillation and mortality	138

Conditions	Dose	Cardiovascular effects	Reference
Isolated rat hearts (Langendorff prep.), treated for 15 min before and after LAD occlusion	0.5 or 1.0%; 2.0 or 4.0%	Little effect at low conc., at 2.0 or 4.0% increased incidence of ventricular fibrillation; dose-dependent decrease in peak left ventricular pressures	138
Pressor response to nitric oxide synthase inhibitor, L-NNA	4% induction + 1.5% maint.	Pressor response attenuated more than with enflurane	139
IV bolus of L-NNA (32 mg/kg)	4% induction + 1.5% maint.	Increased mean aortic pressure only 3 ± 2 mmHg when anesthetized, when conscious increased pressure 51.3 mmHg	140
Measured cerebral plasma volume (CPV)	1 MAC	CPV = 2.96 ± 0.44 ml/100 g brain tissue compared to pentobarbital anesthetized where CPV = 2.1 ± 0.26 ml/100 g	140
Isolated left atrium, decapitated, atrium electrically stimulated	1.5% V/V	Decreased inhibitory concentration of morphine, i.e. increased the potency of morphine, effect probably mediated by opiod receptors	141
Myocardial prep., made permeable by mild homogenization, saponin &/or 2% Triton X-100	1.9 & 9.4 mM	Maximal force decreased, increased Ca^{2+} sensitivity; components assoc. with cellular membrane systems normally modulate force, halothane has complex effects on these components	142
Intact, awake, responses to hypoxemia	1 MAC	Brain and coronary blood flow increase during hypoxemia in awake rats, decreased in anesthetized; no response to hypoxemia in renal, GI or total hepatic blood flows in awake rats, decreased significantly with anesthesia and hypoxemia	143
Ten min. of bilateral carotid artery occlusion with simultaneous hypotension; halothane with normothermia vs halothane with hypothermia; after 3 days survival histopathological injury evaluated	1.3 MAC	Moderate to severe injury to observed portions of brain, no difference between normo- & hypo-thermia groups or normothermia isoflurane group	144

Conditions	Dose	Cardiovascular effects	Reference
Pressor response to N^G-nitro-L-arginine (L-NNA) a nitric oxide synthase inhibitor	1 MAC	Markedly attenuated pressor response to L-NNA compared to conscious rats	**139**
Compared normo- and hypo-capnia in halothane and isoflurane anesthetized (2 X 2 factorial design)	1.05 %, inspired	Hypocapnia decreased global cerebral blood flow (CBF) by 30% in both halothane and isoflurane groups; CBF was greater in 3 cortical samples in both normo- and hypo-capnic groups anesthetized with halothane than with isoflurane	**145**
Isolated heart (Langendorff) with constant pressure head, heart arrested with tetrodotoxin, coronary flow reserve defined as the difference between coronary flow prior to and during administration of a maximally dilating dose of adenosine	0 - 3 MAC	Dose-dependent decrease in magnitude of coronary vascular resistance and of coronary flow reserve; latter the same as with isoflurane but significantly more than with sevoflurane	**146**
Normocapnic, normothermic	0.75 MAC + 60% N_2O	Cerebral blood flow associated with major electrocorticogram changes and sustained depolarization, same as with Isoflurane /N_2O, as were isoelectricity, incidence of sustained depolarization; in rats subjected to cardiac arrest and to carotid occlusion time to depolarization was longer in isoflurane/N_2O; cortical cerebral metabolic rate for glucose was decreased with isoflurane/N_2O	**147**

7.1:4 Halothane-Guinea pigs	Dose	Cardiovascular effects	Reference
Isolated papillary muscles after stunning with a blow to the head	0.5 to 4% in 5% CO_2 and 95% O_2	Concentrations $\geq 1\%$ inhibited slow Na^+, Ca^{2+} channels; negative inotropic effects may be due, in part, to decreased Ca^{2+} influx; negative inotropy with 0.5% concentrations, wherein slow actions potentials are unaffected, suggests additional mechanisms not involving the slow channels	83
Decapitated, isolated SA node preparations	1 & 2 MAC equivalents	Significant decrease in HR, slope of phase 4 and phase and a decrease in action potential duration; at 2 MAC there was a significant decrease in action potential amplitude and overshoot; no changes in threshold potential; maximum diastolic potentials decreased only with 2 MAC concentrations	84
Isolated papillary muscle preps.; analyzed effects of halothane on action potential elicited by field stimulation and upon isoproterenol-induced slow action potentials	0.5-4% in 95% O_2 and 5% CO_2	Concentrations of 0.5, 1 and 2% decreased twitch tension for both types of action potentials; Vmax of normal AP not depressed by $\geq 3\%$ concentrations but amplitude and duration of the AP decreased; on slow AP's concentrations of $\geq 1\%$ caused a dose-dependent decrease in Vmax amplitude and duration; results suggest that negative inotropy of halothane is due, in part, to inhibition of the slow Na^+, Ca^{2+} channels plus a possible depression of internal Ca^{2+} release	85
IP ketamine + decapitation, isolated papillary muscle prep.	0.65 & 1.15%	Dose-dependent decrease in inotropy closely related to decreased Ca^{2+} transients	148
Isolated heart prep. (Langendorff), compared to effects of N_2 & N_2O exposures	Dose-response	Dose-dependent decrease in left ventricular pressure, positive and negative dP/dtmax, myocardial oxygen consumption, HR and % O_2 extraction; no change in coronary flow or oxygen diffusion rate	148

7.1:5 Halothane-Rabbits	Dose	Cardiovascular effects	Reference
In vitro SA nodal fibers	2%	Caused a significant decrease in overshoot and repolarization was slightly prolonged; no marked changes in resting potential or amplitude of the action potential	4
In vitro SA nodal fibers	1%	Moderate decrease in rate, slightly reduced rate of slow diastolic depolarization and an increase in threshold potential	4
Same as above	2%	Decreased rate from reduced rate of phase 4 depolarization and increased threshold potential	4
Same as above	4%	Progressive decrease in maximum diastolic potential, overshoot and amplitude with eventual fiber arrest	4
Anesthetized with pentobarbital (about 45 mg/kg,IV); heart excised, right ventricular papillary muscle isolated preparation	0.6 & 1%	Data suggest that negative inotropic effects are caused by a combination of quantitatively similar effects of the anesthetic on the transsarcolemmal and intracellular sources of activator Ca^{2+}	86
Mechanically disrupted myocardial fiber preparations; hearts were excised after cervical dislocation	1-4%, dose-response	Increasing doses significantly shifted the relationship between Ca^{2+} and tension towards higher Ca^{2+} concentrations and depressed the maximum Ca^{2+} activated tension; concluded that halothane slightly, but significantly, decreased the interactions of contractile proteins and, to a lesser degree, Ca^{2+} activation of the regulatory proteins	87
Isolated heart prep.	1 X 10-4, 1 X 10^{-3} and 5 X 10^{-3} mol/l	Dose-dependent decrease it heart rate and inotropy	89
Isolated lung prep.	Dose-response	Enhanced lipid peroxide tertiary butyl-hydroperoxide-induced pulmonary vasoconstrictions	150

7.1:6 Halothane-Pigs	Dose	Cardiovascular effects	Reference
Anesthetized with halothane to effect, open chest, total and right heart bypass	0.5% additional to anesthetic level	Decreased stroke volume, myocardial oxygen consumption during normoxia; during hypoxia myocardial O2 consumption increased; decreased coronary blood flow, lactate extraction and myocardial pO_2 and pCO_2	89
Induced with halothane, intubated, positive pressure ventilation, closed chest	0.05-1.7 vol% end-tidal in 60% N_2O and remainder O_2	Dose-dependent decrease in aortic pressure, cardiac output, peak LV dP/dt, Vmax and ejection fraction; non-dose-dependent decrease in HR and circumferential fiber shortening rate; no effect on LV compliance	90
Induced with thiamylal, maintained with N_2O (60%), positive pressure ventilation, open chest, extracorporal constant pressure perfusion between the femoral and right coronary arteries	0.8% local conc., 0.5% systemic conc.	Coronary vasodilation with subsequent increased flow during constant perfusion pressure, accompanied by a decrease in dP/dt	91
Right and total heart by-pass, acute instrumentation, compared regional conduction anesthesia between morphine (10 mg/kg) and halothane	0.5%, inspired	Direct depression of myocardial function independent of changes in filling pressure, arterial pressure and HR; during normoxia depression was accompanied by a decrease in myocardial oxygen consumption, during cyanosis halothane decreased myocardial function more than morphine or regional block; hypoxic depression was accompanied by an increase in myocardial oxygen consumption	89
Newborn pigs, intact, awake, previously instrumented	0.5, 1.0 & 1.5 MAC	Decreased heart rate, mean aortic pressure and cardiac index	151
Hepatic ischemia-reperfusion model, induction with methohexitol (20 mg/kg,IM) + pancuronium (0.1 mg/kg)	0.9%, end-expired	Provided less protection from hepatic ischemia-reperfusion injury than isoflurane or fentanyl, same amount of protection as enflurane or pentobarbital	152

Conditions	Dose	Cardiovascular effects	Reference
Intact, awake, previously instrumented piglets; < 2 mos of age; pressor & depressor tests (phenylephrine & nitroprusside) to construct stimulus-response curves of mean aortic pressure to HR	0.45, 0.9 & 1.35%	Dose-dependent decrease in baroreflex sensitivity, decreased resting heart rate and decrease limits and narrowed the range of the baroreflex HR response; decreased resting blood pressure, decreased lower limit and widened the span of the baroreflex blood pressure range	153
Acutely instrumented, compared halothane to pentobarbital anesth.	Dose-response	Dose-dependent decrease in left ventricular pressure, LV dP/dtmax and cardiac output; no appreciable effect upon occlusion-induced arrhythmias when compared to pentobarbital anesthesia in pigs	138
Surgical preparation enabling stepwise decrease in hepatic blood flow without hepatic hypoperfusion	0.9% end-expired	Decreased hepatic oxygen delivery the most compared to isoflurane, enflurane, fentanyl and pentobarbital; decreased hepatic lactate uptake when hepatic flows were lowered	154
Sedated with 120 mg azaperidone IM, anesthetized with 150 mg metomidate, IV, intubated & maintained with oxygen:N_2O (1:2) & 1% halothane	1% halothane (added to previous)	Decreased HR, cardiac output, LV dP/dt, mean aortic pressure, peripheral resistance, left ventricular blood flow, left ventricular oxygen delivery and LV oxygen consumption	155
7.1:7 Halothane-Sheep			
In vitro ventricular cell preparation (Purkinje fibers)	2%	Resting potential unchanged, overshoot decreased significantly, action potential duration decreased and effective refractory period shortened	4
In vitro Purkinje fiber preparation	1%	Resting potential increased, overshoot and duration of action potential decreased	4

Conditions	Dose	Cardiovascular effects	Reference
1-3 day old lambs, previously instrumented	0.5 & 1.0 MAC	Decreased total body oxygen consumption, cardiac output & mean aortic pressure; lower concentration had no effect on organ blood flow except muscle which decreased 64%; 1.0 MAC decreased blood flow to brain, heart, kidney, muscle and gut; both concentrations decreased serum catecholamines and prevented hypoxia from increasing serum catecholamines; did not prevent redistribution of blood flow to the heart and brain in hypoxic lambs, nor did it prevent hypoxic pulmonary vasoconstriction	**156**
7.1:8 Halothane-Horses			
Induction by mask, intubation, spontaneous and controlled ventilation, acute instrumentation	Equivalent to 1.0, 1.5 & 2.0 MAC to standard pain stimulus	Dose-dependent decrease in cardiovascular function, less severe during spontaneous ventilation and associated hypercapnia; increased systemic resistance independent of dose	**92**
Sedated with xylazine (0.5 mg/kg), induced with guaifenesin (10%), thiamylal (0.4%) to effect, IV; intubation, varied F_{IO2} (0.3 or >0.85	1.2%, end-tidal	Mean aortic pressure, cardiac output, central venous pressure, pulmonary arterial pressure, arterial pH and arterial base excess not different between groups during 4 hours of anesthesia; end-tidal pCO_2, $PaCO_2$, PaO_2 & alveolar-to-arterial O_2 tension greater in horses exposed to >0.85 F_{IO2}; greater hypoventilation and ventilation/perfusion mismatch in horses breathing higher oxygen concentrations	**157**
Halothane combined with succinylcholine	Halothane to effect, surgical plane	When combined with succinylcholine resulted in malignant hyperthermia in a significant number of cases	**158**

7.1:9 Halothane-Primates (Old World)	Dose	Cardiovascular effects	Reference
1 baboon & 1 chimpanzee, intact, previously instrumented, breathing 100% O_2	1 & 2%, inspired	Concentration-dependent decrease in myocardial contractility, increased left ventricular end-diastolic diameter; at 1% conc., renal vascular resistance decreased; at 2% regional blood flow increased with time	**71**
Baboons, chronic renovascular hypertension, anesth. with Phencyclidine (12 mg,IM), thiopentone (7.5 mg/kg,IV), N_2O (78% in O_2), phencyclidine (3-4 mg,IM/30 min), suxamethonium (50 mg, IM/30 min), positive pressure ventilation	Dose-response	Graded hypotension induced over 5-6 hr by increased concentrations of halothane; cerebral blood flow remained constant until the mean blood pressure decreased to approx. 90 mmHg, at aortic pressures less than 90 mmHg cerebral blood flow was pressure passive, i.e. no longer autoregulated	**93**
Intact, awake, previously instrumented	1 & 2%, end-tidal	Concentration-dependent decrease in LV dP/dt, increase in LV end-diastolic diameter; at 1% decreased renal resistance and increased mesenteric resistance; at 1% regional vascular resistance tended to increase with time, at 2% it tended to decrease with time	**14**
7.1:10 Halothane-Ferrets			
Isolated right ventricular papillary muscle, anesth. with 100 mg/kg pentobarbital, IP; heart excised as soon as surgical plane of anesthesia reached	Dose-response, 0-1.5 MAC in 0.25 MAC increments	Concentration-dependent decrease in developed force; alteration in myofibrillar Ca^{2+} responsiveness is minor relative to decrease in intracellular Ca^{2+} availability	**117**

7.1:11 Halothane-Beaver	Dose	Cardiovascular effects	Reference
Diazepam (0.1 mg/kg) and ketamine (25 mg/kg),IM; compared spontaneously breathing vs positive pressure ventilation	approx. 1% end-expired	Parameters measured after 30, 60, 75 & 90 min of halothane; no change in HR, respiratory rate increased in spontaneously breathing, arterial pH decreased in spontaneously breathing, while $PaCO_2$ decreased, end-tidal CO_2 increased, PaO_2 decreased but no difference in mean aortic pressures between the groups	159
7.1:12 Halothane-Chickens			
Intact, awake	Dose-response	Dose-dependent decrease in respiratory and cardiovascular function	160

Table 7.2: The Cardiovascular Effects of Enflurane

Conditions of the experiment	Dose	Cardiovascular effects	Reference
7.2:1 Enflurane-Dogs			
Previously instrumented, respiration controlled with positive pressure ventilation, succinylcholine (3 mg/kg,IV) vs spontaneous respiration; carotid chemoreceptor stimulation with intracarotid injections of nicotine (8 or 12 µg)	2 & 4 vol%, inhaled	Unanesthetized carotid chemoreceptor stimulation resulted in increased iliac vascular resistance and an increase in cardiac cycle length, i.e. decreased HR; with 2% enflurane the carotid chemoreceptor stimulation responses were attenuated and with 4% they were abolished	94

Conditions	Dose	Cardiovascular effects	Reference
Intact, awake, chronically instrumented and isolated heart-lung preps. from the same dogs	2 & 4 vol%, inspired	Dose-dependent increase in HR, decreases in stroke shortening, maximum velocity of LV fiber shortening, LV systolic pressure, dP/dt and mean aortic pressure; diastolic performance was only moderately affected, i.e. moderate increase in LV end-diastolic pressure at higher concentrations with no change in end-diastolic dimensions; the same effects were seen with spontaneous rather than controlled ventilation and β-adrenergic blockade or combined β- and cholinergic blockade; in the isolated heart-lung preps. there was an increase in LV end-diastolic pressure and diameter; it appears that LV unloading is mandatory in order to prevent acute myocardial failure from higher doses	95
Intact, awake, programmed stimulation of premature atrial beats	1, 1.5 & 2 MAC	Lower concentrations increased the probability of spontaneous premature beats after programmed stimulation; the response was less sensitive than with equal concentrations of halothane; increased concentrations prolonged the atrial effective refractory period and AV nodal functional refractory period; experimental arrhythmias occurred less frequently than with halothane	52
Closed chest, catheterized, awake	1.6 vs 3.2%, end-tidal	Increased concentrations resulted in increased LV end-diastolic pressures, decreases in aortic pressure, cardiac output, stroke volume, LV dP/dt, myocardial blood flow and myocardial oxygen consumption; there was no change in systemic resistance, or in oxygen or lactate extraction by the heart	46
Intact, awake, previously instrumented	2.53, 3.78 & 5.06%, end-tidal	No change in spontaneous cycle length or ventricular specialized conduction; HIS-Purkinje specialized conduction increased at 5.06%, AV nodal conduction increased at 3.78 and 5.06%	13
Intact, awake, atrial pacing	Dose-response	Dose-dependent impairment of AV nodal conduction with minimal effects of HIS-Purkinje conduction	4

Conditions	Dose	Cardiovascular effects	Reference
Positive pressure ventilation, normocapnea, normothermia, HIS bundle electrocardiography with closed chest, response to pancuronium (0.1 mg/ kg,IV) compared to halothane effects	1.25% end-tidal MAC	No change in HIS-Purkinje or ventricular conduction following pancuronium; spontaneous HR increased but less than with halothane, AV nodal conduction decreased but less than with halothane, atrial effective refractory period increased, there was no change with halothane; AV nodal functional refractory period decreased whereas there was no change with halothane	96
Anesthetized with thiopental (15-20 mg/ kg,IV), compared untreated group to pretreatment with Pargyline (100 mg/day/ os-a MAO inhibitor) and pretreatment with Imipramine (25 mg/ day/os- a tricyclic anti-depressant), positive pressure ventilation	2.6%	Response to exogenous dose of epinephrine on arterial pressure; No pretreatment- 90 ± 18 to 168 ± 30 increase Imipramine- 101 ± 31 to 177 ± 22 increase Pargyline- 82 ± 19 to 154 ± 19 increase Was more effective than halothane but less effective than methoxyflurane in protecting against epinephrine induced ventricular disrhythmias	18
Thiopentone (5-10 mg/ kg,IV) vs Ketamine (8-12 mg/kg,IM), intubated, positive pressure ventilation, 40% N_2O & 60% O_2; response to 1.4 µg/kg/ min adrenaline	1 to 5%, inspired	Dose-dependent decrease in aortic pressure; when an arrhythmia occurred the adrenalin infusion was stopped; there was no relationship observed between the inspired concentration or enflurane and the onset of arrhythmias	97
Thiopentone (up to 300 mg), atropine (0.6 mg), intubation, alcuronium (2-5 mg), positive pressure ventilation	0.8 to 2.1%, end-tidal (0.4 to 1.0 MAC)	Dose-dependent myocardial depression, decreased cardiac index and aortic pressure, no change in central venous pressure; there was a sudden decrease in renal function at concentrations greater than 1 MAC	16

Conditions	Dose	Cardiovascular effects	Reference
Anesthetized with pentobarbitone (30 mg/ kg,IV), suxamethonium (100 mg), intubated, positive pressure ventilation adjusted to maintain a constant $PaCO_2$ and PaO_2, open chest, acute instrumentation, left anterior descending coronary artery ligation	1.5%, inspired	Produced a significantly smaller reduction in blood flow in the ischemic vs non-ischemic myocardium in the presence of a 46% decrease in mean aortic pressure. The improvement in oxygen availability/ consumption ratio in the ischemic vs non-ischemic areas was attributed to a 16% decrease in HR	98
Acute preparation, controlled ventilation	1 MAC	Decreased hepatic arterial, portal venous and superior mesenteric arterial blood flows by approx. 35%; decreased mean aortic pressures about 45% and cardiac output approx. 35%; suggests autoregulation within preportal and hepatic vascular beds to cope with decreased perfusion pressures; decrease in hepatic arterial resistance also counteracted by a marked decrease of portal oxygen supply to liver	99
Sarcoplasmic reticulum prep.	0.6 to 2.8%	Stimulated calcium uptake at low concentration of ATP (0.5-2.0 mM), does not alter uptake at 5 & 10 mM ATP; at 2.8% there was a decrease in Km for ATP from approx. 2 mM to 0.25 mM with no change in Vmax of Ca^{2+} uptake	100
Pentobarbital (25 mg/ kg,IV) + pancuronium (0.1 mg/kg + 1-2 mg/ hr)	0.7 MAC	Decreased HR, mean aortic pressure, mean pulmonary arterial pressure, cardiac index, LV stroke work index, LV oxygen delivery & LV oxygen consumption; increased LV oxygen extraction ratio and lactate; no change in right atrial pressure, pulmonary arterial wedge pressure, stroke index, systemic resistance or systemic oxygen consumption	122

Conditions	Dose	Cardiovascular effects	Reference
Intact, awake, previously instrumented	Dose-response	Dose-dependent decrease in blood pressure, LV dP/dt & other measures of myocardial function, stroke volume, increased HR; at 45 mmHg blood pressure cardiac function more depressed than with halothane or isoflurane at equivalent levels of blood pressure; coronary and renal flow well maintained	135
Intact, awake, previously instrumented; studied the effects of decreases and increases in $[Ca^{2+}]$ in blood	2.5%, end-tidal	Hemodynamic effects caused by increases and decreases in $[Ca^{2+}]$ greater than in dogs anesthetized with isoflurane or halothane; depressed responses compared to awake dogs	136
Chronically instrumented, intact, awake, hemorrhagic shock model	3%	Conscious dogs able to tolerate considerably more severe levels of hemorrhage than enflurane anesthetized; response to hemorrhage in conscious dogs primarily from sympathoadrenal system, in anesthetized dogs the renin-angiotensin system predominated; later defense mechanisms not sufficiently powerful to prevent overall hemodynamic deterioration with hemorrhage during anesthesia with enflurane	161
Intact, awake, previously instrumented	1.25 & 1.75 MAC	Increased HR & systemic resistance, decreased mean aortic pressure and myocardial contractility	118
7.2:2 Enflurane-Cats			
Isolated papillary muscle prep.	Dose-response	Dose-dependent decrease in contractile properties	64
Isolated papillary muscle prep.	Conc. equal to MAC for general anesthesia for each individual	Depressed contractility to a greater extent than diethyl ether, cyclopropane, methoxyflurane or halothane	63

7.2:3 Enflurane-Rats	Dose	Cardiovascular effects	Reference
Isolated, cultured myocardial cells from 3-5 day old rats	Dose-response (10,20 & 30 mg%) substrate/ anesthesia	Decreased glucose metabolism but produced a less profound disruption of fatty acid metabolism than did halothane	**80**
Isolated atrial prep. from decapitated rats	Dose-response	Dose-dependent increase in HR, not mediated by β-adrenergic or cholinergic mechanisms	**75**
Two pairs of isolated rat lungs in series, constant pulmonary vascular flow; one of the preps. was made atelectatic by airway occlusion, the other by ventilation with 2% O_2	Dose-response	The increase in pulmonary vascular resistance caused by atelectasis was decreased by the enflurane	**76**
Previously instrumented with an aortic cannula; induced with 4% enflurane	1.5 or 7.5%	Marked protection against mortality and occurrence of kidney lesions following bleeding induced hypotension (30-50 mmHg) for 60 min	**69**
Cremaster muscle prep., measured internal diameter of microvasculature before and after response to hemorrhage to 30 mmHg	2.2 vol%, inspired	First order vessels; decreased approx. 20% at 10 & 20 min after hemorrhage, decreased approx. 36% at 30 min post-hemorrhage. Third order vessels; decreased approx. 3% at 30 min, no change at 10 or 20 min. Fourth order vessels; decreased approx. 85, 88 and 92% at 10, 20 & 30 min, respectively	**71,101**
Previously instrumented, awake, used microsphere technique to measure distribution of blood flow; each rat served as its own control	2.2%	Flow was decreased to the heart and muscle, increased to the liver, spleen and large intestine; no change in blood flow occurred in the brain, lung, skin, kidneys, stomach or small intestine; there was no change in cardiac output	**72**
Isolated atria prep.	Dose-response	Dose-dependent increase in HR, but less negative than response caused by methoxyflurane or diethyl ether	**4**
Awake vs anesth., isotope techniques	1 & 2 MAC	Decreased aortic pressure with no change in cerebral blood flow	**78**

Conditions	Dose	Cardiovascular effects	Reference
Mesocecum prep., direct observation of microvasculature, anesth. with pentobarbitone (30 mg/ kg,IP)	1, 2 & 3%, inspired	Increased vasodilation, venular flow maintained, small modifications in capillary flow an increased vasomotion; sensitivity to norepinephrine decreased	**81**
Pressor response to N^G-nitro-L-arginine (L-NNA- nitric oxide synthase inhibitor)	1 MAC	Markedly attenuated pressor response to L-NNA compared to conscious rats	**139**
Myocardial prep., made permeable by mild homogenization, saponin and/or 2% Triton X-100	3.3 & 16.5 mM	Increased Ca^{2+} sensitivity, no effect on maximal developed force; Complex effects on components assoc. with cellular membrane that normally modulate force	**142**
IV bolus response to L-NNA (32 mg/kg) (nitric oxide synthase inhibitor)	4% induction, 1.5% maint.	Increased mean aortic pressure 22 ± 3 mmHg (conscious 51.3 mmHg)	**139**
Previously instrumented compared to conscious rats	2%	Decreased respiratory rate, aortic blood pressure, HR and cardiac output; respiratory depression rapidly reversed by thyrotropin-releasing hormone	**162**
Pressor response to nitric oxide synthase inhibitor L-NNA	4% induction, 1.5% maint.	Increased aortic pressure response attenuated by the anesthetic	**139**
Compared to intact, awake responses to hypoxemia	1 MAC	Brain & coronary blood flow increased during hypoxemia in awake rats decreased in anesthetized; no response to hypoxemia in renal, GI or total hepatic blood flows in awake rats, decreased significantly with anesthesia + hypoxemia	**143**
7.2:4 Enflurane-Rabbits			
Functionally skinned myocardial fibers	1.0 to 7.5% conc. in bath	Significant but small decrease of maximum Ca^{2+}-activated tension at 5%; no change in $[Ca^{2+}]$ required for half-maximal activation; markedly inhibited Ca^{2+} uptake by sarcoplasmic reticulum at 2.5 to 7.5% (dose-dependent); concluded that myocardial depression was mainly due to inhibition of Ca^{2+} uptake by the sarcoplasmic reticulum	**103**

Conditions	Dose	Cardiovascular effects	Reference
Acute instrumentation under ether anesth.	1, 3 & 5%, inspired	Dose-dependent decrease in aortic pressure, HR, respiratory rate & respiratory amplitude; no change in plasma levels of Na^+, K^+ or Ca^{2+}, no change in ECG pattern	**104**
7.2:5 Enflurane-Guinea pigs			
IP ketamine + decapitation, isolated papillary muscle prep.	1.0 & 2.2%	Dose-dependent decrease in inotropy closely related to decreased Ca^{2+} transients	**148**
Isolated heart prep. (Langendorff), compared to effects of N_2 & N_2O exposures	Dose-response	Dose-dependent decrease in LV peak pressure, +LV dP/dtmax, -LV dP/dtmax, myocardial oxygen consumption, HR & % oxygen extraction; no change in coronary flow or oxygen diffusion	**149**
7.2:6 Enflurane-Pigs			
Thiamylal + 60% N_2O, positive pressure ventilation, open chest, extracorporeal constant pressure perfusion between a femoral artery and the right coronary artery	2% local conc., 1.5% systemic conc.	Coronary vasodilation with increased flow during constant perfusion pressure and with no change in myocardial activity as measured by LV dP/dt	**91**
Surgical prep. which enabled the induction of stepwise decreases in hepatic blood supply without induced hepatic hypoperfusion	2.2% end-expired	Decreased hepatic oxygen delivery and decreased hepatic lactate uptake at lowered hepatic blood flows	**154**
Hepatic ischemia-reperfusion model; induction with methohexital (20 mg/kg,IM) + pancuronium (0.1 mg/kg)	2.2 end-expired conc.	Provided less protection than isoflurane or fentanyl from hepatic ischemia; reperfusion injury same as halothane & pentobarbital	**152**

7.2:7 Enflurane-Ferrets	Dose	Cardiovascular effects	Reference
Isolated right ventricular papillary muscle, anesth. Pentobarbital (100 mg/kg,IP); heart excised as soon as surgical plane of anesth. achieved	Dose-response, 0.1.5 MAC in 0.25 MAC increments	Concentration-dependent decrease in developed force; alteration in myofibrillar Ca^{2+} responsiveness minor relative to decreased intracellular Ca^{2+} availability	117

Table 7.3: The Cardiovascular Effects of Methoxyflurane

Conditions of the experiment	Dose	Cardiovascular effects	Reference
7.3:1 Methoxyflurane-Dogs			
Intact, awake, previously instrumented	Dose-response	Dose-dependent increase in functional refractory period of AV conduction system	4
Intact, vagotomized and trimethadinium pretreated; compared response to saline infusion at 0.76 ml/min vs ouabain equal volume and rate (36 μg/kg/hr)	0.3 & 1.6%	Dose-dependent increase in functional refractory period of AV system, digitalization further increased the AV functional refractory period and increased contractile force; increased time of ouabain infusion was required to produce ventricular disrhythmias; vagotomy decreased time to ouabain-induced arrhythmias; increased digitalis tolerance	15
Anesth. with thiopental and pentobarbital (no doses given), inserted a tracheal divider to ventilate each lung separately	0.5%	Marked decrease in cardiac output; no apparent effect of methoxyflurane on pulmonary vasoconstrictor responses	105
Hexobarbital anesthesia (no dose given), heparin (300 IU/kg), bled to cardiac arrest, isolated perfused lung prep. with lungs ventilated	2.5%	No effect during normotonic perfusion but enhanced pulmonary flow during microembolism-induced pulmonary hypertension	44

Conditions	Dose	Cardiovascular effects	Reference

Thiopental (15-20 mg/ kg,IV), positive pressure ventilation; compared untreated group to a group treated with Pargyline (100 mg/day/os) and another treated with imipramine (25 mg/day/os)	0.28% in 50% N_2	Response to exogenous dose of epinephrine:
		    Control group-aortic pressure increased from 97 ± 27 to 176 ± 42
		    Imipramine- aortic pressure increased from 93 ± 29 to 217 ± 16
		    Pargyline- aortic pressure increased from 107 ± 34 to 204 ± 20
		Methoxyflurane was more effective than enflurane or halothane in protecting against epinephrine induced disrhythmias
			18

In vitro SA nodal prep.	0.5 to 1.0%	Decreased rate leading to arrest of SA nodal activity, associated with loss of maximum diastolic potential, an increase in threshold potential and a loss of excitability; all of this followed an initial increase in rate chiefly due to a slight loss in maximal diastolic potential	4
Purkinje fiber prep.	0.5 and 1.0%	Quiescent fibers showed slightly less negative resting potentials but no automaticity developed; spontaneously active fibers showed a marked increase in rate	4
7.3:2 Methoxyflurane-Cats			
Isolated papillary muscle prep.	0.25 and 0.45% delivered to the bath, actual conc. not measured	Dose-dependent decrease in total developed tension; staircase phenomena and post-extrasystolic potentiation did not seem to be affected; no significant changes in increase of developed tension or in the effective refractory period initiated by high voltage electrical stimulation or tyramine	108
Isolated papillary muscle prep.	Conc. equal to MAC for general anesth. for each individual	Depressed contractility more than diethyl ether and cyclopropane but less than halothane and enflurane	63

7.3:3 Methoxyflurane-Rats	Dose	Cardiovascular effects	Reference
Previously instrumented with aortic cannulae; induced with 2.5% methoxyflurane	0.3 or 0.6%	Marked protection against mortality and occurrence of kidney lesions following bleeding to 30-50 mmHg for 60 min	**69**
Decapitation, isolated atrial prep.	Dose-response	Dose-dependent increase in HR, not β-adrenergic or cholanergically mediated	**75**
7.3:4 Methoxyflurane-Rabbits			
Isolated arterial microsomes	Dose-response	Inhibition of acyl co-enzyme A and cholesterol acyltransferase	**109**
Functionally skinned right ventricular papillary muscles	2, 3 & 4%	Slightly decreased maximum Ca^{2+}-activated tension; submaximum Ca^{2+}-activated tension also decreased; at 3 & 4% decreased the caffeine-induced tension transient at the uptake phase; no change in caffeine-induced tension transient at the release phase; concluded that myocardial depression is partly achieved by decreasing Ca^{2+}-activation of the contractile proteins, but less depressive effect than halothane or enflurane	**110**
7.3:5 Methoxyflurane-Guinea pigs			
Isolated atrial prep.	0.15, 0.25 & 0.45% delivered to bath, actual conc. not measured	Dose-dependent decrease in developed tension but no change in rate of spontaneous beating; no change in staircase phenomena or post-extrasystolic potentiation	**108**
Decapitated, isolated SA nodal prep.	1 & 2 MAC equivalent	Significant decrease in HR, slope of phase 4 and phase 0 and decrease in action potential duration; at 2 MAC significant decrease in action potential amplitude and overshoot, no change in threshold potential	**84**

Table 7.4: The Cardiovascular Effects of Isoflurane

Conditions of the experiment	Dose	Cardiovascular Effects	Reference
7.4:1 Isoflurane-Dogs			
Intact, awake, previously instrumented	1.25 & 2.0%, end-tidal	No significant change in contractility at 1.25% but significant decrease at 2.0%; measured slope of the end-systolic pressure-length relationship; LV peak pressure and LV dP/dt decreased with 1.25% and decreased much more with 2.0%	**106**
Intact, awake, previously instrumented	1.73, 2.58, 3.45%, end-tidal	No change in spontaneous cycle length, HIS-Purkinje or ventricular specialized conduction; at 3.45% AV nodal specialized conduction increased	**13**
Closed chest, catheterized	1.6% & 3.2%, end-tidal	There was a 40-60% decrease in mean aortic pressures, cardiac output, stroke volume, LV dP/dt and systemic resistance without changing HR, LV end-diastolic pressure, myocardial blood flow, myocardial oxygen or lactate extraction by the heart at higher concentration	**46**
Chronic concentric valvular LV hypertrophy created by non-coronary cusp obliteration in 8 week old puppies; instrumented 7-10 days prior to the experiment	1.25 & 2.0%, end-tidal	Significant decrease in peak LV pressure and LV dP/dt but no change in the end-systolic, pressure-volume relationship at 1.25%; at 2.0% all 3 parameters were significantly lowered; there was no change in maximum fiber length shortening	**107**
Sarcoplasmic reticulum prep.	0.6 to 3%	Stimulates Ca^{2+} uptake at low concentrations of ATP, but no effect at high conc. (5 & 10 mM); less effect than enflurane in this regard; at 3% decreased Km for ATP to 0.8 mM; no effect on Vmax of Ca^{2+} uptake	**100**

Conditions	Dose	Cardiovascular effects	Reference
Pentobarbital (25 mg/ kg,IV) + pancuronium (0.1 mg/kg + 1-2 mg/ hr)	0.7 MAC	Decreased HR, mean aortic pressure, cardiac index, LV stroke work index, oxygen delivery, oxygen consumption; increased oxygen extraction ratio; no change in mean pulmonary arterial pressure, right atrial pressure, pulmonary wedge pressure, systemic resistance, mixed venous O_2 saturations, oxygen diffusion or lactate	122
Effect of left circumflex ligation on regional myocardial function	Dose-response	Dose-dependent decrease in fractional shortening and a shift to the right in the end-systolic pressure-length relationship, i.e. a deleterious effect on preexisting myocardial ischemia	163
Isolated cardiac sarcoplasmic reticulum vesicles	2.5 - 4%	Decreased net Ca^{2+} accumulation rate, increased ATP consumption, increased passive Ca^{2+} efflux, decreased Ca^{2+} retention	126
Intact, awake, previously instrumented; induced with thiopentone (5-8 mg/kg,IV), positive pressure ventilation	2.0 MAC	Marked but short-lasting effect on disposition of propranolol due to a decrease in intrinsic clearance	164
Intact, awake, previously instrumented	1.0 & 1.5 MAC	Dose-dependent prolongation of isovolumetric relaxation and decrease in LV diastolic compliance	128
Intact, awake, previously instrumented	1.0 MAC	Increase in coronary blood flow > equal dose of halothane; with autonomic blockade coronary flow still increased with isoflurane exposure; when increase myocardial oxygen demand isoflurane produces only small and transient increases in coronary flow	129
Chronically instrumented, intact, awake, after 30 min of equilibration	To effect, surgical plane	Decreased regional preload recruitable stroke work - end-diastolic segment length relationship (contractility)	165
Chronically instrumented, intact, awake	1.5 & 2.0 MAC	Decreased contractility in dose-dependent manner	130

Conditions	Dose	Cardiovascular effects	Reference
Intact, chronically instrumented, stenosis of left circumflex and total occlusion of LAD	1.6-1.8 & 2.3-2.5%, end-tidal	Decreased mean aortic pressure, peak systolic LV pressure, LV dP/dt$_{50}$; no change in HR; decreased blood flow in normal, stenotic and occluded myocardium but when mean aortic pressure & HR restored to conscious state levels myocardial perfusion also was maintained	**166**
Intact, awake, slow progressive single vessel (LAD) coronary occlusion with good collateral development; mean aortic pressure & HR adjusted to conscious levels following anesthesia using phenylephrine & atrial pacing	2.0 & 3.0%	Dose-dependent decrease in global & regional contractility & arterial pressure; decreased myocardial perfusion in both normal & collateral dependent regions; decreased coronary vascular resistance; decreased major determinants of myocardial oxygen consumption but do not unfavorably alter regional distribution of coronary blood flow in this model	**133**
Intact, awake, previously instrumented; Ameroid constrictor on LAD; 4 groups (control, poor, moderate & well-developed collateral circulation), microsphere injections	2 & 3%	Increased HR, decreased aortic pressure, LV dP/dtmax, regional contractile function; 3% decreased subepicardial, subendocardial & transmural blood flow in both normal and collateral-dependent regions; myocardial perfusion back to awake levels when aortic pressure and HR adjusted back to awake levels	**167**
Chronically instrumented, intact, awake, ganglionic, cholinergic & β-adrenergic blockade + a calcium channel stimulator	2%	Significant attenuation of the increase in aortic pressure after bolus administration of phenylephrine & azepexole (a selective α2 agonist); non-selective reduction of pressor response to both α1- and α2-adrenergic receptor stimulation, apparently not mediated by inhibition of transmembrane Ca^{2+} flux	**134**
Intact, awake, previously instrumented	Dose-response	Dose-dependent decrease in aortic pressure, LV dP/dt, myocardial thickening fraction & stroke volume, increase in HR; during profound hypotension (pressure 45 mmHg) cardiac function maintained better than with halothane or enflurane, coronary and renal blood flows well maintained even at 45 mmHg pressure	**135**

Conditions	Dose	Cardiovascular effects	Reference
Intact, awake, previously instrumented; studied the effects of decreases and increases of $[Ca^{2+}]$ in the blood	1.6 % end-tidal	Hemodynamic effects caused by increases and decreases in $[Ca^{2+}]$ less depressed in isoflurane anesthetized vs halothane or enflurane; all responses depressed compared to awake state	136
Anesthetized with fentanyl & pentobarbital (no doses given); isolated coronary artery prep., *in situ*, open thorax, perfusion pressure maintained constant	0.5, 1.0 & 2.0%	A direct, concentration-dependent vasodilatory effect on coronary vascular smooth muscle; at higher concentrations increased coronary blood flow to nearly maximal while decreasing local myocardial oxygen requirements	168
Measured effects of theophylline on cerebral blood flow & cerebral oxygen utilization	1.4%	The adenosine receptor antagonist theophylline partially reversed the cerebral depressant effects of isoflurane, i.e. increased cerebral blood flow & oxygen metabolic rate	169
Intact, awake, previously instrumented	1.25 & 1.75 MAC	Increased HR, systemic vascular resistance, and diastolic coronary blood flow velocity; decreased mean aortic pressure, myocardial contractility, and coronary vascular resistance at 1.75 MAC; after autonomic blockade still increased coronary velocity	118
Intact, awake, previously instrumented, pharmacologic autonomic blockade	1.0 & 1.5 MAC	Dose-dependent decrease in myocardial contractility	170
Intact, awake, previously instrumented	1.2, 1.4, 1.75 & 2.0 MAC	Decreased mean aortic pressure, stroke volume, systemic vascular resistance, LV dP/dt & wall thickness, dose-dependent for mean aortic pressure, stroke volume and LV dP/dt but not dose-dependent for systemic resistance; HR increased but not dose-dependent; increased coronary flow and decreased coronary resistance, both dose-dependent; hepatic flow increased slightly, hepatic resistance decreased, no change in combined hepatic and portal flow; no change in renal flow but renal resistance decreased	116

Conditions	Dose	Cardiovascular effects	Reference
Anesth. with fentanyl (40 µg/kg + 20 µg/kg/hr) and pentobarbital (10 mg/kg + 1 mg/kg/hr); mechanical ventilation, open thorax; vecuronium bromide (0.1 mg/kg + 0.05 mg/kg/hr)	Isoflurane conc. sufficient to decrease mean aortic pressure 30%	Decreased mean aortic pressure, aortic flow, LV dP/dtmax, stroke volume; increased HR; no change in systemic vascular resistance or arterial blood gases; venous blood gases unchanged except for a decrease in oxygen saturation and an increase in oxygen extraction; decreased endo/epi blood flow ratio; decreased myocardial oxygen consumption & extraction; increased coronary sinus pO_2, O_2 saturation and O_2 content	171
7.4:2 Isoflurane-Cats			
Chronically instrumented for direct stimulation of CNS pressor sites (hypothalamic)	1.5, 2.5 & 3.0%, inspired	Dose-dependent attenuation of pressor responses, heart rate responses and infra renal aortic blood flow responses	172
7.4:3 Isoflurane-Rats			
Previously instrumented, compared to conscious rats	1.4%	Decreased respiratory rate, no change in blood pressure, heart rate or cardiac output	162
Measured cerebral plasma volume (CPV)	1 MAC	CPV = 3.06 ± 0.44 ml/100 g brain tissue, compared to pentobarbital where CPV = 2.1 ± 0.76 ml/100 g	140
α-chloralose (2 mg/100 g/hr,IV), positive pressure ventilation	0.96 & 2.43 vol%	Lower concentration- decreased mean aortic pressure to 70 mmHg, also decreased HR, cardiac output, systemic resistance and LV rate-pressure product; increased cerebral blood flow; no change in total hepatic blood flow or renal blood flow but myocardial flow decreased: Higher concentration- decreased mean aortic pressure to 50 mmHg, reduced other parameters accordingly, decreased hepatic and renal blood flow and a very significant decrease in myocardial blood flow	173

Conditions	Dose	Cardiovascular effects	Reference
Myocardial preparation made permeable by mild homogenization, saponin and/or 2% Triton X-100	1.6 & 8.1 mM	Increased Ca^{2+} sensitivity, no effect on maximal developed force, complex effects on components associated with cellular membrane that normally modulate force	**142**
Instrumented with isoflurane anesthesia, awake for 2 hours then compared awake and anesthetized states	0, 1 & 2%	Blood-brain transfer coefficient was less in 11 of 13 brain regions in both 1 & 2% than in control group; blood flow was less in the cortex and greater in the medulla and pons in anesthetized vs control; regional cerebral blood flow not affected in 9 of 13 brain regions	**174**
Compared anesthetized to awake responses to hypoxemia	1 MAC	Brain and coronary blood flow increased in response to hypoxemia in awake rats, in anesthetized rats it decreased; hypoxemia did not change blood flow to kidneys, GI tract or total hepatic blood flow in awake rats but decreased these parameters significantly in the anesthetized animals	**143**
Intact, awake, previously instrumented, microsphere injections, blood pressure increased with phenylephrine and decreased with ganglionic blockade and hemorrhage to study 5 different ranges of aortic pressure	1.0 & 2.0 MAC	Autoregulation seen in all tissues in awake rats at all levels of blood pressure; autoregulatory coefficient ($\Delta Q/\Delta P$) increased in midbrain and spinal cord at 1 MAC and in all tissues during 2 MAC isoflurane; in normal blood pressure ranges (90-130 mmHg) at 1 MAC cortex flow decreased, subcortex, midbrain and spinal cord increased; at 2.0 MAC blood flow increased in all portions of the brain that were measured	**175**

Conditions	Dose	Cardiovascular effects	Reference
Ten min of bilateral carotid artery occlusion with simultaneous hypotension; halothane with normothermia vs halothane with hypothermia compared to isoflurane + normothermia; after 3 days survival histopathological evaluation of injury	1.3 MAC	No difference in grading of lesions between the 3 groups; all showed moderate to severe histomorphologic injury	**144**
Compared normo- and hypo-capnia in halothane and isoflurane anesthetized rats (2 X 2 factorial design)	1.38%, inspired	Hypocapnia decreased global cerebral blood flow (CBF) by 30% in both anesthetic groups; CBF was greater in 3 cortical samples in both normo- and hypo-capnic groups anesthetized with halothane than with isoflurane	**145**
Isolated heart (Langendorff) with constant pressure, heart arrested with tetrodotoxin, coronary flow reserve defined as the difference between coronary flow prior to and during administration of a maximally dilating dose of adenosine	0 - 3 MAC	Dose-dependent decrease in magnitude of coronary vascular resistance & of coronary flow reserve; latter the same as with halothane but significantly greater than with sevoflurane	**146**
Normocapnic, normothermic, combined N_2O with the isoflurane	0.75 MAC + 60% N_2O	Cerebral blood flow associated with major electrocardiogram changes and sustained depolarization, isoelectricity and incidence of sustained depolarization all the same as in rats anesthetized with halothane/N_2O; in rats subjected to cardiac arrest and to carotid occlusion time to depolarization was longer than in halothane/N_2O rats, cortical cerebral metabolic rate for glucose decreased more than halothane/N_2O group	**147**

7.4:4 Isoflurane-Pigs	Dose	Cardiovascular effects	Reference
Intact, awake, previously instrumented with and without N_2O	1.45% (1 MAC), 2.18%(1.5 MAC), 0.95% with N_2O (1 MAC), 1.68% with N_2O (1.5 MAC)	Mean aortic pressure decreased, dose-dependent; cardiac output decreased only during 1.5 MAC; no changes in heart rate; dose-dependent increase in brain blood flow and decrease in myocardial blood flow; adrenal gland blood flow increased at 1.5 MAC; splenic blood flow increased, decreased blood flow to stomach, small intestine, diaphragm, skeletal muscle and fat; no change in renal, hepatic arterial and cutaneous blood flows	111
Newborn pigs, intact, awake, previously instrumented	0.5, 1.0 & 1.5 MAC	Decreased HR, mean aortic pressure and cardiac index	151
Hepatic ischemia-reperfusion model; induction with methohexital (20 mg/kg,IM) + pancuronium bromide (0.1 mg/kg)	1.5% end-expired conc.	Provided more protection from hepatic ischemia-reperfusion injury than halothane, enflurane or pentobarbital	152
Previously instrumented	1.2 MAC by mask then intubated and maintained	Decreased peripheral resistance, cardiac output and stroke volume index; increased HR	176
Surgical preparation which enabled the stepwise decrease in hepatic blood flow without hepatic hypoperfusion	1.5% end-expired	Decreased hepatic O_2 delivery and decreased hepatic lactate uptake at lowered hepatic blood flows	154
7.4:6 Isoflurane-Rabbits			
Cerebral blood flow measured with microspheres; compared effects of 3 different vasopressors, angiotensin II, norepinephrine & phenylephrine	1.0 MAC	Baseline total cerebral blood flow, hemispheric cerebral blood flow & posterior fossa blood flow the same; results indicate norepinephrine and phenylephrine result in indirect vasodilation or angiotensin II has intrinsic vasoconstrictor effects	177

7.4:7 Isoflurane-Guinea pigs, conditions	Dose	Cardiovascular effects	Reference
Ketamine (IP) + decapitation, isolated papillary muscle prep.	0.77 & 1.6%	Dose-dependent decreased inotropy not closely related to decreased Ca^{2+} transients but less than halothane or enflurane; some dissociation between Ca^{2+} and negative ionotropy with isoflurane	148
Isolated heart preparation (Langendorff), compared to N_2 & N_2O exposures	Dose-response	Dose-dependent decrease in peak LV pressure, + LV dP/dtmax, - LV dP/dtmax, myocardial oxygen consumption, HR and % oxygen extraction; no change in coronary flow or oxygen diffusion rates; least severe depression compared to enflurane and halothane	149
7.4:8 Isoflurane-Sheep			
Intact, awake, pregnant females, instrumented fetuses, compared fetal asphyxia with mother awake and under isoflurane anesthesia; asphyxia by maternal uterine artery occlusion	1%	Fetal asphyxia + anesthesia increased regional and total brain, heart and adrenal blood flows, decreased flow to spleen and skeletal muscle; asphyxia alone and asphyxia + isoflurane decreased sagittal sinus pH, base excess, pO_2 & oxygen saturation; $[H^+]$ & pCO_2 increased; cerebral oxygen consumption decreased; no change in cerebral oxygen delivery; the balance of fetal cerebral oxygen supply-to-demand is maintained during maternal anesthesia with isoflurane	178
7.4:9 Isoflurane-Ferrets			
Isolated RV papillary muscle, anesthetized with pentobarbital (100 mg/kg,IP), heart excised as soon as surgical plane of anesthesia reached	Dose-response, 0.1.5 MAC in 0.25 MAC increments	Concentration-dependent decrease in developed force; alteration in myofibrillar Ca^{2+} responsiveness minor compared to decreased intracellular Ca^{2+} availability	117
7.4:10 Isoflurane-Ducks			
Intact, awake	Dose-response	Dose-dependent decrease in cardio-pulmonary function	179

7.4:11 Isoflurane- Sandhills crane, conditions	Dose	Cardiovascular response	Reference
Intact, awake	Dose- response	Dose-dependent decrease in cardiovascular and respiratory function	**180**

Table 7.5: The Cardiovascular Effects of Desflurane

Conditions of the experiment	Dose	Cardiovascular Effects	Reference
7.5:1 Desflurane- Dogs			
Intact, awake, previously instrumented	1.0 & 1.5 MAC	Dose-dependent prolongation of isovolumetric relaxation and decreased LV diastolic compliance	**128**
Review article, many sources	Range of doses	Increased HR; decreased mean aortic pressures, systemic resistance, systemic, coronary, renal, hepatic & cerebral flows; decreased indices of LV systolic and diastolic function; may cause coronary vasodilation but no evidence of "coronary steal" in a model of multivessel coronary artery disease; depresses ventilation; dose- dependent decrease in tidal volume and increase in respiratory rate, $PaCO_2$, dead space/tidal volume ratio and intra-pulmonary shunt fractions	**181**
Intact, awake, previously instrumented	1.25 & 1.75 MAC	Increased HR & systemic resistance; decreased mean aortic pressure & myocardial contractility; better preservation of myocardial function than halothane, isoflurane or enflurane; increased diastolic coronary blood flow velocity and decreased diastolic coronary vascular resistance except after autonomic blockade	**118**
Intact, awake, previously instrumented	1.2, 1.4, 1.75 & 2.0 MAC	Dose-dependent decrease in mean aortic pressure, stroke volume & LV dP/dt; systemic resistance decreased but not dose-dependent; dose- dependent increase in coronary flow and decrease in coronary resistance; no change in hepatic flow or resistance at lower concentrations but 2 highest concentrations resulted in a decrease in hepatic resistance; no change in renal flow or resistance	**116**

Conditions	Dose	Cardiovascular effects	Reference
Intact, awake, previously instrumented, pharmacologic autonomic blockade	1.0 & 1.5 MAC	Dose-dependent decrease in myocardial contractility	**170**
7.5:2 Desflurane-Pigs			
Previously instrumented	1.2 MAC by mask then intubated and maintained	Decreased peripheral resistance, cardiac index, stroke volume index and increased HR	**176**

Table 7.6: The Cardiovascular Effects of Sevoflurane

Conditions of the experiment	Dose	Cardiovascular Effects	Reference
7.6:1 Sevoflurane-Rats			
Isolated heart, constant pressure (Langendorff), heart arrested with Tetrodotoxin; coronary flow reserve defined as the difference between coronary flow prior to & during administration of a maximally dilating dose of adenosine	0-3 MAC	Dose-dependent decrease in the magnitude of coronary vascular resistance and of coronary flow reserve; decreased coronary flow reserve significantly less than with halothane or isoflurane	**146**
Intact, awake	0.5, 1.0, 1.2 & 1.5 MAC	12% decrease in mean aortic pressure at 1.5; arterial pCO_2 increase was dose-related; cerebral and spinal cord blood flows increased at 1.2 & 1.5 MAC; coronary and renal blood flows, no change; portal tributary blood flow and preportal resistance, no change; hepatic arterial flow increased at 1.5 MAC but total liver blood flow did not change	**182**

Conditions	Dose	Cardiovascular effects	Reference
α-chloralose (2 mg/100 g/hr,IV, positive pressure ventilation	1.66 vol% & 3.95 vol%	Lower concentration decreased mean aortic pressure to 70 mmHg, decreased HR, cardiac output, systemic resistance & LV rate-pressure product; increased cerebral blood flow; no change in total hepatic flow or renal blood flow, myocardial blood flow decreased; Higher concentrations reduced mean aortic pressures to 50 mmHg and reduced other parameters accordingly; decreased hepatic and renal blood flow; large decrease in myocardial blood flow; all responses were more sever than isoflurane at the same aortic pressures	173
7.6:2 Sevoflurane-Pigs			
Newborn pigs, intact, awake, previously instrumented	0.5, 1.0 & 1.5 MAC	Decreased HR, mean aortic pressure & cardiac index	151

Table 7.7: The Cardiovascular Effects of Diethyl Ether

Conditions of the experiment	Dose	Cardiovascular Effects	Reference
7.7:1 Ether-Dogs			
Hexobarbital (no dose given), heparin (300 IU/kg), bled to cardiac arrest, isolated heart-lung prep., lungs perfused and ventilated but heart in arrest	6-8 vol%	No effect during normoxic perfusion or during increased pulmonary flow; stabilized elevated vascular tone during microembolism-induced pulmonary hypertension	44
7.7:2 Ether-Cats			
Isolated papillary muscle prep.	Conc. equal to MAC for general anesth., as determined for each individual animal	Depressed contractility but least of cyclopropane, methoxyflurane, halothane or enflurane	63

7.7:3 Ether-Rats	Dose	Cardiovascular effects	Reference
Previously instrumented with aortic cannulae	22.5 ml/hr with airflow of 54 l/hr (induction) + 12 ml/hr with airflow of 54 l/hr for maint.	Provided protection against mortality and kidney lesions following bleeding to 30-50 mmHg for 60 min.; protection was significant but less than that achieved with pentobarbital, enflurane, halothane or methoxyflurane	**69**
Previously instrumented, decapitation at various intervals following treatment for renin activity	Inhalation to loss of righting reflex and no pain response	Marked and sustained increase in plasma renin activity; sustained decrease in arterial pressure mediated through β-adenoreceptors	**112**
Two pairs of isolated lungs in series at constant pulmonary vascular flow; 1 lung made atelectatic by airway occlusion subsequent to ventilation with 95% O_2, other lung atelectatic by ventilation with 2% O_2	Dose-response	Increase in pulmonary vascular resistance was decreased in a dose-dependent manner	**76**
Isolated atrial prep.	Dose-response	Dose-dependent increase in HR, not mediated by catecholamine release	**4**
Isolated atrial prep., killed by decapitation	Dose-response	Dose-dependent increase in HR, not mediated by β-adrenergic or cholinergic mechanisms	**75**
Coronary artery ligation, α-chloralose (80 mg/ kg,IV)	Ether to effect	High incidence of ventricular tachycardia or fibrillation	**183**
7.7:4 Ether-Pigs			
Anesthetized with a combination of diethyl ether + halothane, compared to isoflurane	1.3 MAC of combination	Fatal anesthetic ratio was 3.12 compared to 1.7 for halothane alone; higher mean aortic pressure than in isoflurane anesthetized group; general depression of the central circulation with no sign of a decrease in contractility	**184**

Table 7.8: The Cardiovascular Effects of Nitrous Oxide

Conditions of the experiment	Dose	Cardiovascular Effects	Reference
7.8:1 Nitrous oxide-Dogs			
Hexobarbital (no dose given), heparin (300 IU/ kg), bled to cardiac arrest, heart-lung prep. with arrested heart, lungs perfused with constant flow and lungs ventilated	80%	No effect during normoxic perfusion, during enhanced pulmonary blood flow or during microembolism-induced pulmonary hypertension	**44**
Chronically instrumented, intact, previously anesthetized with either isoflurane or sufentanil	70%, 30% O_2	Decreased regional preload recruitable stroke work: end-diastolic segment length relationship (contractility)	**165**
Intact, awake, previously instrumented, induced with thiopentone (5-8 mg/kg,IV), positive pressure ventilation; combined with fentanyl (0.75 µg/kg/min for 20 min + 0.22 µg/kg/min) + atracurium (o.1 mg/kg every 30 min); 1 hr of anesthesia prior to measurements	67%, 33% O_2	Marked but short-lasting effect on disposition of propranolol due to a decrease in intrinsic clearance	**164**
7.8:2 Nitrous oxide-Rats			
Induced with diethyl ether, cannulated femoral artery and vein, suxamethonium, positive pressure ventilation	70%, 30% O_2	Conscious animals developed less blood-brain barrier dysfunction than anesthetized animals; largest difference was seen after injections of amphetamine, smallest differences seen after epinephrine injections	**113**
Anesthetized with halothane, tubocurarine (1.5 mg/kg,IV), acute instrumentation	70%, 30% O_2	Decreased phenylalanine influx to the brain due to alterations in circulating neutral amino acid patterns; little, if any, direct effects on neutral amino acid transport processes	**70**

Conditions	Dose	Cardiovascular effects	Reference
Intact, awake	70%, 30% O$_2$	Produces cerebrovasodilation not related to a change in metabolic demand; plasma catecholamines did not change during 60 min of N$_2$O exposure, indicated increased cerebral blood flow not due to a general stress response	185
7.8:3 Nitrous oxide-Pigs			
Intact, awake, previously instrumented	50%, 50% O$_2$	Attenuated hypotensive effects of isoflurane; cardiac output was maintained near awake control values because the heart rate increased; there was a larger increase in brain blood flow when combined with isoflurane; no change in myocardial blood flow, no change in adrenal gland blood flow	111
Thiopental (2 mg/ kg,IV), fentanyl (20 μg/ kg,IV + 10 μg/kg/hr); halothane (0.5%), pancuronium (0.1 mg/kg + 0.15 mg/kg/hr,IV)	30, 50 & 70%	No change in myocardial contractility; decrease in arterial capacitance but not dose-dependent	186
Anesthesia with desflurane or isoflurane	60%	No changes with desflurane; with isoflurane increased systemic resistance, decreased cardiac output and stroke volume, no change in HR or preload	176
7.8:4 Nitrous oxide-Rabbits			
Isolated lung prep.	Dose-response	Enhanced lipid peroxide tertiary butyl-hydroperoxide-induced pulmonary vaso-constrictions	150

7.8:5 Nitrous oxide-Guinea pigs	Dose	Cardiovascular effects	Reference
Isolated right ventricular papillary muscle prep.	50% with 45% O_2/5% CO_2	Resulted in myocardial depression (negative inotropy) independent of concurrent hypoxic effects; pattern and magnitude of contractile depression similar to that caused by 0.5% halothane	187
7.8:6 Nitrous oxide-Ferrets			
Isolated right ventricular papillary muscle prep.	20,30 & 50% in O_2	Concentration-dependent decrease in contractility under all loading conditions; minor changes in relaxation due to decreased Ca^{2+} availability with no effect on myofibrillar responsiveness to Ca^{2+}	188

Table 7.9: The Cardiovascular Effects of Cyclopropane, Chloroform, Fluroxene and Trichloroethylene

Conditions of the experiment	Dose	Cardiovascular Effects	Reference
7.9: Cyclopropane-Dogs			
Hearts excised from dogs anesthetized with 33% cyclopropane in oxygen or pentobarbital (30 mg/kg,IV); isolated Purkinje fiber preparations from right ventricular papillary muscle and endocardial surface preparations from right atrial strips	6-8 vol%, equivalent to approx. 300-400 mmHg partial pressure	Concentrations of approximately 350 mmHg partial pressure in plasma have been shown to produce spontaneous cardiac arrhythmias in dogs; Purkinje fibers showed a significant increase in rate of repolarization during phase 2 while rate during phase 3 decreased; time required to repolarize to -60 mV was decreased, duration of terminal phase of repolarization and of the total action potential were enhanced	114

Conditions	Dose	Cardiovascular effects	Reference
Anesthetized with 33% cyclopropane or pentobarbital (30 mg/kg,IV); isolated papillary muscle preps. with false tendons containing Purkinje fibers; electrically stimulated at 95 beats/min	Perfused in bath with 6-8 vol%	Acceleration of repolarization during the plateau of the action potential, an apparent Ca^{2+}-dependent phenomena	**115**
7.9:2 Cyclopropane-Cats			
Isolated papillary muscle prep.	Concentration equal to MAC for general anesthesia for each individual	Depressed contractility more than diethyl ether but less than methoxyflurane, halothane or enflurane	**63**
7.9:3 Cyclopropane-Rabbits			
Isolated lung preparation	Dose-response	Enhanced lipid peroxide tertiary butyl hydroperoxide-induced pulmonary vasoconstrictions	**150**
7.9:4 Chloroform-Rats			
Decapitation; isolated atrial preparation	Dose-response	Dose-dependent decrease in HR; not β-adrenergic or cholinergically mediated	**75**
7.9:5 Fluoroxone-Rats			
Decapitation; isolated atrial preparation	Dose-response	Dose-dependent but slight decrease in HR at low concentrations; not β-adrenergic or cholinergically mediated	**75**

7.9:6 Trichloroethylene- Rats	Dose	Cardiovascular effects	Reference
Previously instrumented with aortic cannulae	12 ml/hr with airflow at 60 l/hr during induction and 4.5 ml/hr with airflow at 120 l/hr during maintenance	Little or no protection against mortality and kidney lesions following bleeding to 30-50 mmHg for 60 min	69
Decapitated; isolated atrial preparation	Dose-response	Marked increase in HR, mechanism does not involve stimulation of β-adrenergic or cholinergic receptors	75

References

1.   Parker, J.L., Adams, H.R. The influence of chemical restraining agents on cardiovascular function: a review, *Lab Anim Sci*, 28:575-583, 1978.

2.   Vatner, S.F. Effects of anesthesia on cardiovascular control mechanisms, *Environ Health Perspect*, 26:193-206, 1978.

3.   Price, H.L., Ohnishi, S.T. Effects of anesthetics on the heart, *Fed Proc*, 39:1575-1579, 1980.

4.   Pratila, M.G., Pratila, V. Anesthetic agents and cardiac electromechanical activity, *Anes*, 49:338-360, 1978.

5.   Zimpfer, M., Sit, S.P., Vatner, S.F. Effects of anesthesia on the canine carotid chemoreceptor reflex, *Circ Res*, 48:400-406, 1981.

6.   Eastham, C.L., Moyers, J.R., Carter, J.G., Brooks, L.A., Marcus, M.L. Effects of halothane on the coronary circulation, *Am Heart Assoc Monograph*, 1981.

7.   Smith, N.T., Ingels, N.B. Jr., Daughters, G.T., Wexler, L. Contribution of asynergic contraction to halothane-induced myocardial depression, *Anesth Analg*, 59:178-185, 1980.

8.   Bagshaw, R.J., Cox, R.H. Effects of incremental halothane levels on the reflex responses to carotid hypotension in the dog, *Acta Anaes Scand*, 25:180-184, 1981.

9.   Seagard, J.L., Hopp, F.A., Donegan, J.H., Kalbfleish, J.H., Kampine, J.P. Halothane and the carotid sinus reflex: evidence for multiple sites of action, *Anesth*, 57:191-202, 1982.

10.   Beattie, C., Todd, E.P., Wright, B.D., Davis, J.B. Halothane in dogs with left ventricular hypertrophy, *Anesth*, 53 (Suppl 3):S98, 1980.

11.   Vatner, S.F., Smith, N.T. Effects of halothane on left ventricular function and distribution of regional blood flow in dogs and primates, *Circ Res*, 34:155-167, 1974.

12.   Priano, L.L. Comparative renal vascular effects of thiopental, diazepam, ketamine and halothane, *Anesth*, 57:A34, 1982.

13.   Atlee, J.L., Peterson, M.L. Halothane, isoflurane, enflurane and A-V conduction: Awake vs. anesthesia, *Anesth*, 57:A15, 1982.

14.   Vatner, S.F., Smith, N.T. Effects of halothane on left ventricular function and distribution of regional blood flow in dogs and primates, *Circ Res*, 34:155-167, 1974.

15.   Morrow, D.H., Haley, J.V., Logic, J.R. Anesthesia and digitalis VII. The effect of pentobarbital, halothane and methoxyflurane on the A-V conduction and inotropic responses to ouabain, *Anesth Analg (Cleveland)*, 51:430-438, 1972.

16.   Hunter, J.M., Jones, R.S., Snowdon, S.L., Utting, J.E. Cardiovascular and renal effects of enflurane and halothane in the dog, *Res Vet Sci*, 31:177-181, 1981.

17. Vance, J.P., Brown, D.M., Smith, G., Thorburn, J. Canine coronary blood flow responses to hypoxemia the influence of halothane, *Br J Anaesth*, 51:193-198, 1979.

18. Wong, K.C., Puerto, A.X., Puerto, B.A., Blatnick, R.A. Influence of imipramine and pargyline on the arrhythmogenicity of epinephrine during halothane, enflurane or methoxyflurane anesthesia in dogs, *Anesth*, 53 (Suppl 3):S25, 1980.

19. Kapur, P.A., Flacke, W.E. Verapamil halothane epinephrine arrhythmias and cardiovascular function, *Anesth*, 53 (Suppl 3):S132, 1980.

20. Kapur, P.A., Flacke, W.E. Epinephrine induced arrhythmias and cardiovascular function after verapamil during halothane anesthesia in the dog, *Anesth*, 55:218-225, 1981.

21. Smith, E.R., Dresel, P.E. Site of origin of halothane-epinephrine arrhythmia determined by direct and echocardiographic recordings, *Anesth*, 57:98-102, 1982.

22. Seagard, J.L., Hopp, F.A., Bosnjak, Z.J., Elegbe, E.O., Kampine, J.P. Extent and mechanism of halothane sensitization of the carotid sinus baroreceptors, *Anesth*, 58:432-437, 1983.

23. Chamberlain, J.H., Swan, P.C., Wedley, J.R. Hypotension and myocardial metabolism. Drug-induced hypotension and the heart: a comparison between halothane and nitroprusside, *Anesth*, 35:962-971, 1980.

24. Wilkinson, P.L., Tyberg, J.V., Moyers, J.R., White, A.E. Correlates of myocardial oxygen consumption when afterload changes during halothane anesthesia in dogs, *Anesth Analg*, 59:233-239, 1980.

25. Turner, L.A., Zuperku, E.J., Purtock, R.V., Kampine, J.P. *In vivo* changes in canine ventricular cardiac conduction during halothane anesthesia, *Anesth Analg (Cleve)*, 59:327-334, 1980.

26. Nielsen, N.C., Rusy, B.F. Effect of sodium nitroprusside on directly measured myocardial oxygen consumption during phenylephrine induced hypertension in dogs anesthetized with halothane, *Anesth Analg*, 59:835-838, 1980.

27. Verrier, E.D., Edelist, G., Consigny, P.M., Robinson, S., Hoffman, J.I.E. Greater coronary vascular reserve with halothane, *Anesth*, 51 (Suppl 3):S63, 1979.

28. Lowenstein, E., Foex, P., Francis, C.M., Davies, W.L., Yusuf, S., Ryder, W.A. Regional ischemic ventricular dysfunction in myocardium supplied by a narrowed coronary artery with increasing halothane concentration in the dog, *Anesth*, 55:349-359, 1981.

29. Ahlgren, I., Aronsen, K.F., Bjorkman, I., Wetterlin, S. The hemodynamic effect of halothane in the normovolemic dog, *Acta Anaes Scand*, 22:83-89, 1978.

30. Ingemar, F., Ahlgren, H. The effect of halothane anesthesia on heart function during normovolemia and hypovolemia in the dog, *Acta Anaesth Scand*, 22:93-99, 1978.

31. Wilkinson, P.L., Stowe, D.F., Glantz, S.A., Tyberg, J.V. Heart rate systemic blood pressure relationship in dogs during halothane anesthesia, *Acta Anaesth*, 24:181-186, 1980.

32. Zink, J., Sasyniuk, B.I., Dresel, P.E. Halothane-epinephrine-induced cardiac arrhythmias and role of heart rate, *Anesth*, 43:548-555, 1975.

33. Slogoff, S., Keats, A.S., Hibbs, C.W., Edmonds, C.H., Bragg, D,A,; Failure of general anesthesia to potentiate propranolol activity, *Anesth*, 47:504-508, 1977.

34. Ammendrup, P., Atlee, J.D. Mechanical hyperventilation: effect on specialized atrioventricular conduction, supraventricular refractoriness, and experimental atrial arrhythmias in dogs anesthetized with pentobarbital or pentobarbital-halothane, *Anesth Analg (Cleveland)*, 59:839-846, 1980.

35. Logic, J.R., Morrow, D.H. The effect of halothane on ventricular automaticity, *Anesth*, 36:107-118, 1972.

36. Hantler, C.B., Clifford, B.D., Kroll, D.A., Knight, P.R. Verapamil does have prolonged interactions with halothane, *Anesth*, 57 (Suppl 3):A2, 1982.

37. Atlee, T.L. III, Ammendrup, P., Malkinson, C.E. Halothane and hypocapnia effects on electrically stimulated atrial arrhythmias in digitalized dogs, *Anesth Analg*, 60:302-305, 1981.

38. Bernstein, K.J., Gangat, Y., Verosky, M., Vulliemoz, Y., Triner, L. Halothane effect on β-adrenergic receptors in canine myocardium, *Anesth Analg*, 60:401-405, 1982.

39. Blanck, T.J., Thompson, M. Calcium transport by cardiac sarcoplasmic reticulum: modulation of halothane action by substrate concentration and pH, *Anesth Analg (Cleveland)*, 60:390-394, 1981.

40. Fargas-Babjak, A., Forrest, J.B. Effect of halothane on the pulmonary vascular response to hypoxia in dogs, *Can Anaesth Soc J*, 26:6-14, 1979.

41. Boyce, J.R., Cervenko, F.W., Wright, F.J. Effects of halothane on the pharmacokinetics of lidocaine in digitalis toxic dogs, *Can Anaesth Soc J*, 25:323-328, 1978.

42. Smith, G., Rogers, K., Thorburn, J. Halothane improves the balance of oxygen supply to demand in acute experimental myocardial ischaemia, *Br J Anaesth*, 52:577-583, 1980.

43.   Yasuoka, M. Effects of halothane on the left coronary perfusion pressure-flow relationship and the distribution of blood flow in the ischemic canine left ventricle, *Tokushima J Exp Med*, 25:107-118, 1978.

44.   Dubikaitis, A.Y., Beliakov, N.A., Simbirtsev, S.A. Pulmonary vascular responses to inhalation anesthesia in isolated dog lungs, *Cor Vasa*, 22:384-392, 1981.

45.   Tinker, J.H., Harrison, C.E. Protection from myocardial ischemia, role of anesthetics, *Anesth*, 51 (Suppl 3):S58, 1979.

46.   Merin, R.G. Are the myocardial functional and metabolic effects of isoflurane really different from those of halothane and enflurane?, *Anesth*, 55:398-408, 1981.

47.   Atlee, J.L., Rush, B.F. Halothane depression of A-V conduction studied by electrograms of the bundle of HIS is dogs, *Anesth*, 36:112-118, 1972.

48.   Jackson, S.H., Smith, N.T. Acetate fails to reverse myocardial depression in dogs anesthetized with halothane, *Anes Analg (Cleveland)*, 57:395-403, 1978.

49.   Loarie, D.J., Wilkinson, P., Tyberg, J., White, A. The hemodynamic effects of halothane in anemic dogs, *Anesth Analg (Cleveland)*, 58:195-200, 1979.

50.   Rao, T.L.K., Jacobs, K., Salem, M.R., Santos, P. Deliberate hypotension and anesthetic requirements of halothane, *Anesth Analg*, 60:513-516, 1981.

51.   Pavlin, D.J., Ferens, J., Allen, D.R., Cheney, F.W. Pulmonary arteriovenous shunts during halothane anesthesia in dogs, *Br J Anaesth*, 52:763-768, 1980.

52.   Atlee, J.L. III, Rusy, B.F., Kreul, J.F., Eby, T. Supraventricular excitability in dogs during anesthesia with halothane and enflurane, *Anesth*, 49:407-413, 1978.

53.   Mergner, G.W., Gilman, R.W., Woolfe, W.A., Patch, J.H. Effect of halothane and fentanyl on myocardial infarct size and regional blood flow distribution, *Anesth*, 57:A17, 1982.

54.   Maze, M., Smith, C.M. Halothane decreases arrhythmogenic threshold for epinephrine through α- and β-adrenoceptor mechanisms, *Anesth*, 57:A16, 1982.

55.   Cox, R.H., Bagshaw, R.J. Effects of anesthesia on carotid sinus reflex control of arterial hemodynamics in the dog, *Am J Physiol*, 239:H631-H691, 1980.

56.   Wilkinson, P.L., Tyberg, J.V., Moyers, J.R., White, A.E. Changes in myocardial oxygen consumption, efficiency and haemodynamics when systemic pressure in increased during morphine and added halothane anaesthesia in dogs, *Can J Anaesth Soc*, 27:230-237, 1980.

57.   Bagshaw, R.J., Cox, R.H. Baroreceptor reflexes and pulmonary hemodynamics during halothane and halothane-nitrous oxide anesthesia in the dog, *Anesth Analg (Clevland)*, 60:701-709, 1981.

58.   Wilkinson, P.L., Tyberg, J.V., Moyers, J.R., White, A.E. Changes in myocardial oxygen consumption efficiency and hemodynamics when systemic pressure is increased during morphine and added halothane anesthesia in dogs, *Can Anaesth Soc J*, 27:230-237, 1980.

59.   Larsen, R., Drobnik, L., Teichmann, J., Radke, J., Kettler, D. The effects of halothane induced nitroprusside induced and trimethaphan induced hypotenion on cerebral blood flow and intracranial pressure, *Can Anesth Soc J*, 27:230-237, 1980.

60.   Morrow, D.H., Gaffney, T.E., Holman, J.E. The chronotropic and myotropic effects of halothane, *Anesth*, 22:915-917, 1961

61.   Gerson, J.I., Hickey, R.F., Bainton, C.R. Treatment of myocardial ischemia with halothane or nitroprusside propranolol, *Anesth Analg*, 61:10-14, 1982.

62.   Roy, R.C., Stullken, E.H. Electroencephalographic evidence of arousal in dogs from halothane after doxapram, physostigmine or naloxone, *Anesth*, 55:392-397, 1981.

63.   Brown, B.R. Jr., Crout, J.R. A comparative study of the effects of five general anesthetics on myocardial contractility: I Isometric conditions, *Anesth*, 34:236-245, 1971.

64.   Hohle, R., Siepmann, H.P. The influence of adrenaline on the effects of halothane and enflurane on the myocardium. Papillary muscle of the cat (author's translation), *Anaesth*, 29:172-180, 1980.

65.   Condouris, G.A., Kopia, G.A. Cardiac arrhythmias induced by guanethidine in cats anesthetized with halothane, *Eur J Pharmacol*, 68:257-267, 1980.

66.   Gangat, Y., Vulliemoz, Y., Verosky, M., Danilo, P., Bernstein, K., Triner, L. Action of halothane on myocardial adenylate cyclase of rat and cat, *Proc Soc Exp Biol Med*, 160:154-159, 1979.

67.   Rusy, B.F. Effect of halothane on decay of the potentiated state in cat papillary muscle, *Circ (Suppl)*, 58:11-18, 1978.

68.   Penna, M., Boye, A., Novakovic, L. Effect of halothane on contractile function and reactivity of myocardium, *Eur J Pharmacol*, 10:151-160, 1970.

69.   Peters, J.M., van der Meer, C., Czanky, J.C., Spierdijk, J. Effect of anesthetics on mortality and kidney lesions caused by hypotension, *Arch Int Pharmacodyn Ther*, 238:134-153, 1979.

70. Hawkins, R.A., Mans, A.M., Biebuyck, J.F. Amino-acid supply to individual cerebral structures in awake and anesthetized rats, *Am J Physiol*, 242:E1-E11, 1982.
71. Longnecker, D.E., Ross, D.C. Influence of anesthetic on microvascular responses to hemorrhage, *Anesth*, 51(Suppl 3):S142, 1979.
72. Miller, E.D. Jr., Kistner, J.R., Epstein, R.M. Distribution of blood flow with anesthetics, *Anesth*, 51 (Suppl 3):S124, 1979.
73. Belghiti, J., Blanchet, L., Lebrec, D. Effects of general anesthesia on portal venous pressure in the rat, *Eur Surg Res*, 13:285-289, 1981.
74. Muller, E.D. Jr., Longnecker, D.E., Peach, M.J. Renin response to hemorrhage in awake and anesthetized rats, *Circ Shock*, 6:271-276, 1979.
75. Krishna, G., Paradise, R.R. Mechanisms of chronotropic effects of volatile inhalational anesthetics, *Anesth Analg (Cleveland)*, 56:173-181, 1977.
76. Bjertnaes, L., Mudal, R., Hauge, A., Nicolaysen, A. Vascular resistance in atelectatic lungs effects of inhalation anesthetics, *Acta Anesth Scand*, 24:190-218, 1980.
77. Bernstein, K., Gangat, Y., Vulliemoz, Y., Verosky, M., Triner, L. Halothane dobutamine myocardial β-adrenoceptors, *Anesth (Suppl 3)*, 52:A31, 1979.
78. Ray, K.F., Kohlenbergeb, R.W., Shapiro, H.M. Local cerebral blood flow and metabolism during halothane and enflurane, *Anesth (Suppl 3)*, 51 :S10, 1979.
79. Peyton, R., Christian, C. II, Fagraeus, L., van Trigt, P., Spray, T., Pellom, G., Pasque, M., Wechsler, A. Halothane and myocardial protection, *Anesth (Suppl 3)*, 57 :A9, 1982.
80. Miletich, D.J., Holshouser, S.J., Seals, C.F., Albrecht, R.F. Differential effects of halothane or enflurane on heart cell utilization of glucose and fatty acids, *Anesth (Suppl 3)*, 57 :A19, 1982.
81. Novelli, G.P. Effects of enflurane and halothane on the microcirculation, *Acta Anaes Scand (Suppl)*, 0:64-68, 1979.
82. Bjertnaes, L.J. Hypoxia-induced vasoconstriction in isolated perfused lungs exposed to injectable or inhalation anesthetics, *Acta Anaesth Scand*, 21:133-136, 1977.
83. Lynch, C., Vogel, S., Sperelakis, N. Halothane depression of myocardial slow action potentials, *Anesth*, 55:360-368, 1981.
84. Bosnjak, Z.J., Kampine, J.P. Effects of halothane, enflurane and isoflurane on the SA node, *Anesth*, 58:314-321, 1983.
85. Lynch, C., Vogel, S., Sperelakis, N. Halothane inhibits slow action potentials in heart muscle, *Fed Proc*, 39:#2496, 1980.
86. Komai, H., Rusy, B.F. Effect of halothane on rested-state and potentiated-state contractions in rabbit papillary muscle: relationship to negative inotropic action, *Anesth Analg (Cleveland)*, 61:403-409, 1982.
87. Su, J.Y., Kerrick, W.G.L. Effects of halothane on calcium ion activated tension development in mechanically disrupted rabbit myocardial fibers, *Eur J Physiol*, 375:111-118, 1978.
88. Kaukinen, S. the combined effects of antihypertensive drugs and anaesthetics (halothane and ketamine) on the isolated heart, *Acta Anaes Scand*, 22:649-657, 1978.
89. Moores, W.Y., Weiskopf, R.B., Dembitsky, W.P., Utley, J.R. Comparative effects of halothane and morphine anesthesia on myocardial function and metabolism during cyanosis in swine, *Surg Forum*, 30:221-223, 1979.
90. Brower, R.W., Merin, R.G. Left ventricular function and compliance in swine during halothane anesthesia, *Anesth Suppl 3)*, 53:409-415, 1979.
91. Sawyer, D.C., Ely, S.W., Scott, J.B. Halothane and ethrane effects on the coronary circulation, *Anesth (Suppl 3)*, 53:S129, 1980.
92. Steffy, E.P., Howland, D. Jr. Comparison of circulatory and respiratory effects of isoflurane and halothane anesthesia in horses, *Am J Vet Res*, 41:821-825, 1980.
93. Fitch, W., Jones, J.V., Graham, D.I., MacKenzie, E.T., Harper, A.M. Effects of hypotension induced by halothane on the cerebral circulation in baboons with experimental renovascular hypertension, *Br J Anaesth*, 50:119-126, 1978.
94. Beck, A., Zimpfer, M., Raberger, G. Inhibition of the carotid chemoreceptor reflex by enflurane in chronically instrumented dogs, *Arch Pharmacol*, 321:145-148, 1982.
95. Zimpfer, M., Gilly, H., Krosl, P., Schlag, G., Steinbereithner K; Importance of myocardial loading conditions in determining the effects of enflurane on left ventricular function in the intact and isolated canine heart, *Anesth*, 58:159-169, 1983.
96. Kreul, J.F., Atlee, J.L. Pancuronium enhances atrio-ventricular conduction in anesthetized dogs, *Anesth (Suppl 3)*, 51:S86, 1979.

97.   Krivosic, R., Besse, M.D., Bosznai, Z., Moreau, J.D. Compatibility of enflurane and adrenaline -
      experiments in the dog, *Acta Anaesth Scand (Suppl)*, 71:52-58, 1979.
98.   Smith, G., Evans, D.H., Asher, M.J., Bentley, S. Enflurane improves the oxygen supply demand
      balance in the acutely ischemic canine myocardium, *Acta Anaesth Scand*, 26:44-47, 1982.
99.   Andreen, M., Irestedt, L. Effects of enflurane on splanchnic circulation, *Acta Anaesth Scnd
      (Suppl)*, 0:48-51, 1979.
100. Blanck, T.J.J., Thompson, M. Stimulation of canine cardiac sarcoplasmic reticulum calcium
      uptake by enflurane and isoflurane, *Fed Proc (3 Part 1)*, 40:#2897, 1981.
101. Longnecker, D.E., Ross, D.C., Silver, I.A. Anesthetic influence on arteriolar diameters and tissue
      oxygen tension in hemorrhaged rats, *Anesth*, 57:177-182, 1982.
102. Lynch, C., Vogel, S., Pratila, M.G., Sperelakis, N. Enflurane depression of myocardial slow action
      potentials, *J Pharm Exp Ther*, 222:405-409, 1982.
103. Su, J.Y., Kerrick, W.G.L. Effects of enflurane on functionally skinned myocardial fibers from
      rabbits, *Anesth*, 52:385-389, 1980.
104. Mohareb, A., El-Koussi, A., Osman, F., Afifi, A., Ali, H. Evaluation of cardiovascular and
      respiratory effects of different concentrations of Ethrane in rabbits, *Pharma Res Comm*, 11:745-
      747, 1979.
105. Marin, J.L.B., Carruthers, B., Chakrabarti, M.K., Sykes, M.K. Preservation of the pulmonary
      vasoconstrictor response to alveolar hypoxia during the administration of methoxyflurane, *Br J
      Anaesth*, 50:629-637, 1978.
106. Christian, C. II, Fagraeus, L., van Trigt, P. III, Pasque, M., Rellom, G., Frame, J., Wechsler, A.
      The effects of isoflurane on global ventricular mechanics, *Anesth (Suppl 3)*, 57:A13, 1982.
107. Fagraeus, L., Christian, C., van Trigt, J., Pasque, M., Frame, J., Neglen, P., Pellon, G., Wechsler,
      A. Inotropic effects of isoflurane on the hypertrophied left ventricle in dogs, *Anesth (Suppl 3)*,
      A14, 1982.
108. Redondo, J., Novakovic, L., Olivari, F. The effects of methoxyflurane on myocardial contractility
      and reactivity, *Anesth*, 34:450-457, 1971.
109. Bell, F.P., Hubert, E.V. Membrane active agents effect of various anesthetics and chlorpromazine
      on arterial lipid metabolism, *Atherosclerosis*, 39:517-526, 1981.
110. Su, J.Y., Bell, J.G. Effects of isoflurane on functionally skinned myocardial fibers from rabbits,
      *Anesth (Suppl 3)*57:A11, 1982.
111. Lundeen, G., Manohar, M., Parks, C. Systemic distribution of blood flow in swine while awake
      and during 1.0 and 1.5 MAC isoflurane anesthesia with or without 50% nitrous oxide, *Anesth
      Analg*, 62:499-512, 1983.
112. Leenen, F.H.H., Provoost, A.P. Maintenance of blood pressure by β-adrenoceptor mediated renin
      release during different forms of anesthesia in rats, *Can J Physiol Pharm*, 59:364-370, 1981.
113. Johansson, B.B. Effect of an acute increase of the intravascular pressure on the blood brain
      barrier; a comparison between conscious and anesthetized rats, *Stroke*, 9:588-590, 1978.
114. Davis, L.D., Temte, J.V., Helmer, P.R. *et al.* Effect of cyclopropane and of hypoxia on
      transmembrane potentials of atrial, ventricular and Purkinje fibers, *Circ Res*, 18:692-704, 1966.
115. Temte, J.V., Helmer, P.R., David, L.D. Effects of calcium and cyclopropane on Purkinje fibers,
      Anesth, 28:354-362, 1967.
116. Merin, R.G., Bernard, J.-M., Doursout, M.-F., Cohen, M., Chelly, J.E. Comparison of the effects
      of isoflurane and desflurane on cardiovascular dynamics and regional blood flow in the
      chronically instrumented dog, *Anesth*, 74:568-574, 1991.
117. Baele, P., Housmans, P.R. The effects of halothane, enflurane, and isoflurane on the length-
      tension relation of the isolated ventricular papillary muscle of the ferret, *Anesth*, 74:281-291,
      1991.
118. Pagel, P.S., Kampine, J.P., Schmeling, W.T., Warltier, D.C. Comparison of the systemic and
      coronary hemodynamic actions of desflurane, isoflurane, halothane, and enflurane in the
      chronically instrumented dog, *Anesth*, 74:539-551, 1991.
119. Deegan, R., He, H.B., Wood, A.J., Wood,M; Effects of anesthesia on norepinephrine kinetics.
      Comparison of propofol and halothane anesthesia in dogs, *Anesth*, 75:481-488, 1991.
120. Hunt, G.B., Ross, D.L. Comparison of effects of three anesthetic agents on induction of
      ventricular tachycardia in a canine model of myocardial infarction, *Circ*, 78:221-226, 1988.
121. Halliwill, J.R., Billman, G.E. Effect of general anesthesia on cardiac vagal tone, *Am J Physiol*,
      262:H1719-H1724, 1992.
122. van der Linden, P., Gilbart, E., Engelman, E., Schmartz, D., Vincent, J.L. Effects of anesthetic
      agents on systemic critical O_2 delivery, *J Appl Physiol*, 71:83-93, 1991.

123. Nyhan, D.P., Chen, B.B., Fehr, D.M., Rock, P., Murray, P.A. Anesthesia alters pulmonary vasoregulation by angiotensin II and captopril, *J Appl Physiol*, 72:636-642, 1992.

124. Fehr, D.M., Nyhan, D.P., Chen, B.B., Murray, PA; Pulmonary vasoregulation by cyclooxygenase metabolites and angiotensin II after hypoperfusion in conscious, pentobarbital-anesthetized, and halothane-anesthetized dogs, *Anesth*, 75:257-267, 1991.

125. Chen, B.B., Nyhan, D.P., Fehr, D.M., Goll, H.M., Murray, P.A. Halothane anesthesia causes active flow-independent pulmonary vasoconstriction, *Am J Physiol*, 259:H74-H83, 1990.

126. Frazer, M.J., Lynch, C. III; Halothane and isoflurane effects on Ca^{2+} fluxes of isolated myocardial sarcoplasmic reticulum, *Anesth*, 77:316-323, 1992.

127. Johnson, D., Mayers, I., Hurst, T. Halothane inhibits hypoxic pulmonary vasoconstriction in the presence of cyclooxygenase blockade, *Can J Anaesth*, 37:287-295, 1990.

128. Pagel, P.S., Kampine, J.P., Schmeling, W.T., Warltier, D.C. Alteration of left ventricular diastolic function by desflurane, isoflurane, and halothane in the chronically instrumented dog with autonomic nervous system blockade, *Anesth*, 74:1103-1114, 1991.

129. Kenny, D., Proctor, L.T., Schmeling, W.T., Kampine, J.P., Warltier, D.C. Isoflurane causes only minimal increases in coronary blood flow independent of oxygen demand, *Anesth*, 75:640-649, 1991.

130. Pagel, P.S., Kampine, J.P., Schmeling, W.T., Warltier, D.C. Comparison of end-systolic pressure-length relations and preload recruitable stroke work as indices of myocardial contractility in the conscious and anesthetized, chronically instrumented dog, *Anesth*, 73:278-290, 1990.

131. Kim, Y.D., Danchek, M., Myers, A.K., Burke, T.A. *et al.* Anaesthetic modification of regional myocardial functional adjustments during myocardial ischaemia: halothane vs fentanyl; *Br J Anaesth*, 68:286-292, 1992.

132. Kochi, T., Ide, T., Mizuguchi, T., Nishino, T. Halothane does not depress contractile function of fresh or fatigued diaphragm in pentobarbitone-anesthetized dogs, *Br J Anaesth*, 68:562-566, 1992.

133. Hartman, J.C., Kampine, J.P., Schmeling, W.T., Warltier, D.C; Volatile anesthetics and regional myocardial perfusion in chronically instrumented dogs: halothane versus isoflurane in a single-vessel disease model with enhanced collateral development, *J Cardiothorac Anesth*, 4:588-603, 1990.

134. Kenny, D., Pelc, L.R., Brooks, H.L., Kampine, J.P. *et al.* Calcium channel modulation of alpha 1- and alpha 2-adrenergic pressor responses in conscious and anesthetized dogs, *Anesth*, 72:874-881, 1990.

135. Hysing, E.S., Chelly, J.E., Doursout, MF, Merin RG; Comparative effects of halothane, enflurane, and isoflurane at equihypotensive doses on cardiac performance and coronary and renal blood flows, *Anesth*, 76:979-984, 1992.

136. Hysing, E.S., Chelly, J.E., Jacobson, L., Doursout, M.F., Merin, R.G. Cardiovascular effects of acute changes in extracellular ionized calcium concentration induced by citrate and $CaCl_2$ infusions in chronically instrumented dogs, conscious and during enflurane, halothane, and isoflurane anesthesia, *Anesth*, 72:100-104, 1990.

137. Roth, S. The effects of halothane on retinal and choroidal blood flow in cats, *Anesth*, 76:455-460, 1992.

138. MacLeod, B.A., McGroarty, R., Morton, R.H., Walker, M.J. Effects of halothane on arrhythmias induced by myocardial ischaemia, *Can J Anaesth*, 36:289-294, 1989.

139. Wang, Y.X., Zhou, T., Chua, T.C., Pang, C.C. Effects of inhalation and intravenous anesthetic agents on pressor response to N^G-nitro-L-arginine, *Eur J Pharmacol*, 198:183-188, 1991.

140. Weeks, J.B., Todd, M.M., Warner, D.S., Katz, J. The influence of halothane, isoflurane, and pentobarbital on cerebral plasma volume in hypocapnic and normocapnic rats, *Anesth*, 73:461-466, 1990.

141. Laorden, M.L., Hernandez, J., Carceles, M.D., Miralles, F.S., Puig, M.M. Interaction between halothane and morphine on isolated heart muscle, *Eur J Pharmacol*, 175:285-290, 1990.

142. Herland, J.S., Julian, F.J., Stephenson, D.G. Effects of halothane, enflurane, and isoflurane on skinned rat myocardium activated by Ca^{2+}, *Am J Physiol*, 264:H224-H232, 1993.

143. Durieux, M.E., Sperry, R.J., Longnecker, D.E. Effects of hypoxemia on regional blood flows during anesthesia with halothane, enflurane, or isoflurane, *Anesth*, 76:401-408, 1992.

144. Sano, T., Drummond, J.C., Patel, P.M., Grafe, M.R. *et al.* A comparison of the cerebral protective effects of isoflurane and mild hypothermia in a model of incomplete forebrain ischemia in the rat, *Anesth*, 76:221-228, 1992.

145. Young, W.L., Barkai, A.I., Prohovnik, I., Nelson, H., Durkin, M. Effect of PaCO$_2$ on cerebral blood flow distribution during halothane compared with isoflurane anaesthesia in the rat, *Br J Anaesth*, 67:440-446, 1991.

146. Larach, D.R., Schuler, H.G. Direct vasodilation by sevoflurane, isoflurane, and halothane alters coronary flow reserve in the isolated rat heart, *Anesth*, 75:268-278, 1991.

147. Verhaegen, M.J., Todd, M.M., Warner, D.S. A comparison of cerebral ischemic flow thresholds during halothane/N$_2$O and isoflurane/N$_2$O anesthesia in rats, *Anesth*, 76:743-754, 1992.

148. Bosnjak, Z.J., Aggarwal, A., Turner, L.A., Kampine, J.M., Kampine, J.P. Differential effects of halothane, enflurane, and isoflurane on Ca^{2+} transients and papillary muscle tension in guinea pigs, *Anesth*, 76:123-131, 1992.

149. Stowe, D.F., Monroe, S.M., Marijic, J., Bosnjak, Z.J., Kampine, J.P. Comparison of halothane, enflurane, and isoflurane with nitrous oxide on contractility and oxygen supply and demand in isolated hearts, *Anesth*, 75:1062-1074, 1991.

150. McShane, A.J., Crowleg, K., Shayevitz, J.R., Michael, J.R. *et al.* Barbiturate anesthetics inhibit thromboxane-, potassium-, but not angiotensin-induced pulmonary vasoconstriction, *Anesth*, 70:775-779, 1989.

151. Lerman, J., Oyston, J.P., Gallagher, T.M. *et al.* The minimum alveolar concentration (MAC) and hemodynamic effects of halothane, isoflurane, and sevoflurane in newborn swine, *Anesth*, 73-717-721, 1990.

152. Nagano, K., Gelman, S., Parks, D., Bradley, E.L. Hepatic circulation and oxygen supply-uptake relationships after hepatic insult during anesthesia with volatile anesthetics and fentanyl in miniature pigs, *Anesth Analg*, 70:53-62, 1990.

153. Palmisano, B.W., Clifford, P.S., Hoffman, R.G., Seagard, J.L., Coon, R.L., Kampine, J.P. Depression of baroreflex control of heart rate by halothane in growing piglets, *Anesth*, 75:512-519, 1991.

154. Nagano, K., Gelman, S., Parks, D.A., Bradley, E.L. Jr. Hepatic oxygen supply-uptake relationship and metabolism during anesthesia in miniature pigs, *Anesth*, 72:902-910, 1990.

155. van Daal, G.J., Lachmann, B., Schairer, W., Tenbrinck, R., van Woerkens, L.J., Verdouw, P., Erdman, W. The influence of different anesthetics on the oxygen delivery to and consumption of the heart, *Adv Exp Med Biol*, 248:527-532, 1989.

156. Cameron, C.B., Gregorym, G.A., Rudolph, A.M., Heymann, M. The cardiovascular and metabolic effects of halothane in normoxic and hypoxic newborn lambs, *Anesth*, 62:732-737, 1985.

157. Cuvelliez, S.G., Eicker, S.W., McLauchlan, C., Brunson, D.B. Cardiovascular and respiratory effects of inspired oxygen fraction in halothane-anesthetized horses, *Am J Vet Res*, 51:1226-1231, 1990.

158. Riedesel, D.H., Hildebrand, S.V. Unusual response following use of succinylcholine in a horse anesthetized with halothane, *J Am Vet Med Assoc*, 187:508-508, 1985.

159. Greene, S.A., Keegan, R.D., Gallagher, L.V., Alexander, J.E., Horari, J. Cardiovascular effects of halothane anesthesia after diazepam and ketamine administration in beavers (Castor canadensis) during spontaneous or controlled ventilation, *Am J Vet Res*, 52:665-668, 1991.

160. Ludders, J.W., Mitchell, G.S., Schaefer, S.L. Minimum anesthetic dose and cardiopulmonary dose response for halothane in chickens, *Am J Vet Res*, 49:929-932, 1988.

161. Mayer, N., Zimpfer, M., Kotai, E., Placheta, P. Enflurane alters compensatory hemodynamic and humoral responses to hemorrhage, *Circ Shock*, 30:165-178, 1990.

162. Schaefer, C.F., Brackett, D.J., Biber, B., Lerner, M.R. *et al.* Respiratory and cardiovascular effects of thyrotropin-releasing hormone as modified by isoflurane, enflurane, pentobarbital and ketamine, *Regul Pept*, 24:269-282, 1989.

163. Chinzei, M., Morita, S., Chinzei, T., Takahashi, H. *et al.* Effects of isoflurane and fentanyl on ischemic myocardium in dogs: assessment by end-systolic measurements, *J Cardiothorac Vasc Anesth*, 5:243-249, 1991.

164. Reilly, C.S., Merrell, J., Wood, A.J., Koshakji, R.P., Wood, M. Comparison of the effects of isoflurane or fentanyl-nitrous oxide anaesthesia on propranolol disposition in dogs, *Br J Anaesth*, 60:791-796, 1988.

165. Pagel, P.S., Kampine, J.P., Schmeling, W.T., Warltier, D.C. Effects of nitrous oxide on myocardial contractility as evaluated by the preload recruitable stroke work relationship in chronically instrumented dogs, *Anesth*, 73:1148-1157, 1990.

166. Hartman, J.C., Kampine, J.P., Schmeling, W.T., Warltier, D.C. Alterations in collateral blood flow produced by isoflurane and a chronically instrumented canine model of multivessel coronary artery disease, *Anesth*, 74:120-133, 1991.

167. Hartman, J.C., Kampine, J.P., Schmeling, W.T., Warltier, D.C. Actions of isoflurane on myocardial perfusion in chronically instrumented dogs with poor, moderate, or well-developed coronary collaterals, *J Cardiothorac Anesth*, 4:715-725, 1990.

168. Crystal, G.J., Kim, S.J., Czinn, E.A., Salem, M.R. *et al.* Intracoronary isoflurane causes marked vasodilation in canine hearts, *Anesth*, 74:757-765, 1991.

169. Roald, O.K., Forsman, M., Steen, P.A. Partial reversal of the cerebral effects of isoflurane in the dog by theophylline, *Acta Anaesthesiol Scand*, 34:548-551, 1990.

170. Pagel, P.S., Kampine, J.P., Schmeling, W.T., Warltier, D.C. Influence of volatile anesthetics on myocardial contractility *in vivo*: Desflurane versus Isoflurane, *Anesth*, 74:900-907, 1991.

171. Abdel-Latif, M., Kim, S.-J., Salem, M.R., Crystal, G.J. Phenylephrine does not limit myocardial blood flow or oxygen delivery during isoflurane-induced hypotension in dogs, *Anesth Analg*, 74:870-876, 1992.

172. Poterack, K.A., Kampine, J.P., Schmeling, W.T. Effects of isoflurane, midazolam and etomidate on cardiovascular responses to stimulation of central nervous system pressor sites in chronically instrumented cats, *Anesth Analg*, 73:64-75, 1991.

173. Conzen, P.F., Vollmar, B., Habazettl, H., Frink, E.J., Peter, K., Messmer, K. Systemic and regional hemodynamics of isoflurane and sevoflurane in rats, *Anesth Analg*, 74:79-88, 1992.

174. Chi, O.Z., Anwar, M., Sinha, A.K., Wei, H.M. *et al.* Effects of isoflurane on transport across the blood-brain barrier, *Anesth*, 76:426-431, 1992.

175. Hoffman, W.E., Edelman, G., Kochs, E., Werner, C. *et al.* Cerebral autoregulation in awake versus isoflurane-anesthetized rats, *Anesth Analg*, 73:753-757, 1991.

176. Weiskopf, R.B., Eger, E.I. II, Holmes, M.A., Yasuda, N., Johnson, B.H., Targ, A.G., Rampil, I.J. Cardiovascular actions of common anesthetic adjuvants during desflurane (I-653) and isoflurane anesthesia in swine, *Anesth Analg*, 71:144-148, 1990.

177. Patel, P.M., Mutch, W.A. The cerebral pressure-flow relationship during 1.0 MAC isoflurane anesthesia in the rabbit; the effect of different vasopressors, *Anesth*, 72:118-124, 1990.

178. Baker, B.W., Hughes, S.C., Shnider, S.M., Field, D.R., Rosen, M.A. Maternal anesthesia and the stressed fetus: effects of isoflurane on the asphyxiated fetal lamb, *Anesth*, 72:65-70, 1990.

179. Ludders, J.W., Mitchell, G.S., Rode, J. Minimal anesthetic concentration and cardiopulmonary dose response of isoflurane in ducks, *Vet Surg*, 19:304-307, 1990.

180. Ludders, J.W., Rode, J., Mitchell, G.S. Isoflurane anesthesia in sandhill cranes (Grus canadensis): minimal anesthetic concentration and cardiopulmonary dose-response during spontaneous and controlled breathing, *Anesth Analg*, 68:511-516, 1989.

181. Warltier, D.C., Pagel, P.S. Cardiovascular and respiratory actions of desflurane: is desflurane different from isoflurane?, *Anesth Analg (Suppl 4)*, 75:S17-S29, 1992.

182. Crawford, M.W., Lerman, J., Pilato, M., Orrego, H. *et al.* Haemodynamic and organ blood flow responses to sevoflurane during spontaneous ventilation in the rat: a dose-response study, *Can J Anaesth*, 39:270-276, 1992.

183. Dai, S. Anaesthetic-related occurrence of early ventricular arrhythmias during acute myocardial ischaemia in rats, *Arch Int Physiol Biochim*, 97:341-346, 1989.

184. Kalman, S., Eintrei, C. Central circulation during halothane-diethyl-ether azeotrope and isoflurane anaesthesia in the pig, *Acta Anaesthesiol Scand*, 35:736-740, 1991.

185. Baughman, V.L., Hoffman, W.E., Miletich, D.J., Albrecht, R.F. Cerebrovascular and cerebral metabolic effects of N_2O in unrestrained rats, *Anesth*, 73:269-272, 1990.

186. Coetzee, A., Fourie, P., Bolliger, C., Badenhorst, E., Rebel, A., Lombard, C. Effect of N_2O on segmental left ventricular function and effective arterial elastance in pigs when added to a halothane-fentanyl- pancuronium anesthetic technique, *Anesth Analg*, 69:313-322, 1989.

187. Lawson, D., Frazer, M.J., Lynch, C. III; Nitrous oxide effects on isolated myocardium: a reexamination *in vitro*, *Anesth*, 73:930-943, 1990.

188. Carton, E.G., Wanek, L.A., Housmans, P.R. Effects of N_2O on contractility, relaxation and the intracellular calcium transient of isolated mammalian ventricular myocardium, *J Pharmacol Exp Thera*, 257:843-849, 1991.

189. Pagel, P.S., Kampine, J.P., Schmeling, W.T., Warltier, D.C. Reversal of volatile anesthetic-induced depression of myocardial contractility by extracellular calcium also enhances left ventricular diastolic function, *Anesthesiology*, 78:141-154, 1993.

8. Cardiovascular effects of hallucinogens, neurolept analgesic/anesthetic combinations and steroid anesthetics

In recent years there has been an upsurge in the use of dissociative analgesics (hallucinogens) and various neurolept analgesic/anesthetic or sedative combinations. Some of this popularity is spillover from human medicine, where, for a variety of reasons, so-called "balanced anesthesia/analgesia" is increasingly popular. In veterinary medicine and in biomedical research, the dissociative anesthetic agents are popular because they usually do not require an intravenous injection and render the animal semiconscious or unconscious with a large safety factor and very little skill needed. These advantages are especially important when working with primates but are useful for other species as well. Some combinations of these agents seem to offer great advantages in the study of the cardiovascular system.

A number of agents, when used in combination, seem to potentiate calming and/or analgesic properties while minimizing problems of ataxia. The latter is particularly important when dealing with very large animals such as horses, or animals which are difficult to restrain physically such as primates and pigs. These combinations frequently include one of the opiods and a tranquilizer (i.e. Innovar, Immobilon) or a hallucinogenic agent and a tranquilizer (i.e. Telazol). The agents may be given as separate injections at the same time, in sequence or, when they are chemically compatible, they may be mixed in the same syringe as a "cocktail". Some combinations produce profound analgesia and sedation which may approach anesthesia (neurolept-analgesia).

Ketamine

One of the most popular agents presently being used is the hallucinogen ketamine. This agent is restricted to use in young children in human medicine because of the high incidence of severely unpleasant hallucinations and flashbacks. In veterinary medicine it is used most frequently in cats and swine, but has been recommended for other species as well, particularly in combination with a variety of tranquilizers. It provides true dissociation and a form of sedation or, at least, lack of purposeful movement. It's analgesic properties are a subject of some debate.

Ketamine has marked effects on the cardiovascular system. It stimulates the heart in the clinically normal subject, manifested as an increase in heart rate, cardiac output and mean aortic pressure. These are probably indirect effects caused by a combination of parasympathetic inhibition and sympathetic stimulation. Subjects with cardiac arrhythmias do not appear to be detrimentally effected but extreme caution is recommended in those with valvular insufficiencies or diseased or traumatized myocardium. There seems to be a direct negative inotropic effect coupled with an increase in cardiac work. The peripheral vasopressor response is considered to be centrally mediated, but there is no reported increase in preload.[1,2] The cardiovascular effects of ketamine are summarized, by species, in Table 8.1.

Table 8.1: The Cardiovascular Effects of Ketamine

Conditions of the experiment	Dose	Cardiovascular effects	Reference
8.1:1 Ketamine-Dogs			
Previously instrumented, intact, awake	8 mg/kg, IV	Increased mean aortic pressure, cardiac index, hepatic arterial flow, portal pressure, portal venular resistance; no change in portal hepatic blood flow or ratio between hepatic arterial blood flow and total hepatic blood flow	3
Previously instrumented, intact, awake	5 mg/kg	Increased mean aortic pressure, heart rate and cardiac output; all parameters remained elevated for 15-30 min; no change in systemic resistance	2
Previously instrumented, intact, awake	5 mg/kg	Significant increases in aortic pressure and renal blood flow; renal vascular resistance significantly increased early then returned to baseline	4
Previously instrumented, intact, awake	5 mg/kg	Increased mean aortic pressure, heart rate, cardiac output, LV dP/dt; LV end-diastolic pressure decreased; latter effect reversed by β-adrenergic blockade	5
Previously instrumented, intact, awake, compared untreated with phentolamine (2 mg/kg)IV and phentolamine + atropine (0.1 mg/kg)IV	5 mg/kg, IV	Untreated; increased heart rate, cardiac output and mean aortic pressure Phentolamine; mean aortic pressure increase less than control, cardiac output and heart rate both increased significantly Phentolamine + atropine; blocked the pressor, the chronotropic and the early part of the cardiac output response	6
Anesthetized with halothane, acute instrumentation, waited approx. 60 min before experiment; another group pretreated with atropine (0.1 mg/kg),IV	5 mg/kg, IV	Increased blood pressure, cardiac output, respiratory rate and minute volume; arterial pO_2 and pH decreased while $PaCO_2$ increased; atropine attenuated the pressor response	7
Anesthetized with halothane	6 mg/kg, IV	Abolished epinephrine-induced ventricular arrhythmias	2

Conditions	Dose	Cardiovascular effects	Reference
Same as above	32 mg/kg, IV	Transient decrease in mean aortic pressure with an increase in heart rate and mean aortic pressure after several minutes	2
Anesthetized with halothane, right-side by-pass preparation with preload controlled	32 mg/kg	Negative inotropic effects, same negative inotropy seen with dogs subjected to bilateral vagotomy and bilateral sectioning of the carotid sinus nerve	2
Anesthetized with pentobarbital (30 mg/kg, IV), positive pressure ventilation with 70% N_2O, arterial pH and $PaCO_2$ maintained at 7.35-7.45 and 34-42 mmHg, respectively	3 mg/kg	Increased mean arterial pressure and heart rate; response was demonstrated to originate at some site in the central nervous system or at a peripheral site other than a baroreceptor mediated phenomena	8
Anesthetized with α-chloralose (100 mg/kg, IV), positive pressure ventilation, acute instrumentation, determinations made after a 30 min wait following completion of the instrumentation	3 mg/kg, IV	Decreased mean aortic pressure and cardiac index; hepatic arterial, portal and total hepatic blood flow were unchanged as were portal pressure and portal vascular resistance	3
Anesthetized with thiopentone (15-20 mg/kg),IV, suxamethonium (100 mg),IV, positive pressure ventilation, trichloroethylene (0.3-0.6%), occasional suxamethonium (50 mg),IM as needed, open chest, acute instrumentation	5 mg/kg, 10 mg/kg boluses and 5 mg/kg followed by infusion of 0.1 mg/kg/min	Decreased mean aortic pressure, increased cardiac output and stroke volume; coronary blood flow and myocardial oxygen consumption increased but not change in myocardial oxygen extraction	9

Conditions	Dose	Cardiovascular effects	Reference
Tolerance to ouabain sufficient to produce ventricular tachycardia and death, positive pressure ventilation with 100% O_2; $PaCO_2$ maintained at approx. 35 mmHg	10 mg/kg + additional as needed	Increased the dose of ouabain required to cause both ventricular tachycardia and LD_{50}; a greater dose of ouabain was required than with pentobarbital treated or untreated controls	10
Anesthetized with pentobarbital (30 mg/kg), open chest, positive pressure ventilation, by-pass from femoral artery to the SA nodal artery, constant pressure of 100 mmHg	30, 100 and 300 µg direct into the perfusate	Positive chronotropic response of SA node to ketamine might be induced by an inhibition of norepinephrine uptake at the adrenergic nerve endings, similar to cocaine effects	11
Selective perfusion of SA nodal artery using femoral arterial blood at a constant pressure of 100 mmHg; anesthetized with pentobarbital (30 mg/kg), positive pressure ventilation, open chest	100 µg to 3 mg into perfusate	Results indicated than an activation of the peripheral adrenergic mechanism plays an important role in the induction of the excitatory effect of ketamine injected into the SA nodal artery	12
Isolated hindlimb preparation; anesthetized with ketamine, thiopental and N_2O	5 mg/kg, IV	Sympathetic mediated vasoconstriction and direct vasodilation in the hindlimb vasculature immediately after injection	13
Same as above	5, 10 &25 mg/kg into the carotid artery	Increased mean aortic pressure, increased perfusion pressure, transient vasoconstriction of the hindlimb vasculature	13
Same as above	5, 50 & 500 µg/ml into perfusate	At 5 µg/ml there was no uptake blockade of tritiated norepinephrine; at 20 & 500 µg/ml the preparation exhibited a cocaine-like effect (i.e. there was a blocked uptake of tritiated norepinephrine); at 50 & 500 µg/ml there was a direct depressant effect of ketamine which predominated	13

Conditions	Dose	Cardiovascular effects	Reference
Intact, awake, acute instrumentation	10 mg/kg, IV	Increased heart rate, mean aortic pressure, cardiac output & LV work; decreased central venous pressure, stroke volume, respiratory rate & minute ventilation; no change in mean pulmonary arterial pressure, systemic resistance, LV stroke work or tidal volume	64
Intact, awake, previously instrumented, autonomic blockade with propranolol (2 mg/kg), atropine (3 mg/kg), hexamethonium (20 mg/kg)	25, 50 & 100 mg/kg/hr, dose-response	Dose-dependent decreases in all measures of myocardial contractility indicating increases in cardiac parameters are due to autonomic stimulation	65
Intact, awake, acepromazine (0.2 mg/kg)	10 mg/kg, IV	Increased heart rate and mean aortic pressure; decreased stroke volume; no change in mean pulmonary arterial pressure, central venous pressure, cardiac output, peripheral resistance, LV work, or LV stroke work	66
Control group anesthetized with Pentobarbital (25 mg/kg), IV + Pancuronium (0.1 mg/kg + 1-2 mg/hr)	5 mg/kg + 0.2 mg/kg/min	Decreased mean aortic pressure, cardiac index, stroke index, LV stroke work index, oxygen delivery and oxygen consumption; no change in heart rate, mean pulmonary arterial pressure, pulmonary arterial wedge pressures or systemic resistance	67
Same as above	5 mg/kg + 0.4 mg/kg/min	Decreased pulmonary arterial wedge pressures, oxygen consumption; no change in heart rate, mean aortic pressure, mean pulmonary arterial pressure, right atrial pressure, cardiac index, stroke index, systemic resistance, LV stroke work index, venous oxygen saturation, oxygen delivery, or lactate production	67
Chronically instrumented, conscious vs anesthetize with autonomic blockade	Dose-response; 25, 50 & 100 mg/kg/hr infusions	Dose-dependent increase in time constant of isovolumetric relaxation and increase in regional passive chamber stiffness, i.e. decreased diastolic compliance	68

8.1:2 Ketamine-Cats, conditions	Dose	Cardiovascular effects	Reference
Intact, awake, previously instrumented	not given	Increased mean aortic pressures, heart rate and cardiac output, no change in systemic resistance	2
8.1:3 Ketamine-Rats			
Previously instrumented with aortic cannulae, awake	80 mg/kg, IP	Little or no protection against mortality and kidney lesions following bleeding to 30-50 mmHg for 60 min	14
Previously instrumented, awake, using a double microsphere technique, each rat served as its own control	125 mg/kg, IM	Flow was increased to the brain, decreased to skeletal muscle, no change in flow to heart, lung, skin, kidneys, liver, spleen, stomach, large intestine or small intestine, no change in cardiac output	15
Awake versus ketamine treated, following 1 hr of hemorrhage to 40 mmHg mean aortic pressure	125 mg/kg, IM	Plasma renin activity was not altered by ketamine but was altered by hemorrhage; concluded that anesthetic influence on survival following severe hemorrhage does not result from anesthetic-induced alterations of the renin-angiotensin system	16
Decerebrated at mid-collicular level under halothane anesthesia and then allowed to recover for at least 90 min prior to the study	5 mg/kg, IV	Decreased heart rate and blood pressure, decreased respiratory rate, decreased carotid occlusion and tilt-induced baroreceptor responses and sodium cyanide induced chemoreceptor responses	17
Acute instrumentation, positive pressure ventilation, using spontaneously hypertensive rats; compared effects of ketamine in combination with antihypertensive drugs and hemorrhagic shock	100 mg/kg, IP + 60 mg/kg/hr	With respect to hemorrhagic shock tolerance hydralazine and methyldopa, and to a lesser extent clonidine, have a favorable effect on the circulation while rats are anesthetized with ketamine, β-adrenergic blockade may be harmful under these circumstances	18

Conditions	Dose	Cardiovascular effects	Reference
Isolated atrial preparation	5 X 10⁻⁵ M to 2 X 10⁻⁴ M	Increased inotropic response to noradrenergic nerve stimulation and to exogenous noradrenaline; Results were consistent with the hypothesis that ketamine causes a post-junctional sympathomimetic super-sensitivity combined with an increase in the available noradrenaline as a result of blockade of neuronal re-uptake	19
Isolated atrial and isolated portal vein preparations	2.5 µg/ml to 1.2 mg/ml	Depression of atrial rate and amplitude of myogenic activity in the portal vein preparation; the reaction was Ca^{2+}-dependent but qualitatively different than the response to thiopentone in the same preparation	20
Cremaster muscle preparation, mean arterial pressure lowered to and maintained at 30-35 mmHg	125 mg/kg, IM + 30 mg/kg, as needed	Diminished the constrictor response to hemorrhage compared to enflurane anesthesia, no tissue hypoxia was noted	21
Cremaster muscle preparation, measured internal diameter of the arteries and their response to hemorrhage down to a mean aortic pressure of 30 mg/kg	125 mg/kg, IM + 30 mg/kg as needed	1st order vessels; decreased internal diameter approximately 20% at 10, 20 & 30 min. No changes in 3rd order vessels; 4th order vessels showed an approximate 20% increase in diameter but only at 30 min.	22
Killed by cervical dislocation, isolated Langendorff preparation	Dose-response	Dose-dependent inhibition of norepinephrine uptake by both neuronal and extraneuronal processes	23
Coronary artery ligation	150 mg/kg, Sub Q	Lower incidence of ventricular arrhythmias than rats anesthetized with pentobarbital, urethane or ether + chloralose	69
IV bolus response to L-NNA (32 mg/kg)	125 mg/kg, IP + 20 mg/kg/30 min, IV	Increased mean aortic pressures 57 ± 4 mmHg versus the response in conscious rats which was approx. 51 mmHg	70
Previously instrumented, conscious	60 mg/kg/ hr, IV	No change in respiratory rate, mean aortic pressure; decrease in heart rate and cardiac output	71

8.1:4 Ketamine-Rabbits, conditions	Dose	Cardiovascular effects	Reference
Intact, awake, previously instrumented	35 mg/kg, IM	Decreased aortic pressure, respiratory rate and heart rate, the latter only slightly	24
Isolated heart preparation	2×10^{-5}, 1×10^{-4} & 5×10^{-4} M	Dose-dependent decrease in spontaneous rate and inotropy, increase in coronary flow	25
Isolated heart preparation	500 µg/ml in perfusate	When combined with isoproterenol or dopamine decreased LV dP/dt compared with the amines alone; the effect was less apparent at temperatures lower than $35^{\circ}C$; these results indicate ketamine may be a catecholamine uptake inhibitor, similar to cocaine	26
Isolated aortic and pulmonary artery strips	1.1×10^{-5} to 3.7×10^{-4} M	Potentiated adrenaline-contraction, potentiation not impaired by pretreatment with reserpine, 6-hydroxydopamine or cocaine; potentiation blocked by catechol-methyltransferase inhibitors or extraneuronal uptake inhibitors; ketamine potentiated responses to catecholamines but not to phenylephrine, methoxamine or synephrine (relaxation); potentiated responses to tyramine (cocaine inhibited), decreased rate at which aortic strips inactivated adrenaline; inhibits extraneuronal uptake in vascular smooth muscle	27
Functional skinned muscle fiber prep.	0.5-10 mM	Increased submaximal Ca^{2+}-activated tension development; concentrations greater than or equal to 5 mM decreased maximum tension; concentrations between 1-10 mM decreased sarcoplasmic reticulum Ca^{2+} uptake but did not change sarcoplasmic reticulum Ca^{2+} release as a result of exposure to 25 mM caffeine; conclusion was that ketamine-induced myocardial depression may be due to the inhibition of Ca^{2+} uptake by the sarcoplasmic reticulum and inhibition of the maximum Ca^{2+}-activated tension	28

8.1:5 Ketamine-Goats, conditions	Dose	Cardiovascular effects	Reference
Intact, awake, previously instrumented, compared respiratory paralyzed and mechanically ventilated group; pancuronium (0.05 mg/kg,IV) to unparalysed group	5 mg/kg, IV	No significant effect on cerebral blood flow, only a slight decrease in cerebral metabolic rate when ventilation was controlled; data suggests that the observed increase in cerebral spinal fluid pressures could be minimized with adequate ventilation; if $PaCO_2$ and mean aortic pressures were held constant there were decreased effects from the ketamine infusion	29
Previously instrumented, intact, awake vs anesthetized with pentobarbital (25-30 mg/kg, IV), positive pressure ventilation	0.1 to 4 mg directly into the CNS via a temporal artery	In the awake animals there was an immediate increase in mean systemic blood pressure, cardiac output and heart rate and there were variable changes in cerebral blood flow; in the pentobarbital anesthetized group no changes in any of the cardiovascular parameters were observed	30
Same as above	2 mg/kg, IV	Awake; increase in aortic pressure, cardiac output, heart rate, cerebral blood flow and arterial $PaCO_2$; Anesthetized; no change in any of the parameters; concluded that ketamine produces peripheral sympathomimetic effects, primarily by direct stimulation of CNS structures, when CNS anesthetized peripheral effects are removed	30
Intact, awake, previously instrumented vs pentobarbital anesthetized	No dose given	Increase in cardiac output, heart rate and mean aortic pressure; responses were prevented when anesthetized first with pentobarbital	2

8.1:6 Ketamine-Sheep, Conditions of the experiment	Dose	Cardiovascular Effects	Reference
Both fetus and dam instrumented acutely under anesthesia, then allowed 24 hours for recovery	0.7 mg/kg, IV into dam	Maternal effects: Increased mean aortic pressure, heart rate, cardiac output and $PaCO_2$, decreased systemic resistance and arterial pH; The uterine artery showed a decrease in flow within 1 min then increased for 5-30 min; tone in the artery increased within 3 min then decreased to baseline over 30 min Fetal effects: Mean aortic pressure increased within 1 min then decreased to baseline within 30 min; there was no change in fetal arterial pH or $PaCO_2$; fetal PaO_2 increased within 5 min, persisted for more than 30 min; maternal norepinephrine and epinephrine values significantly decreased during the period that the cardiovascular effects were most pronounced	31
8.1:7 Ketamine-Cattle			
Intact, awake, local anesthesia used for acute catheterization (Buffalo calves)	2 mg/kg, IV	Increased heart rate, mean aortic pressure, cardiac output and systemic resistance; central venous pressure decreased until approx. 30 min then returned to baseline; preanesthetic treatment with chlorpromazine (2 mg/kg, IM) increased the duration of analgesia, increased standing and recovery times and the degree of muscle relaxation but no report on the cardiovascular effects of chlorpromazine pretreatment	32
Myosin B and sarcoplasmic reticulum isolated from carotid arteries taken from cattle at slaughter	not given	No effects on superprecipitation and the ATP-ase activity of arterial myosin B, but a significant increase in Ca^{2+} uptake; suggests the effect of ketamine on the contraction-relaxation of vascular smooth muscle is performed through the change in Ca^{2+} uptake by sarcoplasmic reticulum	33

8.1:8 Ketamine-Pigs, Conditions of the experiment	Dose	Cardiovascular Effects	Reference
Anesthetized with halothane, acute instrumentation, metocurine (0.2 mg/kg + supplementation as needed), positive pressure ventilation, measurements made after end-tidal halothane conc. reduced to <0.05 mmHg, blood volume reduction by 30% with and without ketamine	6.6 ± 0.5 mg/kg, IV	No significant difference in the cardiovascular parameters monitored as a result of ketamine; hemorrhage produced increases in plasma catecholamines, decreased mean aortic pressure, cardiac output, systemic resistance and oxygen consumption and increased lactate concentrations as would be predicted	34
8.1:9 Ketamine-Monkeys (macaca mulatta)			
Intact, instrumented under thiamylal anesthesia just prior to the experiment but allowed to regain consciousness before the ketamine was administered	7 mg/kg, IM	No change in respiratory rate, arterial pH, PaO_2, $PaCO_2$ or PvO_2; a significant increase in PvO_2 30 min after the ketamine was injected	35
8.1:10 Ketamine-Chickens			
Isolated hearts from 4 & 7 day old embryos	2×10^{-4} M	Decreased rate and force of contraction by 50% of control	36
Ketamine-Ferrets,			
Isolated, electrically stimulated papillary muscle preparations	10^{-6} to 3×10^{-4} M	Positive inotropic effects, max. @ 1×10^{-4} M; apparent mechanism of action to inhibit norepinephrine uptake at the neuroeffector junction	72

Ketamine-Tranquilizer Combinations

Because of the apparent central stimulatory and catecholamine uptake blockade induced by ketamine a variety of combinations with various tranquilizers have been suggested. Although the cardiovascular effects of these combinations have not been systematically studied in all species some information is available. Combinations have been physically mixed, in the same syringe, and given as a "cocktail". This practice is not appropriate for all agents since chemical interactions can and do occur. This can result in precipitation, sludging or other, less visible but still chemically neutralizing reactions. Even if two agents mixed together do not visibly change in color, consistency or viscosity, it is not always possible to determine if some chemical change has or has not occurred. The cardiovascular effects of those combinations that have been studied are summarized in the following tables.

Table 8.2: Cardiovascular Effects of Ketamine-Phenothiazine Type Tranquilizer Combinations:

Conditions of the experiment	Drug combination and Dose	Cardiovascular effects	Reference
8.2:1 Ketamine, Promazine-Dogs			
Intact, awake, previously instrumented	Acepromazine (0.2 mg/kg), Ketamine (10 mg/kg), IV	Increased heart rate, effective alveolar volume, alveolar-arterial PO_2 gradient (transient), venous admixture (transient), $PaCO_2$ & $PvCO_2$ (transient); decreased stroke volume, minute ventilation, physiological dead space, arterial & venous PO_2 (transient)	66
8.2:2 Ketamine, Promazine-Cats			
Anesthetized with halothane, instrumented, 36 hrs later conducted experiment	Acepromazine (0.13 mg/lb), Ketamine (13.0 mg/lb), in same syringe, IM	Decrease aortic pressure, increased heart rate for 5 min then decreased; respiratory rate, arterial pH and PaO_2 decreased; increased $PaCO_2$	37
Same as above	Acepromazine (0.5 mg/lb), Ketamine (15 mg/lb) admin. separately, IM	Aortic pressure decreased from acepromazine, prior to ketamine, heart rate increased at 5 min then decreased to baseline prior to ketamine; after ketamine heart rate decreased more; respiratory rate increased prior to ketamine then increased after it was administered	37

Conditions	Drug combination and dose	Cardiovascular effects	Reference
No details given	Acepromazine (0.11mg/kg), IV, Ketamine (11 mg/kg), IV	Does not prolong duration of action, smooths recovery and aids muscle relaxation; no hypotensive effects from acepromazine at this dosage (this is questionable, supposedly get some degree of α-adrenergic blockade)	2
Intact, awake, previously instrumented	Acepromazine (0.5 mg/kg), Ketamine (20 mg/kg), IM	Ten minutes post-injection heart rate was increased, mean aortic pressure was decreased and respiratory rate was decreased	38
Anesthetized with pentobarbital (30 mg/kg, IP), acute instrumentation, still under light pentobarbital anesthesia when studies conducted	Promazine (7.5 mg/ml), Centrine (0.0625 mg/ml), Ketamine 100 mg/ml), all mixed together and given at the rate of 15 mg/kg Ketamine with	Decreased mean aortic pressure, respiratory rate, arterial pH and PaO_2; increased $PaCO_2$	39

Table 8.3: Cardiovascular Effects of Ketamine-Xylazine Combinations:

Conditions of the experiment	Drug combination and dose	Cardiovascular effects	Reference
8.3:1 Ketamine, Xylazine-Dogs			
Acutely instrumented, non-sedated, intact, awake	Xylazine (1.0 mg/kg), Ketamine (10 mg/kg), IV	Increased heart rate, mean aortic pressure, systemic resistance and tidal volume; decreased central venous pressure, stroke volume, left ventricular stroke work, respiratory rate and minute volume; no change in mean pulmonary arterial pressure or left ventricular work	74

Conditions	Drug combination and dose	Cardiovascular effects	Reference
Intact, awake, previously instrumented, pretreated with atropine (0.04 mg/kg)	Xylazine (1.0 mg/kg), Ketamine (11 mg/kg), IV	Increased heart rate, mean aortic pressure, left atrial pressure, systemic resistance; decreased cardiac index and a very large decrease in LV dP/dt from approx. 1400 to 110 (mmHg/sec)	**77**
Intact, awake, previously instrumented	Xylazine (1.0 mg/kg), IV (pretreatment) then Ketamine (10 mg/kg), IV	Increased heart rate (transient), cardiac output, alveolar-arterial PO_2 gradient and venous admixture (transient), arterial PCO_2 (transient); decreased stroke volume (transient), LV stroke work (transient), effective alveolar ventilation, PaO_2 and O_2 content	**74**
Intact, awake, previously instrumented	Xylazine (1.1 mg/kg) + Ketamine (11.0 mg/kg), IM; or same doses with Ketamine given 5 min after Xylazine and given IV	Consistently produced systemic and pulmonary hypertension and decreased cardiac index and arterial oxygen tension	**107**
8.3:2 Ketamine, Xylazine-Cats			
Anesthetized with halothane, instrumented and allowed to recover for 36 hrs prior to the experiment	Xylazine (0.94 mg/lb), Ketamine (9.4 mg/lb), in same syringe, IM	Emesis in 2 of 10 cats within 4 minutes; aortic pressure decreased along with heart rate, respiratory rate, pH and PaO_2; $PaCO_2$ increased	**37**
Same as above	Xylazine (0.3 mg/kg), wait 10 min, Ketamine (12.8 mg/lb), IM	Emesis in 7 of 10 cats within 3-7 min.; aortic pressure decreased prior to the ketamine, increased slightly and then decreased again. Heart rate, respiratory rate, and arterial pH all decreased; $PaCO_2$ decreased slightly then increased; PaO_2 decreased prior to ketamine then decreased more	**37**

8.3:3 Ketamine, Xylazine-Rabbits, conditions	Dose	Cardiovascular effects	Reference
Intact, awake, previously instrumented	Xylazine (5 mg/kg), IM, Ketamine (35 mg/kg), IM	Decreased heart rate which stayed depressed for 120 min; decreased respiratory rate, stayed depressed for 120 minutes, decreased rectal temperature which stayed depressed	76
Intact, awake, previously instrumented	Xylazine (5 mg/kg), IM Ketamine (35 mg/kg, IM)	Decreased aortic pressure which lasted at least 3.5 hrs, also decreased heart rate and respiratory rate	24
Intact, awake, previously instrumented	Xylazine (5 mg/kg), IV, Ketamine (25 mg/kg, IV)	Decreased PaO_2, hypercapnia, respiratory acidosis	77
8.3:4 Ketamine, Xylazine-Horses			
Intact, awake	Xylazine (1.1 mg/kg), wait 3 min then Ketamine (2.7 mg/kg), followed by atropine sulfate (0.02 mg/kg), IV	Within 22 sec after Xylazine all 6 horses had some degree of 2nd degree A-V block; during the next 3 min heart rate decreased by 30%; within 12 sec after ketamine there was a more severe 2nd degree A-V block with premature ventricular contractions which was abolished by atropine; within 1 min and 30 sec following ketamine the 2nd degree A-V block was abolished in 4 of 6 horses, heart rate remained decreased 17% of baseline	40
Intact, awake	Xylazine (1.1 mg/kg), slow IV over 2 min, wait 2 min then Ketamine (2.2 mg/kg), IV	Measurements not made until after the animals were down and immobilized; the time frame is not clear; no apparent change in mean aortic pressure, respiratory rate, heart rate, PaO_2 or $PaCO_2$	41
Intact, awake, previously instrumented	Xylazine (1.1 mg/kg),IV + Ketamine (2.2 mg/kg), IV	No change in cardiac output, mean aortic pressure, pulmonary arterial pressure, central venous pressure or pulmonary arterial wedge pressures; respiratory acidosis with time	78

8.3:5 Ketamine, Xylazine-Pigs,	Dose	Cardiovascular effects	Reference
Intact, awake, previously instrumented	Xylazine (1.0 mg/kg), Ketamine (10 mg/kg), IV	No change in mean aortic pressure, pulmonary arterial pressure, arterial pH, $PaCO_2$, plasma glucose and lactate; decreased cardiac output and PaO_2; systemic vascular resistance increased	81
8.3:6 Ketamine, Xylazine-Cattle			
Intact, awake	Xylazine (0.2 mg/kg), IM, Ketamine (5 mg/kg),IV or (10 mg/kg),IM	Respiratory rates and heart rates decreased after xylazine and increased again after ketamine	82
Intact, awake	Xylazine (0.088 mg/kg), Ketamine (4.4 mg/kg), IM in same syringe	No change in heart rate, central venous pressure, mean pulmonary arterial pressure, cardiac output; mean aortic pressure decreased after 15 min; respiratory rate increased and PaO_2 decreased	83
8.3:7 Ketamine, Xylazine-Monkeys (Macaca mulatta)			
Intact, instrumented under thiamylal just prior to the experiment but allowed to regain consciousness	Xylazine (0.6 mg/kg), IM, Ketamine (7 mg/kg), IM	Decreased aortic pressure and heart rate within 30 min, along with a decrease in PvO_2; no change in respiratory rate, PaO_2, arterial pH or $PaCO_2$	35

Ketamine combined with other agents

Ketamine has been combined with other tranquilizers and sedatives in an apparent attempt to identify some combination of agents that can be administered easily, result in smooth induction and recovery, of moderate duration anesthesia and have minimal effects on the cardiovascular and respiratory systems. Two of these combinations are summarized in the following table.

Table 8.4: Cardiovascular Effects of Ketamine in Combination with Other Agents

Conditions of the experiment	Drug combination and dose	Cardiovascular effects	Reference
8.4:1 Ketamine, Diazepam-Dogs			
Intact, awake	Diazepam (0.5 mg/kg, IV) then Ketamine (10 mg/kg), IV	Less cardiovascular stimulation than when ketamine given alone; increased respiratory depression	**73**
8.4:2 Ketamine, Diazepam-Sheep			
Previously instrumented, spontaneously breathing, intact, awake	Diazepam (0.375 mg/kg), Ketamine (7.5 mg/kg), IV + 0.188 and 3.75 mg/kg every 15 min for 105 min	Good anesthesia but hypoventilation; respiratory acidosis; increased systemic resistance and pulmonary arterial resistance	**79**
8.4:3 Ketamine, Medetomidine-Pigs			
Intact, awake, chronically instrumented	Medetomidine (0.2 mg/kg) (an α_2-adrenoceptor agonist); Ketamine (10 mg/kg), directly into the left atrium, mixed in the same syringe	Increased mean arterial pressure followed by bradycardia; rate of increase in LV pressure and LV wall thickening decreased (worsening of LV function); systemic vascular resistance increased; cardiac output decreased; LV end-diastolic pressure initially increased then returned to control level in 5 min; respiratory rate increased but $PaCO_2$ increased and PaO_2 and arterial pH decreased; rectal temperature decreased; all of above changes were transient and returned to baseline within the 2 hours of the experiment; epinephrine levels were markedly decreased and stayed down for the entire time of monitoring, norepinephrine decreased for 10 min and then returned to baseline levels;	**98**

Guaifenesin (Glycerol guiaculate)

Guaifenesin has been in use in equine veterinary practice for many years. It provides very smooth immobilization and recovery but, for the most part, there is very little truly useful information concerning its cardiovascular effects. We have one report where it was used alone in intact, awake, acutely instrumented horses. These animals were previously catheterized, using local anesthesia. Twenty to 30 minutes was allowed for the animals to stabilize before the guaifenesin was infused and the measurements made. The guaifenesin was infused rapidly, IV, at a dosage of 134 ± 34 mg/kg, to effect. There was no change recorded in heart rate, respiratory rate, right atrial pressure, pulmonary artery pressure, cardiac output, arterial pH or $PaCO_2$. Mean, systolic and diastolic aortic pressures all decreased, along with PaO_2 at 5 minutes after the infusion.[59] The same authors reported effects in the same model with xylazine (1.1 mg/kg, IV) used prior to the guaifenesin which was then used at a reduced dosage of 88 ± 10 mg/kg, IV. They found that, with this regimen, the heart rate and respiratory rates returned to baseline 5 minutes after the guaifenesin infusion. Central venous pressure increased, aortic pressures decreased as did PaO_2.[59] One word of caution, when guaifenesin has been used in mules and zebras, a high incidence of long term to permanent paresis has been seen. We have had personal experience with two mules in this regard, both of whom never could regain their feet after immobilization with guaifenesin. Consultation with other veterinarians has confirmed this experience both in zebras and mules.

Table 8.5: Cardiovascular Effects of Ketamine, Xylazine, Guaifenesin Combinations

Conditions of the experiment	Drug combination and dose	Cardiovascular effects	Reference
8.5:1 Ketamine, Xylazine, Guaifenesin-Dogs			
Acute instrumentation with halothane/nitrous oxide, baseline recordings after recovery	Ketamine (1 mg/ml), Xylazine (0.25 mg/ml), Guaifenesin (50 mg/ml) infused @ 2.2 ml/kg/hr, IV for 2 hrs	No change in heart rate, systemic vascular resistance, mean aortic pressure, rate-pressure product or PaO_2; decrease in cardiac index	84

8.5:2 Ketamine, Xylazine, Guaifenesin- Horses, Conditions of the experiment	Drug Combination and Dose	Cardiovascular Effects	Reference
Previously instrumented, mixture used for induction only animals maintained with halothane	Ketamine (2 mg/kg, IV), Xylazine (0.3 mg/kg, IV), Guaifenesin (100 mg/kg, IV)	No changes in aortic pressures, blood gases or pH; significant ataxia from guaifenesin	**80**

Table 8.6: Cardiovascular Effects of Ketamine Combined with Chloral Hydrate, Ethyl-(1-methyl-propyl) malonyl-thio-urea salt (EMTU), Xylazine + Diazepam, and Xylazine + Acetylpromazine

Conditions of the experiment	Drug combination and dose	Cardiovascular effects	Reference
8.6:1 Ketamine, Chloral hydrate- Rabbits			
Intact, awake, previously instrumented	Ketamine (20 mg/kg, IM), wait 10 min then Chloral hydrate (250 mg/kg, IV)	Increased heart rate with return to baseline and maintain from 90-120 min; decreased respiratory rate with return to baseline by 120 min; no significant change in rectal temperature	76
8.6:2 Ketamine, EMTU- Rabbits			
Intact, awake, previously instrumented	Ketamine (35 mg/kg, IM), wait 10 min then EMTU (25-54.5 mg/kg), IV to effect	Initial increase in heart rate, return to baseline then increased with time; decrease in respiratory rate with return to baseline with time; decrease in rectal temperature	76

8.6:3 Ketamine, Xylazine, Acetylpromazine- Rabbits, Conditions of the experiment	Dose	Cardiovascular Effects	Reference
Intact, awake, previously instrumented	Xylazine (5 mg/kg, SQ) wait 10 min then Ketamine (35 mg/kg, IM) + Acetyl-promazine (0.75 mg/kg, IM)	Decreased heart rate, stayed depressed for 120 min; decreased respiratory rate, stayed depressed for 120 min; large continuous decrease in rectal temperatures	**76**
8.6:4 Ketamine, Xylazine, Diazepam- Horses			
Previously instrumented, used for induction only then maintained with halothane	Ketamine (2 mg/kg, IV), Xylazine (0.3 mg/kg, IV), Diazepam (0.1 mg/kg, IV)	No changes in aortic pressures, blood gases or arterial pH	**80**

Tranquilizer-Opiod Combinations

Combinations of tranquilizers and opiods have been increasingly used as neurolept analgesics. One particular combination, droperidol, a buterophenone tranquilizer, and fentanyl, a synthetic opiod, has been especially popular. This combination has been marketed in the USA under the trade name Innovar[R], and as Thalamonal[R] and other trade names elsewhere. The combination of these agents potentiates their calming and/or analgesic properties, while minimizing problems of ataxia. The latter is particularly important when dealing with very large animals such as horses, or animals which are difficult to restrain physically, such as primates or pigs. The usual concentration for Innovar is 0.4 mg/ml fentanyl and 20 mg/ml droperidol.

We have had considerable experience using the combination of fentanyl and droperidol, along with pentobarbital, for diagnostic cardiovascular catheterization procedures in dogs. It is often not feasible to use inhalation anesthesia during diagnostic catheterization, because of the high levels of inhaled oxygen, unless compressed air is used to drive the anesthetic machine. The barbiturate anesthetics given alone usually result in abnormally high heart rates and cardiac outputs. The usual dosage we use under these circumstances is 0.05 ml/kg Innovar, followed as soon as possible by 15-20 mg/kg pentobarbital, both IV, but as separate injections. This anesthetic regimen produces a good level of surgical anesthesia for 20-30 minutes. Normal sinus arrhythmia is maintained, normal to slow heart rates are maintained along with normal blood gases. One disadvantage of this regimen is that it usually results in increased gastrointestinal motility and tone with resulting defecation and flatulence. Another disadvantage is that when the animal starts to awaken, arousal is frequently very sudden, especially after an external stimulus. After about 15 minutes of anesthesia, the depth of anesthesia must be monitored closely and frequently. Additional doses of pentobarbital may be necessary, given to effect.

Another particularly useful combination has been used extensively in the United Kingdom and Western Europe for neurolept analgesia and restraint in horses.   The combination of Etorphine and Acepromazine is marketed as Immobilon[R]. Telazol is a 1:1 combination of tiletamine, a cyclohexamine anesthetic-hallucinogenic agent (similar to Ketamine), and zolazepam, a benzodiazepine tranquilizer which is more potent than Valium.

A systematic evaluation of the cardiovascular effects of "balanced anesthesia", that is the mixing of different anesthetic and/or analgesic agents, has not been completed.   This is understandable because the number of possible combinations in all species would present an almost infinite list.   A word of caution should be injected. When a number of different pharmacological agents are used, usually in lower doses than are required individually for the same analgesic/anesthetic effect, that does not insure that the cardiovascular effects are reduced. If some, previously unstudied, combination of agents is contemplated, a systematic analysis of effects should be conducted, preferably in intact, awake, previously instrumented animals of the same species to be used in the experiments of primary interest.

Table 8.7: Cardiovascular Effects of Innovar (Fentanyl-Droperidol)

Conditions of the experiment	Drug combinations and dose	Cardiovascular Effects	Reference
8.7:1 Innovar-dogs			
Intact, awake, previously instrumented, effects of acute coronary occlusion	0.05 ml/kg of the standard combination	Apparent decrease in heart rate and aortic pressure; no change in cardiac output, stroke volume or systemic resistance; there were no alterations in response to coronary occlusion	**41**

Conditions	Drug combinations and dose	Cardiovascular Effects	Reference
Intact, awake, previously instrumented	1 ml/12 kg of the standard combination	No change in heart rate; systolic aortic pressure increased at 5 min, decreased at 30 min; Diastolic aortic pressure was unchanged at 5 min, decreased at 15 and 30 min; mean aortic pressure was increased at 5 min, decreased at 15 min and 30 min; there was an increase in LV dP/dt max at 15 and 30 min, but no changes were seen in cardiac output, stroke volume, coronary flow or coronary resistance; systemic resistance increased at 5 min but was unchanged from baseline at 15 or 30 min	42
Intact, awake, previously instrumented	0.088 ml/kg of the standard combination as an IV infusion over 30 sec	No change in mean aortic pressure or $PaCO_2$; arterial pH decreased at 5, 15 and 30 min	43
Intact, tolerance to ouabain-induced ventricular arrhythmias, after induction were intubated and positive pressure ventilated with 100% O_2; $PaCO_2$ maintained at approx. 35 mmHg; compared to pentobarbital anesthetized controls	2 to 4 ml of the standard combination, additional doses as need to maintain anesthesia	Innovar increased the dose of ouabain required to cause both ventricular tachycardia and LD_{50}; a greater dose of ouabain was required than with either pentobarbital or the untreated controls	10

Conditions	Drug combinations and dose	Cardiovascular Effects	Reference
Intact, awake, previously instrumented; atropine sulfate (0.02 and 0.04 mg/kg)	1 ml/12 kg of the standard combination	There was a dose-dependent (atropine) increase in heart rate; there was an increase then a decrease in mean, systolic and diastolic aortic pressures which was not dependent on the atropine dose; LV dP/dt max increased, cardiac output increased at 5 min with the low atropine dose only; dose-dependent decrease in stroke volume; systemic resistance was increased at 5 min with high atropine dose, decreased at 30 min with low dose; coronary flow increased at 5 min, coronary resistance decreased	42
Intact, awake, previously instrumented; compared long term effects of hemorrhagic shock in Innovar treated, Innovar + Thalamonal, Droperidol alone, Fentanyl alone and saline treated controls	Droperidol (0.65 mg/kg), Fentanyl (0.0125 mg/kg), IV	In dogs hemorrhaged to 45-50 mmHg aortic pressure there was an immediate increase in pressure with a return to about 50 mmHg within the first hour; LV dP/dt and heart rate increased; there was 100% survival in the Innovar + Thalamonal treated group; 1 of 5 survived in the Droperidol treated group, all 5 died in the saline treated and Fentanyl treated groups	45
Intact, awake, previously instrumented, anesthesia with nitrous oxide (1:3, O_2:NO_2)	Droperidol (2 mg/kg), Fentanyl (40 μg/kg)	No change in basic electrocardiographic intervals or refractoriness; ventricular tachycardia remained inducible in 9 of 10 dogs with no significant change in cycle length or the number of extra stimuli required	85
Intact, awake, previously instrumented	Standard combination (0.088 ml/kg)	No change in mean aortic pressure or $PaCO_2$; increase in arterial pH	86
Intact, awake, previously instrumented	Standard combination (0.005 ml/kg)	Decreased heart rate, mean aortic pressure, LV dP/dt and PaO_2; No change in arterial pH or on response to coronary artery occlusion; $PaCO_2$ increased	87

Conditions	Drug combinations and dose	Cardiovascular effects	Reference
Intact, awake, previously instrumented and ischemic myocardium created by ligation of LAD and the 1st diagonal branch of the LAD; 2 weeks of recovery allowed	Standard combination (0.1 ml/kg)	No change in basic ECG intervals or refractoriness; able to induce ventricular tachycardia in 9 of 10 dogs with no significant change in cycle length or number of extra stimuli required	**88**
8.7:2 Innovar-Rabbits			
Halothane anesthesia, acute instrumentation, allowed to recover for 2 hours, physically restrained	Standard combination (0.2 ml/kg)	Decreased heart rate, mean aortic pressure, LV dP/dt; respiratory rate decreased to approx. 50% of control; no change in PaO$_2$; after 45 min all variables were equal to baseline values except for the mean aortic pressure which was decreased for about 90 min	**47**
Same as above	Standard combination (0.5 ml/kg)	A greater decrease in heart rate and respiratory rate but no change in mean aortic pressure; LV dP/dt was decreased; PaO$_2$ decreased then returned to baseline within 45 min; other parameters were decreased for up to 135 min	**47**
Instrumented under halothane, 2 hrs to recover, naso-pharyngeal reflex to smoke also tested (i.e. bradycardia and vasoconstrictor response to cigarette smoke)	Standard combination (0.2 ml/kg),IV	Aortic pressure, LV dP/dt max, respiratory rate and heart rate all decreased 5 min after the injection; no change in PaO$_2$; mean aortic pressure did not change in response to smoke inhalation despite a resultant bradycardia	**47**
Same as above	Standard combination (0.5 mg/kg), IV	Decreased heart rate and respiratory rate; no change in mean aortic pressure; LV dP/dt max decreased and there was a dramatic decrease in the smoke stimulus response	**47**

Table 8.8: Other Tranquilizer-Opiod and Opiod + Other Agent Combinations

Conditions of the experiment	Drug combinations and dose	Cardiovascular Effects	Reference
8.8:1 Dogs			
Intact, awake, previously instrumented	Haloanisone (5 mg/kg) Sub Q or IM, Fentanyl (0.1 mg/kg) IV 30 min after Haloanisone	Decreased heart rate; additional doses of 0.05 to 0.1 mg/kg/hr of fentanyl were required for good analgesia in prolonged procedures	**44**
Pentobarbital anesthesia	Midazolam (1.2 mg/kg), IV; Fentanyl (0.05 mg/kg), IV	Decreased the ventricular fibrillation threshold; less of each agent required to achieve the same decrease in ventricular fibrillation threshold produced by each drug alone	**89**
Evaluated vagal tone in intact dogs using time-series analysis of R-R intervals	Morphine (1 mg/kg), Sub Q; α-chloralose (50 mg/kg), IV, Urethane (500 mg/kg), IV	Increased vagal tone	**90**
8.8:2 Cats			
Intact, awake, cannulated 24-48 hrs prior to the experiment; Heparin (500 IU units/kg)	Metomidate (25 mg/kg), Fentanyl (0.025 mg/kg), IM	Cardiac output decreased significantly 15 min post injection then back to baseline; no change in heart rate; blood pressure decreased as did respiratory rate	**46**
Acute instrumentation under Isoflurane and nitrous oxide anesthesia, once instrumented weaned from anesthesia and then given Telazol	9.7, 15.8 and 23.7 mg/kg (sum of 1:1 Tiletamine - zolazepam mixture	Decreased systolic, mean & diastolic aortic pressures at 1 min post injection then increased above baseline with all 3 doses; LV dP/dt and peripheral resistance decreased at 1 min then returned to baseline or above by 10 min.; No significant changes in heart rate, central venous pressure or left ventricular end-diastolic pressures; Respiratory acidosis following highest dose	**108**

8.8:3 Rabbits, conditions of the experiment	Drug combination and dose	Cardiovascular effects	Reference
Intact, awake, previously instrumented	Midazolam (1 mg/kg),IV; Xylazine (1 mg/kg),IV; Alfentanil (0.1 mg/kg), IV	Decreased aortic pressure; hypercapnia and respiratory acidosis	77
8.8:4 Pigs			
Intact, awake, previously instrumented	Etorphine + Acepromazine (Immobilon) (0.00245 mg/kg)	Decreased heart rate, aortic pressure and cardiac output; stroke volume showed an initial increase then a decrease; systemic resistance increased to 4 min, then decreased to 8 min, from 10 min on it had returned to baseline; LV dP/dt decreased, PaO_2 decreased at 30 min; no change in arterial pH	48
Same as above plus atropine sulfate (0.025 mg/kg)	Same as above	Heart rate increased with arrhythmias present; smaller decrease in aortic pressure than without atropine, cardiac output increased, stroke volume increased initially then decreased; systemic vascular resistance decreased to 7 min then increased to 11 min followed by a large decrease; at 30 min arterial pO_2 was decreased but pH was unchanged	48
Acute instrumentation after induction with the same combination, positive pressure ventilation to 11 cm water	Azaperone (2 mg/kg),IM; Atropine sulfate (0.12 mg/kg),IM; Metomidate (4 mg/kg),IV + (8 mg/kg/hr), IV infusion	Good anesthesia provided by metomidate infusion at the rate given; there was an initial decrease in heart rate which then increased back to baseline; aortic pressure decreased approx. 8.5% for 2 h after the azaperone then increased slightly above baseline; cardiac output decreased during the first 3 1/2 hr, probably due to the decrease in heart rate initially but later on due to contractility decreases	49

Conditions	Drug combination and dose	Cardiovascular effects	Reference
Intact, awake, previously instrumented	Azaperone (2 mg/kg),IM; Metomidate (4 mg/kg), IV + (10 mg/kg), IP	Decreased heart rate, respiratory rate, tidal volume; peak response about 10 min post-injections, return to baseline in approx. 1 hr; the aortic pressure decreased to about 80% of the resting value 15 min post-metomidate injection	**50**
Intact, awake, previously instrumented	Etorphine + Acepromazine (Immobilon) (0.00245 mg/kg), IM	Decreased heart rate and mean aortic pressure, stroke volume decreased after an initial increase; systemic resistance increased back to baseline in about 10 min; LV dP/dt max decreased as did PaO_2 and arterial pH; $PaCO_2$ increased	**48**
intact, awake, previously instrumented	Azaperone (2 mg/kg),IV; Metomidate (4 mg/kg),IV into pulmonary artery as a bolus	Mean aortic pressure decreased more than following an IM injection; persisted throughout the experiment; pulmonary arterial pressure increased within 5 min and then decreased; heart rate decreased within 5 min and remained lower than baseline; cardiac index and stroke index decreased within 5 min, then returned to normal; there was a slight hypercapnia	**51**
Intact, awake, previously instrumented	Azaperone (2 mg/kg), IM; Metodmidate (10 mg/kg),IP	Decreased heart rate throughout the experiment; an initial decrease in cardiac index and stroke index with a return to original baseline values and a slight hypercapnia	**51**
8.8:5 Horses			
Intact, awake, previously instrumented with local anesthesia	Acepromazine (100 µg/kg), Etorphine (24 µg/kg), i.e.; Immobilon^R (0.5 ml/100 lbs), IV	Heart rate increased, aortic pressure increased at 5 min post-injection, no change at 15 and 30 min; systemic resistance increased in early stages then decreased; cardiac output increased and stroke volume decreased	**52**
Intact, awake, acute instrumentation with local anesthesia	Acepromazine (0.1 mg/kg), Etorphine (22 µg/kg) given together IM	Blood pressure increased less than with same dose of Etorphine alone; when Acepromazine used 20 min prior to Etorphine initial peak in blood pressure was eliminated	**53**

Conditions	Drug combination and dose	Cardiovascular Effects	Reference
Same as above	Xylazine (3 mg/kg 20 min prior to), Etorphine (22 µg/kg), both IM	Blood pressure initially increased the same as with Etorphine alone, but decreased more rapidly resulting in SA nodal block	53
Same as above	Azaperone (0.7 mg/kg 20 min prior to), Etorphine (22 µg/kg), both IM	Heart rate increased more than with Etorphine alone, same effects on aortic pressure as seen with Acepromazine	53
Intact, awake, acute instrumentation	Acepromazine (0.1 mg/kg), Etorphine (24 µg/kg), IM	Increased heart rate and cardiac output, decreased stroke volume; mean aortic pressure was increased at 5 min post-injection and back to baseline by 15 min; arterial hemoglobin concentration increased at 5 min back to baseline at 30 min; systemic resistance was unchanged initially then decreased at 15 and 30 min	54
Intact, awake, some previously instrumented, others instrumented acutely with local anesthesia	Acepromazine (0.1 mg/kg), Etorphine (24 µg/kg),IV	Increased heart rate, aortic pressure and a slight increase in systemic resistance; there was no significant change in cardiac output but a decrease in stroke volume	52
Intact, awake, acute instrumentation	Azaperone (0.5 mg/kg), IV immediately prior to Metomidate (3.5 mg/kg),IV	All combinations resulted in a smooth induction, heart rate increased about 20%, mean aortic pressure unchanged; venous packed cell volume decreased; no change in $PaCO_2$ but a late decrease in PaO_2 and % saturation, the latter effect was probably from being recumbent, not from the drugs	55
Same as above	Azaperone (0.2 mg/kg),IV immediately prior to Metomidate (3.5 mg/kg),IV	Same as above	55

Conditions	Drug combination and dose	Cardiovascular Effects	Reference
Same as above	Azaperone (0.8 mg/kg),IV 20 min prior to Metomidate (3.5 mg/kg),IV	Same as above	55
Same as above	Azaperone (0.8 mg/kg),IV 30 min prior to Metomidate (3.5 mg/kg),IV	Same as above	55
Intact, awake, acute instrumentation with local anesthesia	Xylazine (0.66 mg/kg), Morphine sulfate (0.12 mg/kg), IV	Decreased heart rate, cardiac output and respiratory rate; central venous pressure increased; transient increase in aortic and pulmonary arterial pressures; no change in $PaCO_2$, PaO_2 or arterial pH	56
Same as above	Xylazine (0.66 mg/kg), Morphine sulfate (0.66 mg/kg), IV	Decreased cardiac output and respiratory rate; no change in heart rate; central venous pressure increased and aortic and pulmonary arterial pressures increased transiently; no change in $PaCO_2$, PaO_2 or arterial pH; improved analgesia with the higher dose of morphine	56
Intact, awake, previously instrumented	Detomidine (10 µg/kg),IV pretreatment then Methadone (0.1 mg/kg),IV	No change in mean aortic pressure, heart rate, PaO_2 or $PaCO_2$	94
Same as above	Detomidine (10 µg/kg),IV pretreatment then Morphine (0.1 mg/kg),IV	Transient increase in mean aortic pressure; no change in heart rate; transient decrease in PaO_2 and increase in $PaCO_2$	94
Same as above	Detomidine (10 µg/kg),IV then Pethidine (1 mg/kg),IV	No change in mean aortic pressure, heart rate or PaO_2; transient increase in $PaCO_2$	94

Same as above	Detomidine (10 µg/kg),IV then Butorphanol (0.05 mg/kg), IV	No change in mean aortic pressure, heart rate, PaO_2 or $PaCO_2$	**94**
Intact, awake, previously instrumented	Acepromazine (0.1 mg/kg), IV, Xylazine (0.4 mg/kg), IV, pretreatment then Methadone (0.1 mg/kg), IV	At 65 min post-methadone injection there was decreased heart rate, aortic pressures, a decrease in the difference between inspiratory and expiratory central venous pressures; decreased respiratory rate, PaO_2 and increased $PaCO_2$	**95**
Intact, awake, previously instrumented	Xylazine (1.1 mg/kg), IV wait 6 min then Butorphanol (0.1 mg/kg), IV	No different than xylazine alone; decreased heart rate and cardiac output; increased diastolic pulmonary artery pressures, mean aortic pressures and central venous pressures; lateral cecal arterial blood flow decreased substantially more than did cardiac output	**96**
Acute instrumentation, intact, awake	Xylazine (1.1 mg/kg),IV + Telazol (tiletamine + zolazepam) (1.1 mg/kg),IV	Increased mean aortic pressure, $PaCO_2$, mean pulmonary artery pressure and central venous pressure; decreased heart rate, respiratory rate, cardiac output, arterial pH and PaO_2	**97**
Same as above	Xylazine (1.1 mg/kg),IV + Telazol (1.65 mg/kg),IV	No change in heart rate or mean aortic pressure; increased mean pulmonary arterial pressures, central venous pressure and $PaCO_2$; decreased respiratory rate, cardiac output, arterial pH and PaO_2	**97**
Same as above	Xylazine (1.1 mg/kg),IV + Telazol (2.2 mg/kg),IV	No change in heart rate, respiratory rate, mean pulmonary arterial pressures; increased central venous pressures, mean aortic pressure and $PaCO_2$; decreased cardiac output, PaO_2 and arterial pH	**97**
Same as above	Xylazine (2.2 mg/kg),IM + Telazol (1.65 mg/kg),IV	Increased heart rate, central venous pressure, $PaCO_2$; decreased respiratory rate, cardiac output, arterial pH, PaO_2; no change in mean aortic pressure or pulmonary arterial pressure	**97**

Conditions	Drug combination and dose	Cardiovascular Effects	Reference
Intact, awake	Xylazine (1.2 mg/kg), IV followed in 5-10 min by Morphine (0.75 mg/kg), IV	Good sedation and analgesia, no cardiovascular data provided	**99**
Intact, awake, previously instrumented	Xylazine (0.66 mg/kg),IV, Morphine (0.12 mg/kg),IV	Decreased heart rate, cardiac output and respiratory rate; increased central venous pressure, transient increased in mean aortic and pulmonary arterial pressures; no change in $PaCO_2$ or PaO_2	**100**
Same as above	Xylazine (0.66 mg/kg), IV, Morphine (0.66 mg/kg),IV	No change in heart rate, all other parameters changed the same as in the lower dose of morphine cited above	**100**
Same as above	Xylazine (0.66 mg/kg), IV, Acepromazine (0.1 mg/kg), IV	Heart rate, cardiac output and respiratory rate all decreased; late decrease in central venous pressure and mean aortic pressure; no change in PaO_2, $PaCO_2$ or arterial pH	**100**
Intact, awake, previously instrumented	Acepromazine (0.11 mg/kg), IV, Methadone (0.11 mg/kg), IV	Duration of effect approximately 1 hr, some effects may persist for as long as 3 days, no cardiovascular effects noted	**101**
Intact, awake, previously instrumented	Chlorproma-zine (2 mg/kg), IV, Promethazine (1 mg/kg), IV, Meperidine (2 mg/kg),IV	Increased heart rate; decreased stroke volume and stroke velocity; cardiac output increased initially and then decreased to near baseline; pulmonary resistance increased about 60% and systemic resistance decreased about 20%	**102**
8.8:6 Pigs			
Intact, awake, previously instrumented and monitored with telemetry	Azaperone (2.0 mg/kg), IV, Atropine (0.08 mg/kg), IV	Heart rate increased about 78%	**103**

Conditions of the experiment	Drug combination and dose	Cardiovascular Effects	Reference
Same as above	Azaperone (0.8 mg/kg),IV, Atropine (2.0 mg/kg),IV	Heart rate increased about 15%	**103**
8.8:7 Cattle			
Acute instrumentation with Isoflurane, recovery and recordings made from awake state	Xylazine (0.1 mg/kg),IV, Telazol (4 mg/kg),IV (Tiletamine: Zolazepam in 1:1 ratio)	No significant changes in LV stroke work index, $PaCO_2$ or arterial pH; mean aortic pressure and systemic resistance increased at 5 min then decreased to below baseline at 40 min; increased pulmonary arterial wedge pressures, pulmonary arterial pressures, central venous pressures and PaO_2 from 5-60 min; increase in stroke volume, stroke index, right ventricular stroke work index from 20-30 min to 60 min; pulmonary resistance increased at 10 min, returned to baseline at 20 min then increased again at 60 min; heart rate, cardiac index and rate pressure product decreased at 5 min and remained depressed for 60 min; cardiac output decreased at 5 min and returned to baseline at 30 min	**91**
8.8:8 Sheep			
Intact, awake, acute instrumentation	Telazol (12 & 24 mg/kg),IV	No change in heart rate, mean aortic pressure, right atrial pressure, pulmonary arterial pressure, pulmonary wedge pressure or pulmonary resistance; decreased cardiac output; increased systemic resistance	**92**
Intact, awake, previously instrumented	Butorphanol (0.5 mg/kg),IV, Telazol (12 mg/kg),IV	Decreased cardiac output, mean aortic pressure; increased systemic resistance; mild respiratory acidosis	**93**

Table 8.9: Cardiovascular Effects of the Steroid Anesthetics and Otherwise Unclassified Agents

Conditions of the experiment	Drug and dose	Cardiovascular effects	Reference
8.9:1 Dogs			
Intact, awake, previously instrumented	Minaxolone (2.5 mg/kg),IV	Immediate and persistent increase in heart rate, decrease in aortic pressure, decrease in systemic vascular resistance and in LV dP/dt max; stroke volume decreased and cardiac output increased immediately and then returned to baseline within 15 min and stayed at that level	58
Previously instrumented using an ultrashort acting barbiturate or α-chloralose anesthesia; instrumentation included ability to monitor cardiac vagal and sympathetic nerve activity	Althesin (Alphaxalone & Alpha-dolone) (0.6 to 1.0 mg/kg),IV slow injection to effect	The slow injection produced a nearly complete block of cardiac vagal efferent activity or reduced it greatly; simultaneous sympathetic activity increased; heart rate and aortic pressure increased	59
Previously instrumented, intact, awake	Pregnenolon e (0.5, 1.0, 2.0 & 4.0 mg/kg),IV dose-response	Cardiac output and heart rate increased from lowest dose and continued with each subsequent dose; mean aortic pressure decreased and LV contractility decreased only at 2 & 4 mg/kg; decreased systemic resistance and increased pulmonary arterial resistance at all doses	104
Same as above	Pregnenolon e (8, 16 & 32 mg/kg), IV	Circulatory shock	104
Intact, awake, compared to control group anesthetized with Pentobarbital (25 mg/kg),IV + Pancuronium (0.1 mg/kg + 1-2 mg/hr),IV	Alfentanil (75 µg/kg + 1 µg/kg/min), IV	Heart rate increased then decreased after 30 min; mean aortic pressure, cardiac index, oxygen delivery and oxygen consumption decreased; no change in mean pulmonary arterial pressure, right atrial pressure, pulmonary wedge pressure, stroke index, systemic resistance, LV stroke work index, venous oxygen saturations, oxygen extraction or lactate levels	67

Conditions	Drug and dose	Cardiovascular Effects	Reference
Same as above	Alfentanil (150 µg/kg + 4 µg/kg/min), IV	Same as above with greater levels of depression	67
Anesthetized with Isoflurane (0.7% ET) + 50% nitrous oxide in oxygen	Sufentanil (20 µg/kg), IV	Decreased mean aortic pressure, cardiac output, cerebral blood flow and cerebral oxygen consumption	105
8.9:2 Rats			
Isolated atrial and portal vein preparations	Althesin (0.3 to 307.2 µg/ml), dose-response	Dose-dependent depression of atrial rate and amplitude of myogenic activity in the portal vein preparation; neither of these negative responses were Ca^{2+}-dependent	20
Induced with Halothane and cannulated; evaluated the pressor response to infusion of the nitric oxide synthase inhibitor L-NNA	Althesin (0.03 ml/kg) + 0.003-0.007 ml/kg/min),IV	Enhanced pressor response compared to conscious rats	70
Cremaster muscle microvascular preparation compared to pentobarbital anesthetized (50 mg/kg, IP + 16 mg/kg, Sub Q or IV)	Etomidate (20 mg/kg + 7.4 mg/kg/hr),IV	Near maximal dilation compared to pentobarbital anesthetized group	106
Cremaster muscle microvascular prep., Pentobarbital anesthetized as above	Etomidate (topical application)	No effect on arteriolar diameters; appears to trigger release of dilator prostaglandins in striated muscle via a central or indirect mechanism	106

8.9:3 Rabbits, conditions of the experiment	Drug and dose	Cardiovascular effects	Reference
Intact, awake	Xylazine (5 mg/kg) Sub Q, wait 10 min then EMTU [ethyl-(1-methyl-propyl) malonyl-thio-urea salt] (12.5 to 47.6 mg/kg), IV to effect	Initial decrease then return to baseline in heart rate; respiratory rate and rectal temperature decreased with time	76
8.9:4 Sheep,			
Intact, awake, previously instrumented	Alphaxolone (9 mg/ml) & Alphadolone (3 mg/ml) [Saffon, Glaxo, CT1341] given at rate of 1.65 to 3 mg/kg, IV, as needed to induce anesthesia	Mild decrease in arterial pH, slight decrease in $PaCO_2$, no change in PaO_2; mean aortic pressure decreased 50% 30 sec after the injection but these responses only lasted for 10 min; prior administration of atropine or mepyramine did not modify the hypotensive response	60
8.9:5 Goats			
Intact, awake, previously instrumented	Althesin (0.1 or 0.2 ml/kg), IV	Heart rate increased 23% with low dose, 6% with high dose; a dose-dependent increase in pulmonary arterial pressure and a decrease in pulmonary arterial flow; stroke volume decreased more with the low dose than with the high dose; most of the measured parameters were back to their baseline values within 5 min; PaO_2 decreased, $PaCO_2$ increased and pulmonary arterial resistance increased; the duration of anesthesia was about 5 min with the low dose and about 7 min with the higher dose	61

8.9:6 Pigs, conditions of the experiment	Drug and dose	Cardiovascular effects	Reference
Intact, awake	Saffon, [Alphaxolone (9 mg/ml), Alphadolone (3 mg/ml)] given 6-8 ml/kg, IM	Good sedation, no cardiovascular parameters were monitored	**62**
Same as above	Saffon (1-4 mg/kg),IM	Mild sedation, no cardiovascular parameters monitored	**62**
Same as above	Saffon (6-8 mg/kg),IM	Deep sedation, unable to stand, no cardiovascular parameters monitored	**62**
8.9:7 Horses			
Intact, awake, previously prepared carotid loops	Saffon Dose-response, 1.9 mg/kg initial	Heart rate increased 2 min after induction, at 5 min still elevated but less so, respiratory rates decreased	**63**

References

1.   Parker, J.L., Adams, H.R. The influence of chemical restraining agents on cardiovascular function: a review, *Lab Anim Sci*, 28:575-583, 1978.
2.   Wright, M. Pharmacologic effects of ketamine and its use in veterinary medicine, *J AVMA*, 180:1462-1471, 1982.
3.   Gelman, S., Mardis, M. Splanchnic circulatory response to ketamine in stressed and unstressed dogs, *Anesth*, 53 (3 Suppl):S53, 1980.
4.   Priano, L.L. Comparative renal vascular effects of thiopental, diazepam, ketamine and halothane, *Anesth*, 57:A 34, 1982.
5.   Traber, D.L., Wilson, R.D., Priano, L.L. The effect of β-adrenergic blockade on the cardiopulmonary response to ketamine, *Anesth Analg (Cleve)*, 49:604-613, 1970.
6.   Traber, D.L., Wilson, R.D., Priano, L.L. The effect of α-adrenergic blockade on the cardiopulmonary response to ketamine, *Anesth Analg (Cleve)*, 50:737-742, 1971.
7.   Traber, D.L., Wilson, R.D., Priano, L.L. A detailed study of the cardiopulmonary response to ketamine and its blockade by atropine, *South Med J*, 63:1077-1081, 1970.
8.   Slogoff, S., Allen, G.W. The role of baroreceptors in the cardiovascular response to ketamine, *Anesth Analg (Cleve)*, 53:704-707, 1974.
9.   Smith, G., Thorburn, J., Vance, J.P., Brown, D.M. The effects of ketamine on the canine coronary circulation, *Anesth*, 34:555-561, 1979.
10. Ivankovich, A.D., El-Etr, A.A., Janeczko, G.F. The effects of ketamine and of Innovar anesthesia on digitalis tolerance in dogs, *Anesth Analg (Cleve)*, 54:106-111, 1975.
11. Nakajima, T., Azumi, T., Yatabe, Y. Mechanism of positive chronotropic response of the canine SA node to selective administration of ketamine, *Arch Int Pharmacodyn Ther*, 234:247-256, 1978.
12. Nakajima, T., Azumi, T., Iwasaki, H., Kaneshiro, S., Yatabe, Y. Biphasic response of the SA node of the dog heart *in vivo* to selective administration of ketamine, *Arch Int Pharmacodyn Ther*, 228:108-117, 1977.
13. Liao, J.C., Koehntop, D.E., Buckley, J.J. Dual effect of ketamine on the peripheral vasculature, *Anesth*, 51:(3 Suppl):S116, 1979.
14. Peters, J.M., van der Meer, C., Czanky, J.C., Spierdijk, J. Effect of anesthetics on mortality and kidney lesions caused by hypotension, *Arch Int Pharmacodyn Ther*, 238:134-153, 1979.

15. Miller, E.D. Jr., Kistner, J.R., Epstein, R.M. Distribution of blood flow with anesthetics, *Anesth*, 51(3 Suppl):S124, 1979.

16. Miller, E.D. Jr., Longnecker, D.E., Peach, M.J. Renin response to hemorrhage in awake and anesthetized rats, *Circ Shock*, 6:271-276, 1979.

17. Sapru, H.N., Krieger, A.J. Cardiovascular and respiratory effects of some anesthetics in the decerebrate rat, *Eur J Pharmacol*, 53:151-158, 1979.

18. Kaukinen, S. Effects of anti-hypertensive medication on the cardiovascular response to ketamine in rats, *Acta Anaesth Scand*, 22:437-444, 1978.

19. Byrne, A.J., Tomlinson, D.R., Healy, T.E. Effects of ketamine on autonomic transmission in rat isolated atria, *Br J Anaesth*, 51:989-990, 1979.

20. Hall, P.J., Pleuvry, B.J. An *in vitro* study of the effects of calcium on the cardiovascular actions of thiopentone, althesin and ketamine in the rat, *J Pharm Pharmacol*, 31:460-465, 1979.

21. Longnecker, D.E., Ross, D.C., Silver, I.A. Anesthetic influence on arteriolar diameters and tissue oxygen tension in hemorrhaged rats, *Anesth*, 57:177-182, 1982.

22. Longnecker, D.E., Ross, D.C. Influence of anesthetic on microvascular responses to hemorrhage, *Anesth*, 51(3 Suppl):S142, 1979.

23. Salt, P.J., Barnes, P.K., Beswick, F.J. Inhibition of neuronal and extraneuronal uptake of noradrenaline by ketamine in the isolated perfused rat heart, *Br J Anaesth*, 51:835-838, 1979.

24. Sanford, T.D., Colby, E.D. Effect of xylazine and ketamine on blood pressure, heart rate and respiratory rate in rabbits, *Lab Anim Sci*, 30:519-523, 1980.

25. Kaukinen, S. The combined effects of antihypertensive drugs and anaesthetics (halothane and ketamine) on the isolated heart, *Acta Anaesth Scand*, 22:649-657, 1978.

26. Hill, G.E., Wong, K.C., Shaw, C.L., Sentker, C.R., Blatnick, R.A. Interactions of ketamine with vasoactive amines at normothermia and hypothermia in the isolated rabbit heart, *Anesth*, 48:315-319, 1978.

27. Lundy, P.M., Frew, R. Ketamine potentiates catecholamine response of vascular smooth muscle by inhibition of extraneuronal uptake, *Can J Physiol Pharmacol*, 59:520-527, 1981.

28. Su, J.Y. Effects of ketamine on functionally skinned myocardial cells from rabbits, *Fed Proc*, 39:#4413, 1980.

29. Schwedler, M., Miletich, D.J., Albrecht, R.F. Lack of cerebral blood flow change during ketamine anesthesia in ventilated goats, *Anesth*, 53(3 Suppl):S129, 1980.

30. Ivankovich, A.D., Miletich, D.J., Reimann, C. *et al.* Cardiovascular effects of centrally administered ketamine in goats, *Anesth Analg (Cleve)*, 53:924-931, 1974.

31. Craft, J.B. Jr., Dao, D.S., Yonekura, M.L., MacKinnon, D.A., Roizen, M., Mazel, P., Gilman, R., Shokes, L. Maternal and fetal catecholamine response to ketamine, *Anesth*, 53 (3 Suppl):S319, 1980.

32. Pathak, S.C., Nigam, J.M., Peshin, P.K., Singh, A.P. Anesthetic and hemodynamic effects of ketamine hydrochloride in buffalo calves *(Bubalus bubalis)*, *Am J Vet Res*, 43:875-878, 1982.

33. Nosaka, S., Yoshikawa, K., Tomi, K., Shibata, N. Effect of ketamine on arterial contraction relaxation system *in vitro*, *Blood Vessels*, 18:222, 1981.

34. Reutlinger, R.A., Karl, A.A., Vinal, S.I., Nieser, M.J. Effects of ketamine HCl-xylazine HCl combination on cardiovascular and pulmonary values of the rhesus macaque *(Macaca mulatta)*, *Am J Vet Res*, 41:1453-1457, 1980.

35. Berry, D.G. Effect of ketamine on the isolated chick embryo heart, *Anesth Analg (Cleve)*, 53:919-923, 1974.

36. Colby, E.D., Sanford, T.D. Feline anesthesia with mixed solutions of ketamine/xylazine and ketamine/acepromazine, *Feline Practice*, 12:16-24, 1982.

37. Beglinger, R., Heller, A., Denac, M. General anaesthesia of cats with ketamine-acepromazine. Effects on respiration and blood circulation, *Schweizer Archiv fur Tierheilkunde*, 119:347-353, 1977.

38. Buyniski, J.P., Christie, G.J. Ketaset Plus. A new combination of anesthetic for cats. 2. Pharmacologic aspects, *Vet Med & Sm An Clin*, 72:559-565, 1977.

39. Purohit, R.C., Mysinger, P.W., Redding, R.W. Effects of xylazine and ketamine hydrochloride on the electroencephalogram and the electrocardiogram in the horse, *Am J Vet Res*, 42:615-619, 1981.

40. Hall, L.W., Taylor, P.M. Clinical trial of xylazine with ketamine in equine anaesthesia, *Vet Rec*, 109:489-493, 1981.

41. Vallance, S.R., Skiner, T.S., Billman, G.E., Fischer, C.L., Randall, D.C., Knapp, C.F., Evans, J.M. Effects of fentanyl droperidol, Innovar, on hemodynamic responses to acute coronary occlusion in intact dogs, *Physiologist*, 24:22, 1981.

42. Buckhold, D.K., Erickson, H.H., Lumb, W.V. Cardiovascular response to fentanyl-droperidol and atropine in the dog, *Am J Vet Res*, 38:479-482, 1977.

43. Turner, D.M., Ilki, J.E., Rose, R.J., Warren, J.M. Respiratory and cardiovascular effects of five drugs used as sedatives in the dog, *Australian Vet J*, 50:260-265, 1974.

44. Marsboom, R.A., Verstraete, D., Thienpont, D., Mattheewos, D. The use of haloanisone and fentanyl for neuroleptanalgesia in dogs, *Br Vet J*, 120:466-468, 1964.

45. DeBie, F.L., Francois, P., Hermans, C., Will, J., Loots, W., Opsteyn, M., Horig, C. Thalamonal, droperidol and fentanyl in hypovolemic shock in the conscious dog, *Anaesth*, 29:78-84, 1980.

46. Erhardt, W., Fritsch, R., Christ, K., Sprenzinger, P., Blumel, G. Anaesthesia with fentanyl-metomidate in the cat and its effects on respiration and circulation, *J Sm An Pract*, 19:401-407, 1978.

47. Brill, R.W., Jones, D.R. On the stability of Innovar, a neuroleptic analgesic, for cardiovascular experiments, *Can J Physiol Pharmacol*, 59:1184-1189, 1981.

48. Becker, M., Beglinger, R. Effects of Immobilon and Revivon on the cardiovascular system and acid base status of the Gottingen minipig, *Res Vet Sci*, 29:21-25, 1980.

49. Lagerweij, E. Anaesthesia in swine for experimental purpose, Doctoral dissertation, *Drukkerij Elinkwijk, Utrecht*, 1973.

50. Jageneau, A.H.M., Bergen, A., Symoens, J. Cardiopulmonary function during azaperone-metomidate anaesthesia in pigs, *Abstracts of Communications to the Third Int Pig Vet Soc Cong*, Lyon, June 12-14, 1974.

51. Orr, J.A., Manohar, M., Will, J.A. Cardiopulmonary effects of the combination of neuroleptic azaperone and hypnotic metomidate in swine, *Am J Vet Res*, 37:1305-1308, 1976.

52. Lees, P., Hillidge, C.J. Neuroleptanalgesia and cardiovascular function in the horse, *Eq Vet J*, 7:184-191, 1975.

53. Bogan, J.A., MacKenzie, G., Snow, D.H. An evaluation of tranquilizers for use with etorphine and neuroleptanalgesic agents in the horse, *Vet Rec*, 103:471-472, 1978.

54. Hillidge, C.J., Lees, P. Influence of etorphine acepromazine and diprenorphine on cardiovascular function in ponies, *Br J Pharmacol*, 56:375P-376P, 1976.

55. Hillidge, C.J., Lees, P., Serrano, L. Influence of anaperone and metomidate on cardiovascular and respiratory functions in the pony, *Br Vet J*, 131:50-64, 1975.

56. Muir, W.W., Skarda, R.T., Sheehan, W.C. Hemodynamic and respiratory effects of xylazine-morphine sulfate in horses, *Am J Vet Res*, 40:1417-1420, 1979.

57. Hubbell, J.A., Muir, W.W., Sams, R.A. Guaifenesin: cardiopulmonary effects and plasma concentrations in horses, *Am J Vet Res*, 41:1751-1755, 1980.

58. Twissell, D.J., Dodds, M.G. The systemic hemodynamic effects of minaxolone: a comparison with other anesthetics in the dog, *Br J Anaesth*, 51:995P-996P, 1979.

59. Kollai, M., Koizumi, K. Steroid anesthetic: vagal depressant, sympathetic excitant, *Fed Proc*, 39: #743, 1980.

60. Waterman, A.E. Evaluation of the actions and use of alphaxalone alphadolone CT-1341 in sheep, *Res Vet Sci*, 30:114-119, 1981.

61. Foex, P., Prys-Roberts, C. Pulmonary haemodynamics and myocardial effects of Althesin (CT 1341) in the goat, *Postgrad Med J*, (June Suppl) 48:24-31, 1972.

62. Cox, J.E., Done, S.H., Lees, P., Walton, J.R. Preliminary studies of the actions of alphaxalone and alphadolone in the pig, *Vet Rec*, 97:497-498, 1975.

63. Eales, F.A. Effects of Saffon administered intravenously in the horse, *Vet Rec*, 99:270-272, 1976.

64. Haskins, S.C., Farver, T.B., Patz, J.D. Ketamine in dogs, *Am J Vet Res*, 46:1855-1860, 1985.

65. Pagel, P.S., Kampine, J.P., Schmeling, W.T., Warltier, D.C. Ketamine depresses myocardial contractility as evaluated by the preload recruitable stroke work relationship in chronically instrumented dogs with autonomic nervous system blockade, *Anesth*, 76:564-572, 1992.

66. Farver, T.B., Haskins, S.C., Patz, J.D. Cardiopulmonary effects of acepromazine and of the subsequent administration of ketamine in the dog, *Am J Vet Res*, 47:631-635, 1986.

67. Van der Linden, P., Gilbart, E., Engelman, E., Schmartz, D., Vincent, J.L. Effects of anesthetic agents on systemic critical O_2 delivery, *J Appl Physiol*, 71:83-93, 1991.

68. Pagel, P.S., Schmeling, W.T., Kampine, J.P., Warltier, D.C. Alteration of canine left ventricular diastolic function by intravenous anesthetics *in vivo*, *Anesth*, 76:419-425, 1992.

69. Dai, S. Anaesthetic-related occurrence of early ventricular arrhythmias during acute myocardial ischaemia in rats, *Arch Int Physiol Biochim*, 97:341-346, 1989.

70. Wang, Y.X., Zhou, T., Chua, T.C., Pang, C.C. Effects of inhalation and intravenous anesthetic agents on pressor response to NG-nitro-L-arginine, *Eur J Pharmacol*, 198:183-188, 1991.

71. Schaefer, C.F., Brackett, D.J., Biber, B., Lerner, M.R. *et al.* Respiratory and cardiovascular effects of thyrotropin-releasing hormone as modified by isoflurane, enflurane, pentobarbital and ketamine, *Regul Pept*, 24:269-282, 1989.

72. Cook, D.J., Carton, E.G., Housmans, P.R. Mechanism of the positive inotropic effect of ketamine in isolated ferret ventricular papillary muscle, *Anesth*, 74:880-888, 1991.

73. Haskins, S.C., Farver, T.B., Patz, J.D. Cardiovascular changes in dogs given diazepam and diazepam-ketamine, *Am J Vet Res*, 47:795-798, 1986.

74. Haskins, S.C., Patz, J.D., Farver, T.B. Xylazine and xylazine-ketamine in dogs, *Am J Vet Res*, 47:636-641, 1986.

75. Kolata, R.J., Rawlings, C.A. Cardiopulmonary effects of intravenous xylazine, ketamine, and atropine in the dog, *Am J Vet Res*, 43:2196-2198, 1982.

76. Hobbs, B.A., Rolhall, T.G., Sprenkel TL, Anthony KL; Comparison of several combinations for anesthesia in rabbits, *Am J Vet Res*, 52:669-674, 1991.

77. Borkowski, G.L., Danneman, P.J., Russell, G.B., Lang, C.M. An evaluation of three intravenous anesthetic regimens in New Zealand rabbits, *Lab Anim Care*, 40:270-276, 1990.

78. Muir, W.W., Skarda, R.T., Milne, D.W. Evaluation of xylazine and ketamine hydrochloride for anesthesia in horses, *Am J Vet Res*, 38:195-201, 1977.

79. Coulson, N.M., Januszkiewicz, A.J., Ripple, G.R. Physiological responses of sheep to two hours anaesthesia with diazepam-ketamine, *Vet Rec*, 129:329-332, 1991.

80. Brock, N., Hildebrand, S.V. A comparison of xylazine-diazepam-ketamine and xylazine-guaifenesin-ketamine in equine anesthesia, *Vet Surg*, 19:468-474, 1990.

81. Trim, C.M., Gilroy, B.A. Cardiopulmonary effects of a xylazine and ketamine combination in pigs, *Res Vet Sci*, 38:30-34, 1985.

82. Waterman, A.E. Preliminary observations on the use of a combination of xylazine and ketamine hydrochloride in calves, *Vet Rec*, 109:464-467, 1981.

83. Rings, D.M., Muir, W.W. Cardiopulmonary effects of intramuscular xylazine-ketamine in calves, *Can J Comp Med*, 46:386-389, 1982.

84. Benson, G.J., Thurmon, J.C., Tranquilli, W.J., Smith, C.W. Cardiopulmonary effects of intravenous infusion of guaifenesin, ketamine and xylazine in dogs, *Am J Vet Res*, 46:1896-1898, 1985.

85. Hunt, G.B., Ross, D.L. Comparison of effects of three anesthetic agents on induction of ventricular tachycardia in a canine model of myocardial infarction, *Circ*, 78:221-226, 1988.

86. Turner, D.M., Ilkiw, J.E., Rose, R.J., Warren, J.M. Respiratory and cardiovascular effects of five drugs used as sedatives in the dog, *Aust Vet J*, 50:260-265, 1974.

87. Vallance, S.R., Fitzovich, D.E., Billman, G.E., Randall, D.C. Effect of Innovar upon the autonomic control of the heart in intact dog, *J Auton Nerv Syst*, 23:47-54, 1988.

88. Hunt, G.B., Ross, D.L. Comparison of effects of three anesthetic agents on induction of ventricular tachycardia in a canine model of myocardial infarction, *Circ*, 78:221-226, 1988.

89. Hess, L., Vrana, M., Vranova, A. The electrostabilizing effect of a combination of anesthetic agents, *Cor et Vasa*, 31:411-418, 1989.

90. Halliwill, J.R., Billman, G.E. Effect of general anesthesia on cardiac vagal tone, *Am J Physiol*, 262:H1719-H1724, 1992.

91. Lin, H.C., Thurman, J.C., Tranquilli, W.J., Benson, G.J., Olson, W.A. Hemodynamic response of calves to tiletamine-zolazepam-xylazine anesthesia, *Am J Vet Res*, 52:1606-1610, 1991.

92. Lagutchik, M.S., Januszkiewicz, A.J., Dodd, K.T., Martin, D.G. Cardiopulmonary effects of a tiletamine-zolazepam combination in sheep, *Am J Vet Res*, 52:1441-1447, 1991.

93. Howard, B.W., Lagutchik, M.S., Januszkiewicz, A.J., Martin, D.G. The cardiovascular response of sheep to tiletamine-zolazepam and butorphanol tartrate anesthesia, *Vet Surg*, 19:461-467, 1990.

94. Clarke, K.W., Paton, B.R. Combined use of detomidine with opiates in the horse, *Eq Vet J*, vol C:331-334, 1988.

95. Nilsfors, L., Kvart, C., Kallings, P., Carlsten, J. Cardiorespiratory and sedative effects of a combination of acepromazine, xylazine and methadone in the horse, *Eq Vet J*, vol C:364-367, 1988.

96. Rutkowski, J.A., Eades, S.C., Moore, J.N. Effects of xylazine-butorphanol on cecal arterial blood flow, cecal mechanical activity and systemic hemodynamics in horses, *Am J Vet Res*, 52:1153-1158, 1991.

97. Hubbell, J.A.E., Bednarski, R.M., Muir, W.W. Xylazine and tiletamine-zolazepam anesthesia in horses, *Am J Vet Res*, 50:737-742, 1989.

98. Vainio, O.M., Bloor, B.C., Kim, C. Cardiovascular effects of a ketamine-medetomidine combination that produces deep sedation in Yucatan mini-swine, *Lab An Sci*, 42:582-588, 1992.

99. Klavano, P.A. Anesthesia-Some developments in equine practice, *Proc Am Assoc Eq Pract*, 21:149-155, 1975.

100. Muir, W.W., Skarda, R.T., Sheehan, W.C. Hemodynamic and respiratory effects of xylazine-morphine sulfate in horses, *Am J Vet Res*, 40:1417-1420, 1979.

101. Booth, N.H. Introduction to drugs acting on the central nervous system. Section 4 in Veterinary Pharmacology and Therapeutics, 5th ed, ed by N.H. Booth and L.E. McDonald, The Iowa State University Press, Ames Iowa, 1982.

102. Goldberg, S.J., Linde, L.M., Wolfe, R.R., Griswold, W., Momma, K. The effects of meperidine, promethazine and chlorpromazine on pulmonary and systemic circulation, *Am Heart J*, 77:214-221, 1969.

103. Buntenkotter, S. Electrocardiography of young pigs during preanaesthetic medication with atropine/azaperone in alternating sequence of application, *Deutsche Tierarztlich Wochenschrift*, 83:207-211, 1976.

104. Hgskilde, S., Wagner, J., Strm, J., Sjntoft, E. *et al.* Cardiovascular effects of pregnenolone emulsion: an experimental study in artificially ventilated dogs, *Acta Anaesthesiol Scand*, 35:669-675, 1991.

105. Werner, C., Hoffman, W.E., Baughman, V.L., Albrecht, R.F, Schulte J; Effects of sufentanil on cerebral blood flow, cerebral blood flow velocity, and metabolism in dogs, *Anesth Analg*, 72:177-181, 1991.

106. Asher, E.F., Alsip, N.L., Zhang, P.Y., Harris, P.D. Prostaglandin-related microvascular dilation in pentobarbital- and etomidate-anesthetized rats, *Anesth*, 76:271-278, 1992.

107. Kolata, R.J. The hemodynamic and ventilatory effects of xylazine and ketamine by difference routes of administration and with acetylpromazine in dogs, *J Vet Critical Care*, 7:11-14, 1984.

108. Hellyer, P., Muir, W.W., Hubbell, J.A.E., Sally, J. Cardiorespiratory effects of the intravenous administration of tiletamine-zolazepam in cats, *Vet Surg*, 17:105-110, 1988.

9. Normal cardiovascular parameters from intact, awake animals

In this chapter resting baseline cardiovascular parameter values for the most commonly used species of animal models are tabulated. Sophistication in collecting data from previously instrumented animals has made more of this information available. Only fairly recent publications are used, based upon a greater level of confidence in the reliability of the measurements obtained.

These data still must be considered with some degree of skepticism. Many species, unless they are very well acclimated by pretraining to the laboratory environment, will be extremely apprehensive and excited due to the strange surroundings and activities. This can lead to high circulating catecholamine levels, hypocapnia (from hyperventilation) and other stress-related artifacts. In spite of these limitations it is possible to see a considerable amount of agreement within many parameters, across species. This is particularly true of arterial and venous pressures, blood flows (normalized by weight of the tissue or by total body weight), and blood gases. Heart rates generally decrease as the size of the animal increases.

A word of caution is also necessary concerning the use of *standard error of the mean* (SEM) rather than the standard deviation in reporting values. The following quotation is appropriate in this regard: "...Most medical investigators summarize their data with the standard error of the mean because it is always smaller than the standard deviation. It makes their data look better. However, unlike the standard deviation, which quantifies the variability in the population, the standard error of the mean quantifies uncertainty in the estimate of the mean. Since investigators are generally interested in knowing about the population, data should never be summarized with the standard error of the mean."[1] Unfortunately, as Dr. Glantz points out, most of the data that follows was reported originally with standard errors. All data have been converted to SD whenever the number of animals was provided.

Another trap exists in reporting means and variance. If the data is skewed or if a few data points are very different from the others the mean and standard deviation will convey a false sense of what the data really represent. In some instances the median value, or the mean and the range, may communicate relationships better.

It is important not to succumb to the temptation of averaging data from many different studies and taking that number as a true representation on the basis of total animals examined. For example many values for diastolic aortic pressure in awake dogs are given in Table 9.1. The numerical averages yields a value of >92 mmHg for the approximately 150 dogs from which data are reported. Common sense should tell us that some of these studies were done with more care than others and that some of the values reported are probably misleading, for a variety of reasons. There is no reason to believe that dogs should be borderline hypertensives with rather high diastolic pressures (i.e >80 mmHg). It is necessary to use some judgement about what data is to be believed.

Table 9.1:1 Dogs; Heart rate (HR), aortic pressures (Pao), pulmonary artery pressures (Ppa) from average sized (15-30 kg) animals. [± = standard deviation]

Heart Rate (b/min)	Pao, mean (mmHg)	Pao, syst. (mmHg)	Pao, diast. (mmHg)	Ppa, mean (mmHg)	n	Reference
102±19.6	111±9.8	-	-	-	6	**2**
76±12	102±9.8	-	-	-	6	**3**
68±9.8	100±9.8	-	-	-	6	**3**
87±31.8	-	-	-	-	6	**4**
80±9	91±6	-	-	-	9	**5**
91.5±34.2	88.2±9.9	111.6±10.2	76.5±9.9	-	8	**6**
115±18.5	-	-	-	-	9	**7**
106±14.1	-	-	-	-	10	**8**
144.9±21.5	-	-	-	-	8	**9**
103±15	105±14	130±17	91±9	-	13	**10**
96±16	99±12	124±23	81±10	-	13	**10**
125±49.7	92±26.5	-	-	-	4	**11**
83.7±10.4	97.6±11.1	-	-	-	19	**12**
94±12	97±16	-	-	-	16	**13**
95±15.5	-	128±15.5	84±11.6	-	15	**14**
72.8±8.9	-	-	-	-	5	**15**
104±4.5	104±15.6	124±11.2	95±15.6	-	5	**16**
-	102±10.1	-	93±11.9	-	13	**17**
-	102±10.1	-	95±16.3	-	15	**17**
-	105±7.6	-	94±12.6	-	11	**17**
111±21	87±18	-	-	-	9	**18**
-	107±6.7	-	-	-	6	**19**
149±21.2	112±15.9	150±21.2	90±15.9	-	7	**20**
93±10.6	-	-	-	-	7	**21**
95±15.9	-	-	-	-	7	**21**
87±4	95±3	-	-	-	17	**22**
80±21	-	118±10	77±10	-	14	**23**
88±11.2	96±8.6	-	-	-	14	**24**
60*	93±8.5	-	-	-	8	**25**

Heart Rate (b/min)	Pao, mean (mmHg)	Pao, syst. (mmHg)	Pao, diast. (mmHg)	Ppa, mean (mmHg)	n	Reference
90±17.6**	95±8.6	-	79±9.0	-	14	**26****
91±16.8**	97±9.3	-	77±11.6	-	14	**26****
92±16.0**	97±7.9	-	-	-	14	**26****
87±18.3**	94±9.3	-	74±12.7	-	14	**26****
83±15.1	100±10.5	-	-	-	15	**27**
91±19	96±18.6	-	-	-	15	**28**
86±10.1	98±7.9	-	-	-	13	**29**
95±12.6	98±12.6	-	-	-	10	**30**
109±4	100±3	-	-	-	15	**31**
-	109.8±2.2	-	-	18.4±0.22	5	**32**
-	124±15.9	-	-	-	7	**33**
98±17.9	96±6.7	155±9	-	-	20	**34**
135±11.3	102±11.3	143±11.3	81±11.3	-	8	**35**
115.5±26.1	-	-	-	12.2±2.4	9	**36*** **
113.9±23.7	-	-	-	13.0±2.7	9	**36*** **
119.2±25.2	-	-	-	13.4±3.0	9	**36*** **
109.9±28.2	-	-	-	12.5±2.4	9	**36*** **
-	115±18.7	-	-	-	14	**37**
87±9.2	92±7.3	-	-	-	10	**38**
114±27	98±17.1	-	-	-	9	**39+**
60±14	99±10	-	-	14±3.1	5	**95**
82±11.3	106±11.3	-	-	-	8	**98**
95±15.9	97±5.3	-	-	-	7	**98**
83±18	106±12	-	-	-	9	**99**
84±18	103±12	-	-	-	9	**99**
93±18	102±12	-	-	-	9	**99**
89±18	103±9	-	-	-	9	**99**
93±24	110±14	-	-	13±4.3	14	**100**
82±7.3	98±7.3	-	-	-	6	**101**

Heart Rate (b/min)	Pao, mean (mmHg)	Pao, syst. (mmHg)	Pao, diast. (mmHg)	Ppa, mean (mmHg)	n	Reference
95±15.9	97±5.3	-	-	-	7	**98**
109±14	-	-	-	-	13	**104++**
116±20	-	-	-	-	13	**104+++**
118±48.1	-	-	-	-	8	**104+++**
79±12	98±9	-	-	-	9	**105**
80±9	96±9	-	-	-	9	**105**
135±15.9	116±7.9	-	-	-	7	**106** (standing)
142±26.4	117±10.6	-	-	-	7	**106** (recumb)
83±8	106±12	-	-	-	9	**99**
93±18	102±12	-	-	-	9	**99**
84±18	103±12	-	-	-	9	**99**
89±18	103±9	-	-	-	9	**99**
123±37	-	126±23	90±20	-	20	**107**
111±30	-	119±24	82±19	-	20	**107**
74±12	94±5	-	-	-	6	**108**
127±36	98.3±9.3	-	-	-	7	**109**
118±14	105±11.4	-	-	-	4	**109**
113±36	100.4±13	-	-	-	5	**109**
79±17.1	99±17.1	-	-	-	6	**110**
90±17	102±14	-	-	11.1±2.0	6	**111**
77±14.1	88±8.5	-	-	-	8	**112**
80±14.1	90±14.1	-	-	-	8	**112**
82±10.6	84±10.6	-	-	-	7	**112**
88±24	100±15	-	-	-	9	**113**
78±15	97±15	-	-	-	9	**113**
88±24	105±24	-	-	-	9	**113**
87±21	101±12	-	-	-	9	**113**
96±27.7	107±6.9	-	-	-	12	**114**
-	93±21.2	138±34.4	67±15.9	-	7	**115**
-	93±31.7	135±47.6	71±29	-	7	**115**
77±13.2	90±13.2	-	-	-	7	**116**

Heart Rate (b/min)	Pao, mean (mmHg)	Pao, syst. (mmHg)	Pao, diast. (mmHg)	Ppa, mean (mmHg)	n	Reference
76±13.2	91±7.9	-	-	-	7	**116**
74±15.8	93±12.6	-	-	-	10	**117**
76±18.9	101±15.8	-	-	-	10	**117**
80±15.8	98±12.6	-	-	-	10	**117**
77±15.8	98±12.6	-	-	-	10	**117**
93±18.5	95±7.9	-	-	-	7	**118**
101±21.2	97±15.9	-	-	-	7	**118**
90±9	89±15	-	-	-	9	**118**
90±17	102±14	-	-	11.1±2.0	5	**118**
79±17	99±17	-	-	-	6	**120**
86±11.3	106±11.3	-	-	-	8	**121**
89±21	112±17	-	-	15.3±4.9	12	**122**
110±34	112.8±10.5	-	-	-	9	**123**

* = Induced complete heart block and paced heart at 60 b/min., ** = Same 14 dogs measured on different days, *** = Same 9 dogs measured at 4 different times, same day

Table 9.1:2 Dogs: Ventricular pressures, atrial pressures, cardiac output, stroke volume and cardiac index from awake, average (15-30 kg) sized animals [± = standard deviation]

Left Ventricular Pressure, Systolic (mmHg)	Left Ventricular Pressure, End-Diastolic (mmHg)	Left Atrial Pressure, mean (mmHg)	Cardiac Output, (ml/min)	Stroke Volume (ml)	Cardiac Index (ml/min/ kg) or (ml/min/ m²)	n	Ref
118±14.7	8±2.4	-	-	-	-	6	**3**
117±9.8	-	-	-	-	-	6	**3**
120±11.2	6±3.7	-	2200±480	33±9	88±19.2	14	**5**
-	4.4±1.1	-	1900±848	23.2±13.8	88±39.6	8	**6**
131.1±19.5	12.9±3.3	-	-	24.2±7.2	-	9	**7**
121±9.4	8.6±2.8	-	-	-	-	10	**8**
105±4.5	8.6±4.8	-	-	-	-	8	**9**

Left Ventricular Pressure, Systolic (mmHg)	Left Ventricular Pressure, End-Diastolic (mmHg)	Left Atrial Pressure, mean (mmHg)	Cardiac Output, (ml/min)	Stroke Volume (ml)	Cardiac Index (ml/min/ kg) or (ml/min/ m^2)	n	Ref
-	-	-	-	-	130±29.8	11	**40**
-	-	3±3	-	-	-	13	**10**
-	-	6±3	-	-	-	13	**10**
-	-	2.1±2.2	2448±479	-	125±24.4	19	**12**
125±15	-	5.4±2.7		-	3900±600 (m^2)	9	**41**
-	7±3.9	-	-	-	-	15	**14**
126±20	10.7±2.2	-	-	-	-	5	**15**
123±6.7	6±2.2	-	3170±726	31±6.6	127±29	5	**16**
140±21		-	4200±1860	-	187±82.5	9	**18**
-	-	-	-	-	7450± 2381 (m^2)	7	**20**
-	-	5±2	-	-	-	14	**23**
126±16.5	9.1±3.4	-	-	-	-	14	**24**
121±14.6	8.3±1.9	-	-	-	-	14	**26***
121±17.2	8.4±0.7	-	-	-	-	14	**26***
117±13.1	-	-	-	-	-	14	**26***
124±14.9	8.4±1.9	-	-	-	-	14	**26***
127±11.9	8.1±2.3	-	-	-	-	14	**27**
120±23.6	8.0±6.5	-	-	-	-	15	**28**
126±13.3	8.8±2.2	-	-	-	-	13	**29**
-	7±3.2	-	-	-	-	10	**30**
-	-	-	2554±157	-	-	15	**31**
-	-	5.9±0.2	2140±22.4	-	112±1.1	5	**32**
-	-	-	3240±132	-	135±55.5	7	**33**
131±29	5±2.2	-	-	-	-	5	**34**

Left Ventricular Pressure, Systolic (mmHg)	Left Ventricular Pressure, End-Diastolic (mmHg)	Left Atrial Pressure, mean (mmHg)	Cardiac Output, (ml/min)	Stroke Volume (ml)	Cardiac Index (ml/min/kg) or (ml/min/m^2)	n	Ref
-	-	-	-	59.5±18.1	7730±1669 (m^2)	8	**35**
-	-	2.3±1.5	2530±444	25±8.7	-	9	**36****
-	-	1.5±1.2	2493±456	24±7.5	-	9	**36****
-	-	3.4±1.2	2388±420	21.4±6.3	-	9	**36****
-	-	2.6±1.2	1975±336	19.6±6.0	-	9	**36****
-	-	-	2620±1085	-	131±54.2	14	**37**
120±12.3	7.3±2.8	-	-	-	-	10	**38**
-	-	2.4±6.6	3300±2973	29.4±21	-	9	**39**
129.2±17.8	11.7±2.8	-	-	-	-	8	**96**
-	-	-	3100±700	-	-	5	**95**
-	3.8±3.3	-	-	-	-	5	**97**
138±14.1	12±2.8	-	2700±1100	35±22.6	-	8	**98**
126±11.3	12±2.6	-	3000±800	31±5.3	-	7	**98**
135±12	11±3	-	2400±600	31±9	-	9	**99**
134±12	10±3	-	2500±1200	30±8	-	9	**99**
129±12	9±3	-	2300±1500	25±15	-	9	**99**
130±12	9±3	-	2500±1200	29±15	-	9	**99**
-	-	-	-	2.0±0.4 (ml/kg)	181±46	14	**100**
-	-	3.3±2.7	2000±500	-	-	6	**101**
126±10.6	12±2.6	-	3000±800	31±5.3	-	7	**98**
122±7.3	9±2.4	-	-	-	-	6	**102**
108±9	13.4±4.4	10.5±2.9	1790±587	15.9±4.5	-	13	**104+**
120±16	12.8±4.8	10.9±4.4	2046±736	16.9±4.0	-	13	**104++**

Left Ventricular Pressure, Systolic (mmHg)	Left Ventricular Pressure, End-Diastolic (mmHg)	Left Atrial Pressure, mean (mmHg)	Cardiac Output, (ml/min)	Stroke Volume (ml)	Cardiac Index (ml/min/ kg) or (ml/min/ m²)	n	Ref
108±19.8	14.3±18.4	11.2±16.4	1724±1089	14±9.9	-	8	**104+**
130±9	10±3	-	2600±600	33±12	-	9	**105**
127±9	9±3	-	2500±600	29±6	-	9	**105**
-	-	-	3610±240	27±2.6	-	7	**106**
-	-	-	2950±610	21±2.6	-	7	**106 +++**
135±12	11±3	-	2400±600	31±9	-	9	**99**
129±12	9±3	-	2300±1500	25±15	-	9	**99**
134±12	10±3	-	2500±1200	29±15	-	9	**99**
130±12	9±3	-	2500±1200	29±15	-	9	**99**
-	-	7.6±4.2	-	-	-	20	**107**
-	-	6.0±3.3	-	-	-	20	**107**
-	-	-	-	-	106±41.6	6	**110**
-	-	-	-	-	145±30	6	**111**
117±8.5	11±2.8	-	2800±800	36±14.1	-	8	**112**
120±11.3	10±2.8	-	2700±600	34±8.5	-	8	**112**
116±7.9	11±2.6	-	3100±800	40±13.2	-	7	**112**
130±27	9±3	-	2690±1000	-	-	9	**113**
124±18	9±6	-	2360±540	-	-	9	**113**
131±18	8±3	-	2770±2100	-	-	9	**113**
123±18	9±3	-	2390±900	-	-	9	**113**
-	-	-	-	-	174±62.4	12	**114**
-	-	-	2250±1000	27.6±0.7	-	6	**115**
-	-	-	2100±200	24.7±0.7	-	6	**115**

Left Ventricular Pressure, Systolic (mmHg)	Left Ventricular Pressure, End-Diastolic (mmHg)	Left Atrial Pressure, mean (mmHg)	Cardiac Output, (ml/min)	Stroke Volume (ml)	Cardiac Index (ml/min/ kg) or (ml/min/ m²)	n	Ref
118±7.9	8±2.6	-	700±800	5±7.9	-	7	**116**
119±7.9	7±2.6	-	2800±1000	37±13.2	-	7	**116**
124±12.6	10±3.2	-	2600±900	36±12	-	10	**117**
131±19	9±3.2	-	2300±900	30±9	-	10	**117**
127±12.6	8±3.2	-	2700±1200	33±12	-	10	**117**
129±15.8	10±3.2	-	2400±900	31±9	-	10	**117**
125±15.9	8±2.6	-	-	-	-	7	**118**
126±15.9	10±2.6	-	-	-	-	7	**118**
117±21	8±2.6	-	-	-	-	9	**118**
-	-	-	-	-	145±30	5	**119**
-	-	-	-	-	106±41.6	6	**120**
136±8.5	10±2.8	-	2900±600	-	-	8	**121**
-	-	-	-	2.0±0.3 (ml/kg)	174±50	12	**122**
-	-	3.6±5.5	-	-	164.3±63	9	**123**

* = Same dogs measured on different days, ** = Same dogs measured at different times in same day
+ = Standing, ++ = Recumbent, +++ = 10-14 years old

Table 9.1:3 Dogs: Indices of myocardial function from awake, average (15-30 kg) sized animals,
[± = standard deviation]

+dP/dt (mmHg/s)	- dP/dt (mmHg/s)	Velocity of Shor-tening (mm/s)	Power	Work	Preload Recruit-able Stroke Work (mmHg•mm)	n	Ref
2970±367	-	67±12.2	-	-	-	6	**3**
2960±245	-	64±9.8	-	-	-	6	**3**
3350±270	-	78±9	-	-	-	9	**5**
2483±240	2631±297	-	-	-	-	8	**6**
3586±534	2814±297	20.7±7.9	35.2±17.7 (x10^4 dynes•cm•sec^{-1})	3.04±1.3 (x10^4 dynes•cm•stroke^{-1})	-	10	**8**
2967±519	-	-	-	-	-	16	**13**
-	-	23.7±12.6	-	-	-	15	**14**
2723±635	-	-	-	-	-	5	**15**
2777±297	-	-	4.4±1.3 (kg•m•min^{-1})	42±13.4 (g•m•beat^{-1})	-	5	**16**
3429±1236	-	-	-	5.32±2.1 (x10^5 kg•m•min^{-1})	-	9	**18**
-	-	-	160±103 (x10^7 ergs •m^{-2})	10.1±3.7 (x10^6 dynes•m^{-2})	-	7	**20**
3338±471	-	-	-	-	-	14	**24***
3491±726	-	-	-	-	-	14	**26***
3541±890	-	-	-	-	-	14	**26***
3051±340	-	-	-	-	-	14	**26***
3517±475	-	-	-	-	-	14	**27**
3531±1068	-	82±35.6	-	-	-	15	**28**
3247±696	-	-	-	-	-	13	**29**
2474±2195	-	-	-	-	-	10	**30**

+dP/dt (mmHg/s)	- dP/dt (mmHg/s)	Velocity of Shor-tening (mm/s)	Power	Work	Preload Recruit-able Stroke Work (mmHg•mm)	n	Ref
3564±467	-	14±4.4	-	-	-	5	**42**
-	-	317±82 (cm• sec^{-1}• m^{-2})	125.7±34.8 (x10^7 ergs •m^{-2})	11.3±3.4 (cm• sec^{-1}• m^{-2})	-	8	**35**
3467±364	-	-	-	-	-	10	**38**
4014±1281	-	-	-	-	-	8	**96**
1875±337	-	-	-	-	249±84.8	8	**98**
1855±262	-	-	-	-	257±92.6	7	**98**
-	-	-	-	-	289±192	9	**99**
3410±495	-	-	-	-	-	6	**101**
1875±337	-	-	-	-	249±85	8	**98**
2612±372	-	-	-	-	-	6	**102**
2923±419	2323±369	-	-	-	-	13	**104 ++**
2948±642	2454±539	-	-	-	-	13	**104 +**
2929±894	2248±486	-	-	-	-	8	**104 +**
2698±537	-	-	-	-	-	9	**105**
2778±585	-	-	-	-	-	9	**105**
1720±273	-	-	-	-	239±192	9	**99**
1740±363	-	-	-	-	323±240	9	**99**
2185±396	-	-	-	-	-	8	**112**
2319±402	-	-	-	-	-	8	**112**
2389±259	-	-	-	-	-	7	**112**
2458±452	-	-	-	-	-	10	**117**
2542±528	-	-	-	-	-	10	**117**
2436±519	-	-	-	-	-	10	**117**
2453±503	-	-	-	-	-	10	**117**
2680±509	-	-	-	-	-	8	**121**

+dP/dt (mmHg/s)	- dP/dt (mmHg/s)	Velocity of Shortening (mm/s)	Power	Work	Preload Recruitable Stroke Work (mmHg• mm)	n	Ref
-	-	-	-	19.6±7.2 mmHg[L /min/kg]	-	12	122
1397±1149	-	-	-	217±45 [ml/min/ kg]•b/ min	-	12	122, 123

* = Readings from same 14 dogs on different days, + = standing, ++ = recumbent

Table 9.1:4 Dogs: Indices of myocardial function from awake, average (15-30 kg) sized animals
[± = standard deviation]

dP/dt$_{50}$ (mmHg/s)	Segmental Shortening (%)	Emax (mmHg/ mm)	Rate Pressure Product (b/min• mmHg• 10^3)	Ejection Fraction (%)	dV/dt (ml/sec)	n	Ref
1737±286	18.6±4.8	-	-	-	-	8	98
1755±198	22.4±6.6	-	-	-	-	7	98
1560±210	18.8±9	42±30	-	-	-	9	99
1689±183	18.5±8.4	21±15	-	-	-	9	99
1737±286	18.6±4.8	-	-	-	-	8	98
-	19±6.1	-	9.6±2.9	-	-	6	102
-	-	-	-	39±6.0	157±56	13	104++
-	-	-	-	42±6.9	185±44	13	104+
-	-	-	-	38±15.8	178±110	8	104+
2061±222	20.8±8.1	-	9.9±1.8	-	-	9	105
2110±312	22.3±10.2	-	10.1±0.9	-	-	9	105
1560±210	18.8±9	21±15	-	-	-	9	99
1630±264	19.2±9	24±12	-	-	-	9	99
-	-	-	15.8±5.6	-	-	20	107
-	-	-	13.2±4.6	-	-	20	107

dP/dt$_{50}$ (mmHg/s)	Segmental Shortening (%)	Emax (mmHg/ mm)	Rate Pressure Product (b/min• mmHg• 10³)	Ejection Fraction (%)	dV/dt (ml/sec)	n	Ref
-	-	-	11.1±2.7	-	-	6	**110**
1902±266	21.1±4.2	-	-	-	-	8	**112**
1923±934	19.4±6.5	-	-	-	-	8	**112**
2031±174	16.3±3.4	-	-	-	-	7	**112**
1991±249	14.4±6.9	-	-	-	-	9	**113**
1836±342	16.0±6.9	-	-	-	-	9	**113**
1954±309	17.6±8.7	-	-	-	-	9	**113**
1877±171	15.5±3.0	-	-	-	-	9	**113**
-	-	-	8.9±1.8	-	-	7	**116**
-	-	-	8.8±1.6	-	-	7	**116**
1997±183	17.9±6	-	9.2±2.2	-	-	10	**117**
2056±243	16.7±5.1	-	10.1±3.5	-	-	10	**117**
2000±313	19.5±3.9	-	10.2±2.5	-	-	10	**117**
1933±224	18.4±4.2	-	9.6±2.5	-	-	10	**117**
2130±291	16.5±7.7	-	-	-	-	7	**118**
2050±291	14.4±4.0	-	-	-	-	7	**118**
2020±300	15.8±5.7	-	-	-	-	9	**118**
-	-	-	11.1±2.7	-	-	6	**120**
2060±311	13.4±3.1	-	11.4±1.4	-	-	8	**121**
-	24.1±2.4	-	-	-	-	10	**8**
-	18.5±1.5	-	-	-	-	15	**14**
-	23±1.8	-	-	-	-	5	**15**
-	34±4	-	-	-	-	5	**16**
-	12.2±1.2	-	-	-	-	20	**34**

+ = Standing, ++ = Recumbent

Table 9.1:5 Dogs: Left ventricular dimensions, diastolic volume, central venous pressure, systemic and pulmonary resistance values from awake, average (15-30 kg) sized animals, [± = standard deviation]

LV End-Diastolic Diameter (mm)	LV End-Systolic Diameter (mm)	LV End-Diastolic Volume (ml)	Central Venous Pressure (mmHg)	Resis-tance, Syst. (dyne•s •cm^{-5})	Resis-tance, Pulmon. (dyne•s •cm^{-5})	n	Ref
36.3±1.3	24.7±1.8	-	-	3032±717	-	9	**5**
-	-	-	-	3272±662	-	19	**12**
-	-	-	-	1899±611	-	7	**20**
34.1±1.5	25.7±1.3	-	-	-	-	14	**24**
37.1±1.4	29.2±1.8	-	-	-	-	15	**28**
-	-	-	-	3124±152	-	15	**31**
-	-	-	-	4142±548	-	7	**33**
-	-	-	-	1500±385	-	8	**35**
-	-	-	-	2394±479	-	9	**39**
33.4±2.7	27.0±2.7	-	-	-	-	6	**3**
32.9±2.4	26.3±2.4	-	-	-	-	6	**3**
-	-	56.2±5.6	-	-	-	9	**7**
-	-	-	-	4094±83	-	5	**32**
-	-	-	-	3300±1046	-	8	**98**
-	-	-	-	2730±608	-	8	**98**
-	-	-	-	3730±1020	-	9	**99**
-	-	-	-	4310±2070	-	9	**99**
-	-	-	-	3650±2010	-	9	**99**
-	-	-	4.8±3.0	2176±616	-	14	**100**
-	-	-	-	2730±608	-	7	**98**

LV End-Diastolic Diameter (mm)	LV End-Systolic Diameter (mm)	LV End-Diastolic Volume (ml)	Central Venous Pressure (mmHg)	Resistance, Syst. (dyne•s•cm^{-5})	Resistance, Pulmon. (dyne•s•cm^{-5})	n	Ref
-	-	41±12.9	-	-	_	13	**104**
-	-	42±12.2	-	-	-	13	**104**
-	-	37.9±22.9	-	-	-	8	**104**
-	-	-	-	3210±780	-	9	**105**
-	-	-	-	3430±720	-	9	**105**
-	-	-	-	2578±271	-	7	**106**
-	-	-	-	3248±567	-	7	**106**
-	-	-	-	3730±1020	-	9	**107**
-	-	-	-	4310±2070	-	9	**107**
-	-	-	-	3650±2010	-	9	**107**
-	-	-	-	3660±1680	-	9	**107**
-	-	59.3±4.4	-	-	-	6	**108**
-	-	-	-	2800±980	-	6	**110**
-	-	-	-0.2±2.8	2204±716	179±57	6	**111**
-	-	-	-	2750±821	-	8	**112**
-	-	-	-	2820±934	-	8	**112**
-	-	-	-	2860±449	-	7	**112**
-	-	-	-	3091±906	-	9	**113**
-	-	-	-	3256±525	-	9	**113**
-	-	-	-	4362±2907	-	9	**113**

LV End-Diastolic Diameter (mm)	LV End-Systolic Diameter (mm)	LV End-Diastolic Volume (ml)	Central Venous Pressure (mmHg)	Resistance, Syst. (dyne•s •cm^{-5})	Resistance, Pulmon. (dyne•s •cm^{-5})	n	Ref
-	-	-	-	4330±1599	-	9	113
-	-	-	-	3439±1963	-	6	115
-	-	-	-	3599±1468	-	6	115
-	-	-	-	2810±1005	-	7	116
-	-	-	-	2840±847	-	7	116
-	-	-	-	3130±1110	-	9	117
-	-	-	-	3410±1020	-	9	117
-	-	-	-	3270±1380	-	9	117
-	-	-	-	3520±810	-	9	117
-	-	-	-0.2±2.8	2204±716	179±57	6	119
-	-	-	-	3060±792	-	8	121
-	-	-	4.5±3.0	-	-	12	122
-	-	-	-	4916±1668	-	9	123

Table 9.1:6 Dogs: Blood flows and other coronary circulation variables from awake, average sized (15-30 kg) animals [± = standard deviation].

Left circumflex late diastolic flow (ml/min)	Left circumflex mean flow (ml/min)	Left circumflex late diastolic coronary resistance (mmHg•min/ml)	Left coronary flow (ml/min/100 g)	Left circ. coronary artery mean diameter (mm)	Left circ. coronary artery internal crosssectional area (mm²)	n	Ref
41±7.3	-	1.91±0.29	-	-	-	6	3
40±7.3	-	1.93±0.24	-	-	-	6	3

Left circum-flex late diastolic flow (ml/min)	Left circum-flex mean flow (ml/min)	Left circum-flex late diastolic coronary resistance (mmHg• min/ml)	Left coronary flow (ml/min/ 100 g)	Left circ. coro-nary artery mean diamet-er (mm)	Left circ. coronary artery in-ternal crosssec-tional area (mm^2)	n	Ref
-	44±14.4	1.63±0.32	-	-	-	13	**5**
-	29.8±14.1	-	-	-	-	8	**6**
-	-	-	135±24	-	-	7	**43**
-	-	-	133±35	-	-	6	**44**
-	-	-	95±6	-	-	4	**11**
-	-	-	80.9±20.9	-	-	19	**12**
-	31±11.6	-	-	-	-	15	**14**
-	47.4±13.3	1.51±0.39	-	-	-	13	**17**
-	45.2±9.3	1.54±0.42	-	-	-	15	**17**
-	45.5±11.9	1.46±0.46	-	-	-	11	**17**
-	-	1.08±0.3 (per 100 g tissue)	95±24	-	-	9	**18**
-	22±5.3	4.75±1.48	-	-	-	7	**21***
-	25±3	4.02±1.06	-	-	-	7	**21+**
-	26.4±16.9	-	-	-	-	8	**25**
38.6±18.3	-	1.94±0.86	-	4.05±1.31	6.54±4.08	14	**26****
36.3±17.6	-	2.01±1.12	-	3.99±1.57	6.40±5.01	14	**26****
45.0±23.6	-	1.59±0.67	-	3.81±0.64	5.74±1.87	14	**26****
33.5±14.2	-	2.06±0.59	-	3.94±1.27	6.29±4.11	14	**26****
28.0±6.9	-	2.83±0.88	-	4.12±0.81	6.75±2.67	15	**27**
-	39±25.6	1.84±1.01	-	-	-	15	**28**
-	34.8±11.9	2.60±0.64	-	3.99±0.54	6.22±1.66	13	**29**
-	32±8.8	2.17±0.51	-	3.65±0.47	5.23±1.42	10	**38**
-	43±29.4	-	-	-	-	6	**101**

Left circumflex late diastolic flow (ml/min)	Left circumflex mean flow (ml/min)	Left circumflex late diastolic coronary resistance (mmHg•min/ml)	Left coronary flow (ml/min/100 g)	Left circ. coronary artery mean diameter (mm)	Left circ. coronary artery internal crosssectional area (mm²)	n	Ref
-	65±11	1.45±0.22	-	3.24±0.25	-	6	**108**
-	40±18	2.54±1.2	-	-	-	9	**114**
-	34±12	2.54±1.2	-	-	-	9	**114**
-	39±18	2.77±2.1	-	-	-	9	**114**
-	40±12	2.39±0.9	-	-	-	9	**114**
-	42±21.2	2.29±1.1	-	-	-	9	**117**
-	41±31.7	2.39±1.3	-	-	-	9	**117**
-	33±7.3 (Hz•10²)	2.64±0.5	-	-	-	9	**117**
-	33±4.9 (Hz•10²)	2.61±0.6	-	-	-	9	**117**
-	34±4.9 (Hz•10²)	2.61±0.3	-	-	-	9	**117**
-	32±13.62 (Hz•10²)	-	-	-	-	7	**118**
-	26±13.2 (Hz•10²)	-	-	-	-	7	**118**
-	32±18 (Hz•10²)	-	-	-	-	9	**118**

* = untrained dogs, ** = same dogs measured on different days, + = partially trained (exercised) dogs

Table 9.1:7 Dogs: Blood flow distribution to the heart in average sized, awake animals. All values are in ml/min/100g of myocardium [± = standard deviation]

Total coronary flow	Flow to the left ventricle	Flow to the septum	Flow to the right ventricle	Flow to the atria	Flow to the LV epicardium	Flow to the LV endocardium	Flow to the LV midwall	Endo/Epicardium flow ratio	n	Ref
116± 14	135± 24	61.5± 8	31.6± 9	12.3± 4	-	-	-	-	7	**43**
-	-	-	53.7± 13.5	-	-	-	-	-	19	**12**
-	-	-	-	-	62± 34.8	67± 54	85± 42.6	1.08± 0.38	15	**14**
-	-	104± 31.7	100± 42.3	-	-	-	121.5 ± 23.8	-	7	**20**
-	140± 20.1	-	-	-	123± 22.4	165± 22.4	159±20.1	1.40± 0.18	5	**34**
-	-	-	-	-	130± 30	166± 40	148± 33.2	1.27± 0.25	25	**34**
-	103± 31.7	-	67± 21.2	-	-	-	-	-	7	**42**
-	-	120± 36.8	81± 31	-	-	-	147± 31	-	8	**35**
-	159± 34	-	-	-	113± 39	184± 42	179± 37	-	7	**118**
-	141± 37	-	-	-	109± 29	163± 45	152± 42	-	7	**118**
-	138± 66	-	-	-	108± 60	152± 70	156± 72	-	9	**118**
-	-	-	-	-	118± 56	138± 65	140± 64	-	20	**107**

Table 9.1:8 Dogs: Non-cardiac blood flow distribution in awake animals in ml/min (± = standard deviation)

Renal	Mesen	Iliac	Bone	Skin	Skel	GI	Liver	Pan	Spleen	Brain	Bron	n	Ref
169 ±11	289 ±21	114 ±8	-	-	-	-	-	-	-	-	-	6	**3**
173 ±24	288 ±46	119 ±15	-	-	-	-	-	-	-	-	-	6	**3**
207 ±45	-	-	79 ±27	86 ±39	832 ± 489	182 ±54	-	32 ±18	73 ±39	64 ± 15	-	9	**2**
440 ± 152	-	-	335 ±83	302 ±131	793 ± 340	360 ±87	207 ± 122	68 ±39	132 ±52	64 ± 13	123 ± 61	19	**12**
145 ±16	-	-	-	-	-	-	-	-	-	-	-	10	**30**
96 ±39	-	-	-	-	-	-	-	-	-	-	-	9	**39**
158 ±10	-	-	-	-	-	-	-	-	-	-	-	17	**22**
92 ±24	-	-	-	-	-	-	-	-	-	-	-	6	**101**
284 ± 136	-	-	-	-	-	-	-	-	-	-	-	7	**109**
293 ±38	-	-	-	-	-	-	-	-	-	-	-	4	**109**
287 ± 103	-	-	-	-	-	-	-	-	-	-	-	5	**109**
117 ±73	-	-	-	-	-	-	624 ± 208	-	-	-	-	6	**115**

R e n a l	M e s e n	I l i a c	B o n e	S k i n	S k e l	G I	L i v e r	P a n	S p l e e n	B r a i n	B r o n	n	Ref
122 ±8 8	-	-	-	-	-	-	626 ± 463	-	-	-	-	6	**115**

Mesen = Mesenteric, Skel = Skeletal muscle, GI = GI tract, Pan = Pancreas, Bron = Bronchial

Table 9.1:9a Dogs: Blood flow distribution per 100 g of tissue (ml/min/100g) and as a percentage of cardiac output ( ) in awake animals (± = standard deviation)

Kidneys	Liver	GI tract	Spleen	Pan	Lungs	Skin	n	Ref
417±96 (14.6± 3.3)	34±17 (6.9± 4.3)	- (12.3± 3.5)	179± 78.5 (4.9± 2.2)	184±91 (2.3± 1.3)	40.4± 19.2 (4.1± 1.7)	11.2± 3.9 (10± 3.9)	1 9	**12**
377±148	38±8	52±16	197±53	-	-	-	7	**20**
-	20±16	71±19	-	173±32	-	-	1 0	**45**
545±140	35±16	33.7±13.2	258±119	64±24	24±8	2.8±1.0	7	**33**
377±130	25±18	56±40	221±90	52±32	54±21	3±2.6	7	**42**
387±116	44±11	54±17	198±48	-	-	-	8	**35**
365±228	35±19	35±30	172±108	49±26	-	-	1 4	**37**
391±220	47±32	-	224±90	217±127	-	13±7.9	7	**106**
354±140	44±24	-	253±100	189±85	-	9±5.3	7	**106**

pan = Pancreas

Table 9.1:9b Dogs: Blood flow distribution per 100 g of tissue (ml/min/100g) and as a percentage of cardiac output ( ) in awake animals (± = standard deviation)

Brain	Bone	Skeletal muscle	Adrenal gland	n	Ref
68.1±14.4 (2.2±0.4)	- (11.4±2.6)	- (25.9±8.7)	-	19	**12**
80±24	-	22±7.9	-	7	**20**
-	-	-	-	10	**45**
55±10.6	-	3.7±1.6	322±180	7	**33**
61±16	8±5.3	3.0±2.6	248±69	7	**42**
80±25	-	24±8.5	-	8	**35**

Brain	Bone	Skeletal muscle	Adrenal gland	n	Ref
38±15	-	3.0±3.7	-	14	**37**
57±21.2	-	60±47.6	-	7	**106***
67±15.9	-	61±31.7	-	7	**106****

* = 1-2 year old dogs, ** = 10-14 year old dogs

Table 9.1:10 Dogs: Blood gases and myocardial oxygen consumption from awake animals [± = Standard Deviation]

Arterial pH	PaO$_2$ (mmHg)	PaCO$_2$ (mmHg)	PvO$_2$ (mmHg) (Cor. sinus)	PvCO$_2$ (mmHg) (Cor. sinus)	Myocard. O$_2$ consump. (ml O$_2$/min/100g	Bicar. (mmol/L)	n	Ref
7.42± 0.03	-	31.9±2.7	-	-	-	-	9	**36**
7.43± 0.03	-	31.3±2.4	-	-	-	-	9	**36**
7.43± 0.06	-	32.1±2.1	-	-	-	-	9	**36**
7.43± 0.06	-	29.7±1.8	-	-	-	-	9	**36**
7.41± 0.03	71.7±8.2	26.6±2.5	-	-	-	-	8	**35**
7.38± 0.01	80.9±2.5	30.0±1.2	-	-	-	-	5	**22**
-	-	-	-	-	3.8±0.27 (untrained)	-	?	**21**
-	-	-	-	-	4.3±0.32 (trained)	-	?	**21**
7.42± 0.02	70.5±2.5	33.4±2.1	27.2±1.9	41.1±2.2	10.5±3.0	-	9	**18**
-	-	-	-	-	10.4±2.6	-	4	**11**
7.43± 0.02	83±6.6	32±3.3	34±6.6	36±6.6	7±3.3 (/kg body wt)	-	11	**40**
-	70±33	34±2	-	-	-	-	5	**95**
7.38± 0.02	-	39.3±2.7	-	43.8±3.3	-	22.1± 2.2	6	**111**
7.44± 0.02	89.8±6.4	30.8±3.1	-	-	-	-	9	**123**

Arterial pH	PaO$_2$ (mmHg)	PaCO$_2$ (mmHg)	PvO$_2$ (mmHg) (Cor. sinus)	PvCO$_2$ (mmHg) (Cor. sinus)	Myocard. O$_2$ consump. (ml O$_2$/ min/100g)	Bicar. (mmo l/L)	n	Ref
7.34± 0.02	404± 85.7 (spon. breath. 100% O$_2$)	42±2.4	-	-	-	-	6	120
7.38± 0.02	103.8± 6.5	39.3±2.7	49.8±2.4	43.8±3.3	4.9±1.6 (/ kg body wt)	22.1± 2.2	6	Ref 119
7.43± 0.03	82±6	32±3.2	-	-	-	-	10	117
7.42± 0.03	81±6	33±2.2	-	-	-	-	10	117
7.39± 0.06	82±9	34±3.2	-	-	-	-	10	117
7.41± 0.07	85±9.5	32±3.2	-	-	-	-	10	117
7.39± 0.03	105±6.9	35±3.5	49±6.9	39±3.5	-	-	12	114

Cor. = Coronary, Myocard. = Myocardial, Bicar. = Bicarbonate

Table 9.1:11 Dogs: Other cardiovascular parameters in awake animals (± = standard deviation)

Parameter	Value	Units	n	Ref
LV end-diastolic longitudinal circumference	19.04±0.6	cm	9	7
LV external major diameter	3.0±1.2	% change	9	7
LV external minor (anterior-posterior) diameter	5.4±1.2	% change	9	7
LV external minor (septal-freewall) diameter	8.5±1.5	% change	9	7
Major axis, change in length	11.4±5.4	% change	8	96

Parameter	Value	Units	n	Ref
Minor axis, change in length	24.9±5.6	% change	8	96
Change in LV wall thickness	24.9±2.3	% change	8	96
Mean systolic ejection rate index	375±100	ml/s/m^2	7	20
	403±11	ml/s/m^2	8	35
Maximum systolic flow index	791±516	ml/s/m^2	7	20
	655±164	ml/s/m^2	8	35
Maximum acceleration index	9.80±6.24	x10^3 cm /s/m^2	7	20
	7.58±2.8	x10^3 cm /s/m^2	8	35
Maximum velocity index	394±257	cm/s/ m^2	7	20
	317±82	cm/s/ m^2	8	35
Stroke volume index	49.7±10.6	ml/m^2	7	20
Arterial lactate levels	1.28±0.57	mM	9	18
Coronary sinus lactate levels	0.75±0.24	mM	9	18
Venous lactate levels (1-2 year old dogs) (10-14 year old dogs)	1.2±0.26 1.4±0.53	vol/ 100ml	7	106
Arterial pyruvate levels	0.15±0.09	mM	9	18
Coronary sinus pyruvate levels	0.07±0.30	mM	9	18
Plasma renin activity	1.95±1.27	ng/ml/ hr	5	32
Left ventricular mass/body wt	4.24±0.60	g/kg	5	97
Right ventricular mass/body wt	1.43±0.40	g/kg	5	97
Total body oxygen consumption (1-2 year old dogs) (10-14 year old dogs)	19.4±3.7 17.1±4.5	ml/kg/ min	7	106
LV preload recruitable stroke length intercept	8.5±1.8	mm	9	99
	8.0±2.4	mm	9	99
	10.5±2.8	mm	8	98
	10.5±2.8	mm	8	98
	11.1±2.6	mm	7	98
	13.5±2.7	mm	9	105
	13.0±3.6	mm	9	105

Parameter	Value	Units	n	Ref
LV preload recruitable stroke work / end diastolic length (slope)	61±11.3	erg/cm^2 x10^3/ mm	8	**98**
	70±23.8	erg/cm^2 x10^3/ mm	7	**98**
Pressure work index	10.2±4.2	ml O$_2$ /min/ 100g	9	**113**
	8.7±1.8	ml O$_2$ /min/ 100g	9	**113**
	10.0±2.7	ml O$_2$ /min/ 100g	9	**113**
	9.0±2.7	ml O$_2$ /min/ 100g	9	**113**
Pulmonary arterial wedge pressures	3.4±3.4	mmHg	6	**119**
End systolic pressure length relation area	151±63	mmHg/ mm	9	**99**
	214±108	mmHg/ mm	9	**99**
	151±63	mmHg/ mm	9	**99**
P-R interval	112±12.2	msec	6	**101**
Duration of diastole	283±218	msec	8	**104**
	352±76	msec	13	**104**
	296±83	msec	13	**104**
LV time constant of relaxation (τ)	28±3.7	msec	13	**104**
	28±3.3	msec	13	**104**
	28±11.9	msec	8	**104**

Table 9.2:1 Cats: Heart rates, aortic, left ventricular and pulmonary arterial pressures and aortic flows from awake animals

Heart rate (beats /min)	Aortic Pres.; mean; sys./ diastol. (mmHg)	LV sys. Pres. (mmHg)	Pul- mon. Art. Pres. (mmHg)	Cardiac Output (ml/min/ kg)	Aortic Flow (infra- renal) (ml/ min)	Resist- ance (infra- renal) (mmHg /ml/ min)	n	Ref
152±5	108±5	-	-	-	-	-	3	47
139±7	-	129±6	-	-	-	-	2	47
-	111±33	-	22±9	78±23	-	-	2 2	48
218± 24	114±17; 150±38/95± 14	-	-	-	107±45 (n=5)	1.14±0. 31 (n=5)	1 2	124
235± 24	111±15; 140±21/96± 12	-	-	-	120±52 (n=4)	1.08±0. 36 (n=4)	9	124
232± 33	98±18; 127±24/83± 15	-	-	-	113±48 (n=4)	1.01±0. 24 (n=4)	9	124

Table 9.2:2 Cats: Blood flow distribution (ml/min/100g) and vascular resistance (mmHg•min•100g•ml^{-1}) in awake animals

Brain	Liver	Kidney	Spleen	Sm. Intestine	LV & Septum	Right Ventricle	Forelimbs	Hindlimbs	n	Ref
48± 6.7	25± 15.6	298± 62.6	198± 62.6	-	154± 51.4	71± 40	2.95± 0.33	3.7± 0.22	5	47
-	-	-	-	100± 23	-	-	-	-	22	48
3.12 ± 1.2	5.34± 2.5	0.45± 0.09	6.1± 2.0	-	7.5± 0.3	14.8± 3.1	34.2± 9.8	29.2± 4.67	5	47

Table 9.2:3 Systemic, pulmonary and mesenteric vascular resistance in awake cats (mmHg•min• kg•ml^{-1})

Systemic	Pulmonary	Mesenteric	n	Ref
1.5±0.46	0.29±0.14	11.1±4.7	22	**48**
0.98±0.5	-	-	8	**132**

Table 9.2:4 Other cardiovascular parameters in awake cats

Parameter	Value	Units	n	Ref
LV dP/dtmax	3427±279	mmHg/sec	2	**47**
Arterial pH	7.40±0.02	pH units	22	**48**
%O$_2$ saturation, arterial	97±1	%	22	**48**

Table 9.3:1 Heart rates, aortic pressures and left ventricular pressures from awake rats

Heart rate (beats/min)	Aortic Pressure, mean (mmHg)	Aortic Pressure, systolic (mmHg)	Aortic Pressure, diastolic (mmHg)	Left Ventricular Pressure, systolic (mmHg)	Left Ventricular Pressure, diastolic (mmHg)	n	Ref
358±31	113±13	-	-	-	-	21	**49**
-	113.4±23.5	-	-	-	-	66	**50**
-	114±12	-	-	-	-	9	**51**
-	113±11	-	-	-	-	8	**51**
398±40	121.8±10.4	132.8±11.5	108.3±10.1	-	-	23	**52***
-	117±15.8	-	-	-	-	10	**53**
361±56	-	122±23.4	74±23.4	-	-	22	**54**
-	114±3	-	-	-	-	11	**55**
-	116±3	-	-	-	-	10	**55**
-	121±2	-	-	-	-	9	**55**
-	129±3	-	-	-	-	10	**55**
-	127±3	-	-	-	-	9	**55**
389±56	-	126±17.9	76±20.1	139±20.1	5±6.7	5	**56**
370±36	-	118±15	75±12	133±9	7±6	9	**56**

Heart rate (beats/min)	Aortic Pressure, mean (mmHg)	Aortic Pressure, systolic (mmHg)	Aortic Pressure, diastolic (mmHg)	Left Ventricular Pressure, systolic (mmHg)	Left Ventricular Pressure, diastolic (mmHg)	n	Ref
378±44	112±22	134±19	93±22	143±15.8	14±6	10	57
395±19.4	140±11.6	-	-	-	-	15	127
365±33	129±16.6	-	-	-	-	11	126
372±34.8	102±11.6	-	-	-	-	15	125
410±23	120±3	-	-	-	-	11	128
472±28.3	127±11.3	-	-	-	-	8	132
-	121±12.6	-	-	-	-	10	131
438±66	112±12.4	-	-	-	-	17	130
394±33.6	120±14.4	-	-	-	-	23	129

* = Brattleboro rats, heterozygous with 50% of normal vasopressin synthesis, i.e. hypertensive

Table 9.3:2 Cardiac output, cardiac index, stroke volume, systemic resistance and central blood volume from awake rats

Cardiac output (ml/min)	Cardiac Index (ml/min/kg)	Stroke Volume (ml)	Systemic Resistance (mmHg•min/ml)	Central Blood Volume (ml/100g)	n	Ref
114±2	404±53	-	-	-	33	49
115±2	405±57	0.32±0.16	-	-	21	49
-	278±91	-	-	-	15	58
77±11.5	381±58.5	0.20±0.05	6.67±1.3	0.96±1.06	23	52*
-	222±58.5 (/m²)	-	-	-	23	52*
-	626±47	1.7±1.3 (ml/kg)	0.25±0.13 (/100g)	-	10	57
112±26	475±267	-	-	-	11	126
132±19.8	614±92	-	-	-	8	132
119±29	563±137	-	-	-	5	134

Table 9.3:3 Blood flow distribution in awake rats (ml/min/100g)

Heart	Skin	Kid-ney	Brain	Liver	Spleen	GI tract	Testes	n	Ref
383±78	-	814± 159	119±2 3	-	-	-	-	33	**49**
380±89	-	-	-	-	-	-	-	21	**49**
464± 188	19.1± 12.3	633.2± 150	103± 34.9	18.2± 2.2	218.9± 69.3	246.3± 61.9	35±6.5	5	**56**
413± 132	-	565.6± 125	-	14.2± 8.4	152.6± 92.1	-	-	9	**56**
-	12± 6.6	678± 292	45± 29.8	40± 39.8	248± 153	-	22±9.9	11	**126**
-	-	260± 120	-	12.0± 7.7	90.0± 58	-	-	15	**127**
-	-	718± 179	124± 76	48±40	260± 133	-	-	11	**128**
-	-	716± 113	113± 19.6	29± 19.6	224± 115.1	-	-	6	**133**
531± 166.9	18± 8.5	763± 130	117±3 1	140± 42.4	164± 39.6	205± 70.7	-	8	**132**

Table 9.3:4 Blood flow distribution in awake rats (ml/min/100g)

Diaphragm	Stomach	Splanchnic Organs (all)	Intestines	Inter-costal muscle	Rectus Abdom. muscle	n	Ref
75±49.7	141±69. 6	106±33	-	11±6.6	-	11	**126**
-	54±62	78±46.5	64±50.3	-	-	15	**127**
89±53	77±46	-	-	-	-	11	**128**
-	93±56.3	-	-	-	-	6	**133**
93±53.7	127±59. 4	-	-	-	18±8.2	8	**132**

Table 9.3:5 Blood flow distribution in awake rats (% cardiac output)

Heart	Skin	Kidney	Brain	Liver	Spleen	GI tract	Testes	n	Ref
-	8.8±3.3	20.1±8.6	1.1±0.7	4.6±4.3	1.8±2.6	32.0±7.0	2.2±1.0	11	**126**
-	-	4.7±1.4	-	2.1±1.9	1.2±1.2	20.5±7.3	-	15	**127**
-	-	17.3±4.8	1.7±0.5	2.2±1.4	1.3±0.5	-	-	23	**129**
-	-	17.2±4.0	1.6±0.2	4.1±2.0	0.7±0.4	-	-	5	**134**
-	-	19.0±3.8	1.5±0.3	1.6±0.9	1.7±0.6	-	-	10	**135**

Table 9.3:6 Blood flow distribution in awake rats (% cardiac output)

Dia-phragm	Stomach	Splanch-nic Organs (all)	Intes-tines	Inter-costal muscle	Pancreas	n	Ref
0.8±0.3	2.4±1.0	32.0±7.0	19.8±3.6	2.5±1.3	3.3±2.0	11	**126**
-	1.6±1.5	-	15.5±11.2	-	-	15	**127**
-	1.4±0.5	18.7±3.3	13.2±2.9	-	0.5±0.1	23	**129**
-	1.1±0.4	15.9±1.3	9.5±1.3	-	0.5±0.2	5	**134**
-	1.4±0.3	19.0±2.2	13.0±1.9	-	1.7±0.6	10	**135**

Table 9.3:7 Other cardiovascular parameters in awake rats

Parameter	Value	Units	n	Ref
Effective renal blood flow	4.3±2.5	ml/min/100g	10	**53**
Glomerular Filtration Rate (GFR)	0.9±0.6	ml/min/100g	10	**53**
Central Venous Pressure (CVP)	0.2±1.6	mmHg	10	**58**
Hematocrit	45±2.8	%	8	**132**
Plasma norepinephrine levels	207±71.4	pg/ml	7	**54**
	218±85	pg/ml	5	**54**
Plasma epinephrine levels	104±103	pg/ml	7	**54**
	147±31.3	pg/ml	5	**54**

Parameter	Value	Units	n	Ref
Plasma renin activity	5.5±3.6	ng/ml/hr	11	**55**
	3.5±1.3	ng/ml/hr	10	**55**
	4.0±3.0	ng/ml/hr	9	**55**
	3.1±1.6	ng/ml/hr	10	**55**
	3.4±1.5	ng/ml/hr	9	**55**
Plasma renin concentration	8.7±4.3	ng/ml/hr	11	**55**
	4.6±2.5	ng/ml/hr	10	**55**
	6.6±3.9	ng/ml/hr	9	**55**
	6.0±2.2	ng/ml/hr	10	**55**
	7.7±5.4	ng/ml/hr	9	**55**
Renal renin concentration	419±189	ng/mg	11	**55**
	385±88.5	ng/mg	10	**55**
	377±90	ng/mg	9	**55**
	336±72.7	ng/mg	10	**55**
	280±72	ng/mg	9	**55**
Plasma aldosterone concentration	83.3±9.5	ng/mg	10	**55**
	97.3±26.7	ng/mg	9	**55**
Arterial lactate/pyruvate ratio	14.8±5.6	ratio	8	**132**
Portal venous flow	119±33.9	ml/min/100g	8	**132**

Table 9.4:1 Heart rates, aortic pressures, systemic resistance, stroke volume, and right atrial pressures from awake rabbits

Heart rate (b/min)	Aortic pressure, mean (mmHg)	Aortic pressure, systolic (mmHg)	Aortic pressure, diastolic (mmHg)	Resistance, systemic (mmHg/ml/min/kg)	Stroke volume (ml)	Right atrial pressure (mmHg)	n	Ref
277± 28.8	87±10.8	104± 14.4	78±10.8	0.44±0.1	2.5±0.4	-	13	**59**
252± 36.4	79±12.4	-	-	-	-	-	15	**60**
-	86±6.7	-	-	-	-	-	5	**61**
-	87±7.9	-	-	-	-	-	7	**61**
-	97±12.7	-	-	0.44±0.2	-	-	18	**62**

Heart rate (b/min)	Aortic pressure, mean (mmHg)	Aortic pressure, systolic (mmHg)	Aortic pressure, diastolic (mmHg)	Resistance, systemic (mmHg/ml/min/kg)	Stroke volume (ml)	Right atrial pressure (mmHg)	n	Ref
228±11.2	91±2.0	-	-	-	-	0.5±0.7	5	**63**
242±13.7	92.8±2.9	-	-	-	-	-3.3±0.8	7	**64**
249±30.2	87.3±6.6	-	-	-	-	-2.8±0.5	7	**64**
261±30.2	84.5±2.6	-	-	-	-	-1.5±1.6	7	**64**
244±30.7	96±8.2	-	-	-	-	-	10	**65**
288±6	90±3	-	-	0.16±0.01	-	-	9	**136**

Table 9.4:2 Cardiac index (ml/min/kg) and flow distribution (ml/min/100g) in awake rabbits

Cardiac Index	Heart	Skin	Kidney	Brain	Liver	Lung	Spleen	n	Ref
207±43.3	338±97.3	12±3.6	462±115	83±32.4	37±32.4	580±288	929±558	13	**59**
254±62.6	462±183	-	-	94±15.6	36±10.1	-	606±320	5	**61**
263±52.9	358±103	-	-	110±34.4	25.9±16.7	-	678±315	7	**61**
232±81	282±148	-	781±263	67±21.2	32.1±37.3	133±225	580±539	18	**62**
219±60.1	-	0.44±0.13*	15.98±6.1*	2.23±1.5*	-	-	-	10	**65***
-	300±94.9	140±6.3	410±94.9	80±31.6	130±19	330±158	420±126.5	10	**66**
375.7±17.2	-	-	-	-	-	-	-	5	**63**
352±127	-	-	-	-	-	-	-	7	**64**
347±30.4	-	-	-	-	-	-	-	7	**64**

Cardiac Index	Heart	Skin	Kidney	Brain	Liver	Lung	Spleen	n	Ref
268±32	-	-	-	-	-	-	-	7	64
281±25.4	-	-	-	-	-	-	-	7	64
274±7.5	-	-	-	-	-	-	-	9	136

* = Reported as ml/g of dry tissue

Table 9.4:3 Blood flow distribution in awake rabbits (ml/min/kg)

Adrenal	Stomach	Small Intest.	Large Intest.	Skeletal Muscle	Fat	Testes	Pancreas	n	Ref
-	80±31.6	70±31.6	40±31.6	100±6.3	52±35	-	60±31.6	10	66
-	-	1.87±0.9*	3.13±1.9	0.29±0.19	-	-	-	10	65*
148±80.6	77±97.6	-	-	8.9±11.9	-	17.1±9.3	-	18	62
-	54±28.8	97±14	52±14.4	11±3.1	23±14	-	68±32.4	13	59
-	151±55.9	-	-	13.2±7.1	-	29.6±9.6	-	5	61
-	267±169	-	-	18.6±11.6	-	29.0±4.5	-	7	61

* = Reported as ml/g of dry tissue

Table 9.4:4 Blood flow distribution in awake rabbits (% of cardiac output)

Heart	Skin	Kidney	Brain	Liver	Lung	Spleen	Stomach	n	Ref
4.3±0.9	9.0±3.8	16.6±6.3	1.5±0.3	2.5±2.8	9.0±6.6	1.2±0.6	4.7±1.3	10	66
3.7±0.7	6.8±2.5	13.0±3.6	1.1±0.4	6.2±6.1	9.6±3.2	2.2±1.4	2.2±1.1	13	59

Table 9.4:5 Blood flow distribution in awake rabbits (% of cardiac output)

Small Intestine	Large Intestine	Skeletal Muscle	Bones	Fat	Testes	Pancreas	n	Ref
6.5±1.9	6.8±3.2	16.0±6.3	12±3.2	1.2±0.6	-	1.3±0.6	10	**66**
5.0±1.4	5.3±1.4	20.5±4.3	-	5.4±2.5	-	0.4±0.4	13	**59**

Table 9.4:6 Other cardiovascular parameters in awake rabbits

Parameter	Value	Units	n	Ref
Arterial pH	7.43±0.06	pH units	10	**65**
	7.37±0.13	pH units	10	**66**
	7.42±0.04	pH units	13	**59**
PaO_2	67±13.3	mmHg	10	**65**
	90±9.5	mmHg	10	**66**
	81±14.4	mmHg	13	**59**
$PaCO_2$	27±5.4	mmHg	10	**65**
	30±3.2	mmHg	10	**66**
	24.8±1.4	mmHg	13	**59**
Bicarbonate	17.7±4.4	meq/L	10	**65**
Oxygen saturation (room air)	95±3.2	%	10	**66**
Arterial blood, lactate	0.6±0.3	mMol/cc	9	**66**
Arterial blood, glucose	9.4±1.8	mMol/cc	9	**66**
Arterial blood, free fatty acids	0.9±0.3	mMol/cc	9	**66**
Arterial blood, inorganic phosphates	1.2±2.1	mMol/cc	9	**66**

Table 9.5:1 Heart rates, aortic, left ventricular and pulmonary arterial pressures from awake sheep

Heart rate (b/min)	Aortic pressure, mean (mmHg)	Aortic pressure, systolic (mmHg)	Aortic pressure, diastolic (mmHg)	Left ventricular pressure (mmHg)	Pulmonary arterial pressure, mean (mmHg)	n	Ref
167±42	98±4.9	-	-	112±4.9	-	6	**67***
120±30.9	89.9±12.5	-	-	-	14.3±2.9	6	**68***

Heart rate (b/min)	Aortic pressure, mean (mmHg)	Aortic pressure, systolic (mmHg)	Aortic pressure, diastolic (mmHg)	Left ventri-cular pressure (mmHg)	Pulmo-nary arterial pressure, mean (mmHg)	n	Ref
77±13.6	86±10.3	-	-	-	-	5	**69**
79±16.3	81±9.2	-	-	-	-	5	**69**
-	-	~105	~80	-	-	3	**70**
-	~100	~125	-	-	~10	11	**71**
113±20.8	98±6.9	-	-	-	20±6.9	12	**72**
95±24.2	105±20.8	-	-	-	14±6.9	12	**73**
-	-	-	-	-	~13±10	4	**74**
111±22.1	99±6.3	-	-	-	20±7.9	10	**75**
81±18	109±6	-	-	-	-	5	**137**
111±41	111±12	-	-	-	-	5	**137**
99±17	82±7.3	-	-	-	-	6	**138**
107±21.2	-	-	-	95±10.6	-	7	**139***
90±13.2	-	-	-	110±7.9	-	7	**139**
78±3.6	-	-	-	-	-	9	**141**
116±9.9	-	-	-	-	-	9	**141***
136±75	70±24	85±3	58±15	-	16±15	9	**142**

* = lambs

Table 9.5:2 Atrial pressures, cardiac output, cardiac index, systemic vascular resistance and pulmonary resistance from awake sheep.

Left Atrial Pressure (mmHg)	Right Atrial Pressure (mmHg)	Cardiac Output (L/min)	Cardiac Index (ml/min/kg)	Systemic Resistance (mmHg/L/min)	Pulmo-nary Resistance (cmH$_2$0/l/min)	n	Ref
-	6±2	5.7±0.9	-	18.7±2.9	1.9±0.8	5	**137**
-	3±2	6.1±1.3	-	18.3±2.3	1.7±0.5	5	**137**
5±12	3±12	-	-	-	-	9	**142***
4.5±2.9	1.5±1.0	-	165±61	-	-	6	**67***
6.2±1.5	2.3±2.2	2.26±0.5	-	41.0±14.4	4.06±2.4	6	**68**
-	-	4.9±2.1	-	16.5±5.8	-	5	**69**
1.4±1.6	-0.3±2.1	5.2±1.4	115.5±30.8	20±4.5	-	12	**72**

	0±0.3	4.7±0.7	117.5±15.2	22±3.5	-	12	**73**
-	-	5.0±2.0	142.8±56	-	-	4	**74**
-	-	5.0±1.3	117.6±29.7	20±4.7	-	10	**75**
-	-	-	194.2±76.5	-	-	9	**147***

* = lambs

Table 9.5:3 Stroke volume, central venous pressure, arterial and venous blood gases in awake sheep.

Stroke volume (ml)	PaO$_2$ (mmHg)	PaCO$_2$ (mmHg)	pH	O$_2$ sat. (%)	PvO$_2$ (mmHg)	PvCO$_2$ (mmHg)	n	Ref
-	83±10.4	36±3.5	7.44±0.03	94±6.9	-	-	12	**72**
53±6	84±6.9	35±3.5	7.46±0.03	-	39±3.5	42±3.5	12	**73**
-	80±12	39±10	7.52±0.04	-	-	-	4	**74**
47±5	84±9.5	36±3.5	7.46±0.03	-	-	-	10	**75**
-	102±9.8	37.1±2.5	7.42±0.02	-	-	-	6	**138**
-	91.4±7.6	30.3±3.1	7.45±0.06	-	-	-	5	**137**
-	88.6±10.3	30.9±4.7	7.42±0.06	-	-	-	5	**137**
1.03±0.78 (ml/kg)	-	-	-	92±6	-	-	9	**142**

Table 9.5:4 Blood flow distribution in awake sheep (all ml/min/100 gm tissue)

Heart	Skin	Kidney	Brain	Spleen	Adren	Diaph	Intest	Skeletal	Intercos	Pancreas	n	Ref
133 ± 50.6	-	687 ±193	60± 9.5	192 ± 72.7	189 ±44.3	13± 2.2	74± 22	-	13± 9.5	184 ± 41	10	**75**
133 ± 48.5	5.6± 2.7	689 ± 170	59± 10.4	90± 55.4	194 ± 52	13.7 ± 2.4	72± 20.8	4.0± 1.1	13.4 ± 8.3	181 ± 41.6	12	**72**
113 ± 26.8	-	722 ± 208	54± 15.6	-	115 ± 55.9	18± 6.7	73± 26.8	-	23± 20.1	-	5	**73**
-	-	-	61.1 ± 12	-	-	-	-	-	-	-	6	**138**

Adren = Adrenal; Intest = Intestine; Intercos = Intercostal muscles

Table 9.5:5 Blood flow distribution within the heart of awake sheep.

Atria (ml/min/100 gm)	Right Ventricle (ml/min/100 gm)	Left Ventricle (ml/min/100 gm)	Left Ventricle endocardial/ epicardial ratio	n	Ref
59±31	109±24	160±62	-	12	**72**
(% of total organ flow)	(% of total organ flow)	(% of total organ flow)	(% of total organ flow)		
5.9±1.5	16.1±2.8	78±3.6	-	12	**72**
5.9±1.6	16.5±2.5	77.6±3.5	1.48±0.13	10	**75**

Table 9.5:6 Blood flow distribution to the CNS in awake sheep.

Cortex (ml/min/100 gm)	Cerebellum (ml/min/100 gm)	Brain stem (ml/min/100 gm)	Thalamus (ml/min/100 gm)	Spinal Cord (ml/min/100 gm)	Dorsal Medulla oblongata (ml/min/100 gm)	Pons (ml/min/100 gm)	Pituitary (ml/min/100 gm)	n	Ref
62±14	69±13.8	50±10.4	49±6.9	-	-	-	-	12	72
-	71±17.1	-	62±9.8	31±14.7	73±9.8	60±12.2	66±19.6	6	138
(% of total organ flow)	(% of total organ flow)	(% of total organ flow)	(% of total organ flow)	(% of total organ flow)	(% of total organ flow)	(% of total organ flow)	(% of total organ flow)		
64.2±3.3	13.8±1.6	13.8±3.4	8.2±3.7	-	-	-	-	12	72
63.5±2.8	13.8±1.3	13.5±3.5	9.0±3.2	-	-	-	-	10	75

Table 9.5:7 Other cardiovascular parameters in awake sheep

Parameter	Value	Units	n	Ref
Left ventricular dP/dt max/P	32±9.0	sec^{-1}	12	72
	33±9.5	sec^{-1}	10	75
Left ventricular dP/dt max	2,097±794	mmHg/sec	7	139
	2,447±574	mmHg/sec	7	139
Left ventricular -dP/dt (min)	2,570±664	mmHg/sec	7	139*
	2,043±402	mmHg/sec	7	139
Left ventricular peak systolic wall stress (end diastolic)	40.0±9.1	gm/cm^2	6	67*
	36±15.9	gm/cm^2	7	139*
	39±21.2	gm/cm^2	7	139
Left ventricular end-diastolic pressure	11±5.3	mmHg	7	139*
	11±5.3	mmHg	7	139
Left ventricular end-diastolic diameter (major axis)	35±2.6	mm	7	139*
Left ventricular end-diastolic diameter (major axis)	52±5.3	mm	7	139

Parameter	Value	Units	n	Ref
Left ventricular end-systolic diameter (major axis)	24±2.6	mm	7	**139***
Left ventricular end-systolic diameter (major axis)	34±5.3	mm	7	**139**
Left ventricular end-diastolic freewall thickness	7±2.6	mm	7	**139***
	10±2.6	mm	7	**139**
Left ventricular end-systolic freewall thickness	10±2.6	mm	7	**139***
	14±2.6	mm	7	**139**
Left ventricular end-diastolic diameter/end-diastolic thickness	4.79±0.58	ratio	7	**139***
	5.10±0.9	ratio	7	**139**
Left ventricular ejection time	225±42.8	msec	7	**139***
	258±26.5	msec	7	**139**
Left ventricular ejection time (corrected for heart rate)	306±26.5	msec	7	**139***
	316±18.5	msec	7	**139**
Left ventricular systolic time	225±18.5	msec	7	**139***
	258±26.5	msec	7	**139**
Left ventricular systolic time (corrected for heart rate)	307±31.7	msec	7	**139***
	317±13.2	msec	7	**139**
Delay (time from end-systole to dP/dt min)	21±5.3	msec	7	**139***
	32±5.3	msec	7	**139**
Left ventricular freewall weight	33.3±6.6	gm	7	**139***
	94.4±12.7	gm	7	**139**
Left ventricular freewall to body weight ratio	2.14±0.29	gm/kg	7	**139***
	1.78±0.18	gm/kg	7	**139**
Left ventricular freewall + LV septum weight	45.7±9.3	gm	7	**139***
	132.0±15.1	gm	7	**139**
LV freewall + LV septum weight to body weight ratio	2.91±0.29	gm/kg	7	**139***
	2.50±0.32	gm/kg	7	**139**
Systemic vascular resistance (normalized for body weight)	504±207	mmHg x kg x min x L^{-1}	9	**142**

Parameter	Value	Units	n	Ref
Left ventricular diastolic myocardial stiffness constant	15.3±6.6	3γ/4	7	**139***
	16.4±6.6	3γ/4	7	**139**
Left ventricular endocardial shortening	31±5.3	%	7	**139***
	33±5.3	%	7	**139**
Right ventricular tension-time index	14.2±5.6	mmHg	6	**67***
Right ventricular stroke work	33.3±10.0	mg x m x beat^{-1}	6	**67***
Right ventricular peak systolic pressure	34±14	mmHg	6	**67***
Pulmonary arterial pressure (mean)	16±15	mmHg	9	**142***
	22.6±3.0	cm H_2O	5	**137**
	19.0±1.6	cm H_2O	5	**137**
Pulmonary arterial wedge pressure	12.3±5.5	cm H_2O	5	**137**
	9.1±2.2	cm H_2O	5	**137**
Pulmonary vascular resistance	1.9±0.8	cmH_2O x L^{-1} x min	5	**137**
	1.7±0.5	same	5	**137**
	79±96	mmHg x kg x min x L^{-1}	9	**142***
Right ventricular freewall weight	15.7±4.0	gm	7	**139***
	45.5±7.9	gm	7	**139**
Right ventricular freewall to body weight ratio	0.99±0.16	gm/kg	7	**139***
	0.85±0.08	gm/kg	7	**139**
Coronary flow; right ventricle/left ventricle	0.73±0.17	ratio	6	**67***
Coronary flow; total	1.19±0.5	ml/min/100 gm	6	**67***
Left ventricular coronary stroke flow	7.73±2.2	ml/gm/beat x 10^{-3}	6	**67***
Right ventricular coronary stroke flow	5.64±2.3	same	6	**67***
Oxygen delivery, left ventricular	15.7±5.9	ml O_2/ min/gm	6	**67***
Oxygen delivery, right ventricular	11.7±5.8	ml O_2/ min/gm	6	**67***
Oxygen delivery, whole body	15.9±9.3	ml O_2/ min/kg	9	**142***

Parameter	Value	Units	n	Ref
Oxygen consumption, whole body	6.7±3.0	ml O$_2$/min/kg	9	142*
	10.1±4.5	ml O$_2$/min/kg	9	147*
Oxygen extraction, whole body	43±12	%	9	142*
Hemoglobin concentration	7.6±2.4	gm/dL	9	147*
	12.2±1.5	gm/dL	5	137
	11.5±1.3	gm/dL	5	137
	9.4±3.0	gm/dL	9	142*
Plasma bicarbonate concentration	24±3.2	mM	6	138

Table 9.6:1 Heart rate, aortic, left ventricular and pulmonary arterial pressures from awake calves.

Heart rate (beats/min)	Aortic pressure, mean (mmHg)	Aortic pressure, systolic (mmHg)	Aortic pressure, diastolic (mmHg)	Left ventricular pressure, end-diastolic (mmHg)	Pulmonary arterial pressure, mean (mmHg)	n	Ref
110±10	105±10	125±15	80±10	-	30±5	6	76
-	95±10	-	-	-	28±4	5	77
111±14.7	112±7.3	-	-	-	-	6	78
119±27.7	108±6.9	-	-	8±3.5	-	12	78
119±27.7	108±6.9	-	-	8±3.5	-	12	79
90±15	117±18	137±9	108±15	-	34±9	9	80
89.5±6.1	123±16.6	-	-	-	18.5±6.1	6	143

Table 9.6:2 Right ventricular pressures, cardiac output, stroke volume, cardiac index and systemic and pulmonary vascular resistance from awake calves.

Right ventric. press., systolic (mmHg)	Right ventric. press., end-diastolic (mmHg)	Resis., systemic (mmHg. min^{-1}. L^{-1})	Resis., pulmon. vascular (mmHg. min^{-1}. L^{-1})	Cardiac output (L/min)	Stroke volume (ml)	Cardiac index (ml/ min/ kg)	n	Ref
-	-	18±1	4±2	7.2±0.5	60±5	102±8	6	76
46±12	7±3	1.04±0.24 (per kg)	0.30±0.06(per kg)	-	-	113±42	9	80
47±6.9	7±3.5	-	-	-	-	-	12	79
47±14.7	7±2.4	-	-	-	-	-	6	78
47±6.9	7±3.5	-	-	-	-	-	12	78
-	-	-	-	4.05± 0.4	-	70±7	5	77
-	-	1168.5± 176.1 (dynes.s. cm^{-5})	73.3± 51.2 (dynes.s. cm^{-5})	8.05± 1.7	91.5± 23.3	4.9±0.7 (L/min/ m^2)	6	143

Table 9.6:3 Indices of myocardial function in awake calves.

Right ventricular systolic pressure-time index (mmHg.sec.min^{-1})	Right ventricular dP/dt max (mmHg. sec^{-1})	Left ventricular systolic pressure-time index (mmHg. sec.min^{-1})	Left ventricular diastolic pressure-time index (mmHg. sec.min^{-1})	Left ventricular dP/dt max (mmHg. sec^{-1})	Left ventricular dP/dt min (mmHg. sec^{-1})	n	Ref
898±107	792±229	3092±558	2767±599	2867±707	-	12	79
898±107	792±229	3092±558	-	2867±707	3567± 1458	12	78

Table 9.6:4 Coronary blood flows in awake calves (ml/min/gm) then as endocardium/epicardium ratio.

RV myo	LV myo	RV out	RV inter	RV pap	RV post	RV free	LV a p	LV lat	LV p p	LV free	Septum	n	Ref
0.6 ± 0.2	1.3 ± 0.2	-	-	-	-	-	-	-	-	-	–	12	**78**
-	-	0.5 ± 0.1	0.4 ± 0.2	0.5 ± 0.2	0.5 ± 0.2	0.5 ± 0.2	1.2 ± 0.2	1.1 ± 0.2	1.1 ± 0.2	1.1 ± 0.2	1.1 ± 0.1	9	**80**
Endo/epi	Endo/epi	Endo/epi	Endo/epi	Endo/epi	Endo/epi	Endo/epi	Endo/epi	Endo/epi	Endo/epi	Endo/epi	Endo/epi		
1.2 ± 0.1	1.2 ± 0.1	-	-	-	-	-	-	-	-	-	-	12	**78**
1.1 ± 0.1	1.2 ± 0.1	-	-	-	-	-	-	-	-	-	-	12	**79**
-	-	1.3 ± 0.1	1.3 ± 0.2	1.0 ± 0.05	1.2 ± 0.3	1.2 ± 0.1	1.3 ± 0.1	1.3 ± 0.2	1.3 ± 0.2	1.3 ± 0.1	1.3 ± 0.2	9	**80**

RV Myo = right ventricular myocardium, LV Myo = left ventricular myocardium, RV out = right ventricular outflow tract, RV inter = Right ventricular intermediated region, RV pap = right ventricular papillary muscle, RV post = right ventricular posterior freewall, RV free = right ventricular freewall, LV a p = left ventricular anterior papillary muscle, LV lat = left ventricular lateral freewall, LV p p = left ventricular posterior papillary muscle, LV free = left ventricular freewall

Table 9.6:5 Other cardiovascular parameters in awake calves.

Parameter	Value	Units	n	Ref
Hemoglobin, arterial	11.0±1.0	gm/dL	12	**78,79**
	11.0±0.15	gm/dL	9	**80**

Parameter	Value	Units	n	Ref
LV rate-pressure product	143±41.6	mmHg.beats. min^{-1}.10^{-2}	12	**78**
	123±15	same	9	**80**
	138.9±30.1	same	6	**143**
Left ventricular weight/body weight ratio	1.91±0.28	gm/kg	12	**79**
	2.42±0.24	same	9	**80**
Left ventricular stroke work index	88.8±26.4	gm.m.m^{-2}	6	**143**
Stroke volume index	56.8±14.4	ml/beat/m^2	6	**143**
Left coronary artery resistance	82.0±9.8	mmHg. ml^{-1}.min.g^{-1}	6	**78**
	99.0±21	same	9	**80**
Left coronary artery resistance, normalized by body weight in kg	41±15	mmHg. ml^{-1}.min.kg^{-1}	9	**80**
Right ventricular weight/left ventricular weight	0.49±0.10	ratio	12	**79**
Right ventricular weight/body weight	0.92±0.24	gm/kg	12	**79**
	1.21±0.12	same	9	**80**
Right ventricular weight/(left ventricular + septal weight)	0.35±0.07	ratio	12	**79**
	0.36±0.03	same	9	**80**
Right ventricular weight/total ventricular weight	0.26±0.03	same	12	**79**
Right coronary artery resistance	164.1±10.3	mmHg. ml^{-1}.min.gm^{-1}	6	**78**
	234±27	same	9	**80**
Right coronary artery resistance, normalized by body weight in kg	194±24	mmHg. ml^{-1}.min.kg^{-1}	9	**80**
Pulmonary arterial wedge pressure	11.0±3.2	mmHg	6	**143**
Right ventricular stroke work index	10.4±6.6	gm.m.m^{-2}	6	**143**
Central venous pressure	7.8±2.9	mmHg	6	**143**
Renal arterial flow	455±112	ml.min^{-1}	5	**77**

Table 9.7:1   Heart rates and pressures from awake pigs.

Heart rate (beats/min)	Aortic pressure, mean (mmHg)	Left ventricular pressure, peak systolic (mmHg)	Left ventricular pressure, end-diastolic (mmHg)	Pulmonary arterial pressure, mean (mmHg)	n	Ref
106±24	-	112±57	12±3	-	9	**81**
114±18	104±12	-	-	15±3	9	**82**
84±9.9	-	-	-	-	11	**40***
103±13.3	-	-	-	-	11	**40****
94±6	107±5	-	-	-	8	**144+**
92±3	111±5	-	-	-	8	**144++**

* = lying down, ** = standing, + = fasted, ++ = fed

Table 9.7:2   Cardiac output, cardiac index, stroke volume, stroke index and resistances from awake pigs.

Cardiac output (L/min)	Cardiac index (ml/min/kg)	Stroke volume (ml)	Stroke index (ml/kg)	Resistance, systemic	Resistance, pulmonary	n	Ref
2.36±0.9	67.4±25.8	20±12	-	-	-	9	**81**
-	134.7±43.2	-	1.2±0.27	0.853±0.30 (mmHg.min. ml^{-1}.kg^{-1})	0.296±0.30 (mmHg.min. ml^{-1}.kg^{-1})	9	**82**
-	75±6.6	-	-	-	-	11	**40***
-	99±19.9	-	-	-	-	11	**40****
-	117±9	-	1.29±0.15	18.8±1.4 (mmHg.min. ml^{-1})	-	8	**144+**
-	128±10	-	1.37±0.10	18.0±1.4 (mmHg.min. ml^{-1})	-	8	**144++**

* = lying down, ** = standing, + = fasted, ++ = fed

Table 9.7:3 Tissue blood flows in ml.min⁻¹.100g tissue⁻¹ in awake pigs.

Stomach, proximal	Stomach, distal	Duoden.	Jejun., prox.	Jejun., distal	Ileum, prox.	Ileum, distal	n	Ref
21±5	44±12	81±23	66±13	55±13	73±21	59±15	8	**144+**
29±7	123±33	108±10	117±18	95±24	93±20	65±19	8	**144++**

+ = fasted, ++ = fed

Table 9.7:4 Tissue blood flows (in ml.min⁻¹.100g tissue⁻¹, unless indicated otherwise) in awake pigs, continued.

Colon, prox.	Colon, distal	Pan-creas	Spleen	Liver	Portal vein (ml. min⁻¹. kg⁻¹)	Hepa-tic artery (ml. min⁻¹. kg⁻¹)	n	Ref
52±8	34±5	157±33	221±47	7±2	24±4	2±1	8	**144+**
45±5	36±3	163±14	209±37	8±3	32±5	2±1	8	**144++**

+ = fasted, ++ = fed

Table 9.7:5 Tissue blood flows (in ml.min⁻¹.100g tissue⁻¹, unless indicated otherwise) in awake pigs, continued.

Total splanchnic flow (ml. min-1.kg-1)	Splanchnic flow (% of cardiac output)	Brain	Lung	Heart	Kid-ney, right	Kid-ney, left	n	Ref
26±4	22±4	84± 15	47±17	120±6	417± 38	413±37	8	**144+**
34±5	27±3	83±6	52±19	141± 13	467± 56	439±58	8	**144++**

+ = fasted, ++ = fed

Table 9.7:6 Tissue blood flows (in ml.min⁻¹.100g tissue⁻¹) in awake pigs, continued.

Adre-nal	Rectus femoris	Biceps femoris	Semi-ten-dinosus	Soleus	Tibid .ant.	Hind -limb	Cre-mas-ter	n	Ref
154±59	9±2	15±4	16±6	14±3	9±2	13±3	10±4	5	**146+**
145±32	5±2	18±4	9±3	31±6	9±3	16±2	5±1	5	**146++**

+ = fasted, + = fed

Table 9.7:7 Other cardiovascular parameters in awake pigs.

Parameter	Value	Units	n	Ref
Left ventricular work	176.7±43.2	kg.mmHg. min^{-1}.kg^{-1}	9	**82**
Right ventricular work	28.3±9.3	kg.mmHg. min^{-1}.kg^{-1}	9	**82**
Total brain blood flow	63.7±18.3	ml. min^{-1}.100g^{-1}	9	**82**
Left ventricular rate pressure product	10.6±1.1	beats.mmHg.min^{-1}	8	**144+**
	10.5±0.6	same	9	**144++**
Left ventricular pre-ejection thickness	10.73±3.12	mm	9	**81**
% left ventricular wall thickening during ejection	18.81±4.5	%	9	**81**
Regional myocardial blood flow	1.03±0.45	ml.min^{-1}.g^{-1}	9	**81**
Endocardial/Epicardial ratio of myocardial blood flow in the left ventricle	1.20±0.45	ratio	9	**81**
Arterial pH	7.38±0.03	pH units	9	**82**
	7.40±0.03	same	9	**40**
	7.45±0.01	same	8	**144+**
	7.46±0.01	same	8	**144++**
Venous pH	7.39±0.03	same	9	**40**
	7.40±0.01	same	8	**144+**
	7.36±0.01	same	8	**144++**
PaO$_2$ (breathing 100% oxygen)	345±114	mmHg	9	**82**
PaO$_2$ (breathing room air)	77±3	mmHg	9	**40**
PvO$_2$ (breathing room air)	37±3	mmHg	9	**40**
PaCO$_2$	30±3	mmHg	9	**40**
	37.5±3.3	mmHg	9	**82**
PvCO$_2$	30±6	mmHg	9	**40**
Oxygen consumption	2.8±0.3	ml O$_2$. min^{-1}.kg^{-1}	9	**40***
	4.4±0.9	same	9	**40****
	7.6±0.4	same	8	**144+**
	8.6±0.6	same	8	**144++**
Mixed venous lactate concentration	0.63±0.12	mM	8	**144+**
	0.92±0.05	same	8	**144++**

Parameter	Value	Units	n	Ref
Mixed venous glucose concentration	3.88±0.46	mM	8	**144+**
	4.13±0.70	same	8	**144++**

* = lying down, ** = standing, + = fasted, ++ = fed

Table 9.8:1 Heart rates, pressures and flow indices from awake ponies (or horses).

Heart rate (b/ min)	Aortic pressure, mean (mmHg)	LV pressure, syst. (mmHg)	LV pressure, end-diast. (mmHg)	RV pressure, syst. (mmHg)	RV pressure, end-diast. (mmHg)	Cardiac index (L.min^{-1}. m^{-2} or L.min^{-1}. kg^{-1})	n	Ref
48±7.3	112±14.7	-	-	38±4.9	7±4.9	4.46±1.37 (/m^2)	6	**83***
-	110.8±20.8	-	-	-	-	3.0±1.0 (/m^2)	12	**84***
49±2	-	-	-	-	-	-	6	**145***
61±6.3	-	122±22.1	29±15.8	-	-	-	10	**146***
50±11.3	110±8.5	-	-	-	-	90±8.5 (/kg)	8	**147***
43±6	96±13	118±15	-	-	-	72±6 (/kg)	4	**148**
40±7	104±10	128±12	-	-	-	72±10 (/kg)	4	**148**
49±7.9	133±10.6	-	-	-	-	53.9±14.3 (/kg)	7	**149***
45.3±6.7	103.3±24.9	138.5±24.3	-	-	-	45.5±8.0 (L/min)	6	**150**
47±7.1	127.7±20.5	155.7±22.9	-	-	-	43.5±6.8 (L/min)	6	**150**

* = ponies (unmarked represent values from full sized horses)

Table 9.8:2 Pulmonary arterial pressures, atrial pressures, stroke volume and stroke index from awake ponies and horses.

Pulmonary arterial press., mean (mmHg)	Pulmonary arterial press., syst. (mmHg)	Pulmonary arterial press., diast. (mmHg)	Central venous press. (mmHg)	Right atrial press. (mmHg)	Stroke index (ml. b^{-1}. m^{-2} or kg^{-1})	Stroke volume (ml)	n	Ref
-	-	-	-	-	93±29	-	6	**83**
25.3±2.1	35±2	19±2	-	5.3±1.2	-	-	8	**145** *
25.4±3.2	-	21.1±3.3	7.9±1.6	-	-	-	4	**148**
20.9±1.8	-	17.0±1.5	6.6±4.9	-	-	-	4	**148**
33.4±2.9	-	-	-	-	-	142± 20.1	7	**149** *
21.6±4.6	-	-	5.1±2.4	-	-	-	6	**150**
23.1±10.9	-	-	8.1±3.3	-	-	-	6	**150**

* = ponies

Table 9.8:3 Indices of myocardial function in awake ponies.

LV Work (kg.m. min^{-1}. m^{-2})	RV Work (kg.m. min-1. m-2)	LV pressure -time index (mmHg. sec. min-1)	RV pressure -time index (mmHg. sec. min-1)	Vmax (sec-1)	LV dP/dt (mmHg/sec)	LV dL/dt (mm/sec)	n	Ref
5.8±1.9	1.1±0.37	2,112± 460	539±105	-	-	-	6	**82***
-	-	-	-	1.5± 0.37	-	-	6	**84**
-	-	-	-	-	1,176± 231	11.3±3.2	10	**146***

* = ponies

Table 9.8:4 Other cardiovascular parameters in awake ponies and horses.

Parameter	Value	Units	n	Ref
Resistance, systemic arterial	2580±593	dynes.sec. cm^{-5}.m^{-2}	6	**83***

Parameter	Value	Units	n	Ref
	164±22.2	mmHg. ml^{-1}.min. kg^{-1}	7	**149***
pH, arterial	7.42±0.03	pH units	12	**85***
.	7.40±0.2	same	8	**147**
	7.42±0.03	same	6	**150**
	7.41±0.03	same	6	**150**
	7.43±0.03	same	10	**146***
PaO$_2$	98±8.5	mmHg	8	**147**
	108.8±13.0	same	6	**150**
	105.7±8.1	same	6	**150**
	88.6±1.7	same	12	**85***
PaCO$_2$	39.6±1.0	mmHg	12	**84***
	40±0.8	same	8	**147***
	39.7±3.2	same	6	**150**
	40.6±4.1	mmHg	6	**150**
HCO$_3$, arterial	24.9±1.7	meq/L	12	**84***
Hemoglobin	9.67±2.5	gm/dL	6	**83***
	10.4±1.1	same	8	**147**
Right ventricular blood flow, total	57±10	ml.min^{-1}. 100 gm^{-1}	6	**83***
	52.6±11.6	same	8	**147***
Right ventricular blood flow, subepicardial	68±22	same	10	**146***
	52±10	same	6	**83***
Right ventricular blood flow, subendocardial	70±16	same	10	**146***
	61±7	same	6	**83***
Right ventricular blood flow, endo/epi ratio	1.05±0.13	ratio	10	**146***
	1.16±0.07	same	6	**83***
Left ventricular blood flow, total	100.6±20.4	ml.min^{-1}. 100gm^{-1}	8	**147***
	133±10	ml.min^{-1}. 100gm^{-1}	6	**83***
Left ventricular blood flow, subepicardial	114±7	same	6	**83***
	93±28	same	10	**146***

Parameter	Value	Units	n	Ref
Left ventricular blood flow, subendocardial	137±7	same	6	**83***
	103±25	same	10	**146***
Left ventricular blood flow, midwall	148±12	same	6	**83***
	106±32	same	10	**146***
Left ventricular blood flow, endo/epi ratio	1.12±0.09	ratio	10	**146***
	1.20±0.12	same	6	**83***
	1.28±0.13	same	10	**146***
Right septal blood flow	68±10	ml.min^{-1}. 100 gm^{-1}	6	**83***
	84±25	same	10	**146***
Middle septal blood flow	134±17	same	6	**83***
	107±35	same	10	**146***
Left septal blood flow	136±24	ml.min^{-1}. 100gm^{-1}	6	**83***
	106±32	same	10	**146***
Septal blood flow, total	93.6±17.5	same	8	**147***
Coronary resistance, right ventricular	200±29.4	mmHg.min.ml^{-1}.gm^{-1}	6	**83***
	211±32.1	same	8	**147***
Coronary resistance, left ventricular	84±12.2	same	6	**83***
	109.3±11.1	same	8	**147***
Cerebral blood flow, total	62±14.5	ml.min^{-1}. gm^{-1}	12	**85***
Cerebral cortex blood flow, left	112.2±24.9	ml.min^{-1}. 100 gm^{-1}	8	**147***
Cerebral cortex blood flow, right	103.9±21.2	same	8	**147***
Adrenal blood flow, left	131.2±56.6	same	8	**147***
Adrenal blood flow, right	123.8±51.5	same	8	**147***
Renal blood flow, left	676.3±126.1	same	8	**147***
Renal blood flow, right	665.0±122.2	same	8	**147***
Diaphragm blood flow	11.5±7.9	same	8	**147***
Intercostal muscles blood flow	6.2±3.7	ml.min^{-1}. 100 gm^{-1}	8	**147***
Arterial hemoglobin oxygen saturation	99.9±0.1	%	8	**147***
Venous hemoglobin oxygen saturation	74.0±2.8	%	8	**147***

Parameter	Value	Units	n	Ref
Oxygen consumption	3.3±0.6	ml.min^{-1}. kg^{-1}	8	**147***
Arterial oxygen content	14.2±1.27	ml O$_2$/dL blood	8	**147***
Arterial-to-mixed venous oxygen content	3.7±0.42	same	8	**147***
Left ventricular systolic shortening	28.9±7.9	%	10	**146***
Left ventricular stroke work	199±82	mmHg.ml. beat^{-1}	10	**146***
Arterial plasma potassium levels	3.7±0.32	mM	10	**146***
Coronary venous plasma potassium levels	3.7±0.32	mM	10	**146***
Arterial plasma lactate levels	0.99±0.69	mM	10	**146***
Coronary venous plasma lactate levels	0.65±0.47	mM	10	**146***
Lactate extraction	36±12.6	%	10	**146***
Arterial plasma norepinephrine levels	114±72.7	pg/ml	10	**146***
Coronary venous plasma norepinephrine levels	239±158	same	10	**146***
Norepinephrine extraction	110±66.4	same	10	**146***
Pulmonary arterial wedge pressure	16.9±2.1	mmHg	7	**149***
Central blood volume	17.0±1.8	ml/kg	7	**149***
Central plasma volume	11.9±1.3	ml/kg	7	**149***

* = ponies

Table 9.9:1 Heart rates, pressures and cardiac index in awake primates.

Heart rate (beats/min)	Aortic pressure, mean (mmHg)	Left atrial pressure, mean (cm H$_2$0)	Right atrial pressure, mean (cm H$_2$0)	Cardiac index (ml.min^{-1}. kg^{-1})	Species	n	Ref
182±10	114±16	-	-	316±70	Rhesus	7	**86**
192±5	122±20	-	-	-	Rhesus	6	**88**
199±3.2	90±1.9	7.2±2.2	-	-	Macaca fasicularis	6	**89**
155±11.2	95±8.9	-	7±2.0	-	same	5	**90**
150±26.8	100± 15.6	-	6.6±2.5	-	same	5	**91**

Heart rate (beats/min)	Aortic pressure, mean (mmHg)	Left atrial pressure, mean (cm H_2O)	Right atrial pressure, mean (cm H_2O)	Cardiac index (ml.min^{-1}. kg^{-1})	Species	n	Ref
283±43	123±9	-	-	3070±0.54 (ml.min^{-1}. m^{-2})	Squirrel	5	**92**
155±12.6	108± 16.9	4.0±4.6 (mmHg)	-	-	Macaca mulatta (7) & papio anubis (4)	11	**93**
-	99±45	-	-	-	Cyno-molgus	12	**94**

Table 9.9:2 Blood gases, systemic resistance, stroke volume index and left ventricular work in awake primates.

PaO_2 (mmHg)	$PaCO_2$ (mmHg)	Art. pH (pH units)	Resis-tance, systemic (mmHg. min./ L/kg)	Stroke volume index (ml./ kg)	Left ventr-icular work (mmHg. min./ L/kg)	Species	n	Ref
99±24.2	29±10.4	7.41± 0.10	-	-	-	Cyno-molgus	12	**94**
87±10	40±3	7.46± 0.03	-	-	-	Rhesus	6	**88**
95±11	-	-	377±101	1.7±0.4	36±10	Rhesus	7	**86**
-	-	-	31.9±7.4 (dynes. sec. cm^{-5}.10^3)	1.2±0.3	-	Squirrel	5	**92**

Table 9.9:3 Other cardiovascular parameters in awake primates.

Parameter	Value	Units	Species	n	Ref
Blood flow to the brain	37±12	ml.min^{-1}. 100gm^{-1}	Cynomolgus	12	**94**
Cardiac output	319±65	ml.min^{-1}	Squirrel	5	**92**
Blood flow to the heart	366±142	ml.min^{-1}. 100gm^{-1}	Rhesus	7	**86**

Parameter	Value	Units	Species	n	Ref
Blood flow to the brain	75±19	same	Rhesus	7	**86**
Blood flow to the kidney	1121±54 4	same	Rhesus	7	**86**
Blood flow to the skin	25±5	same	Rhesus	7	**86**
Blood flow to the skeletal muscle	29±10	same	Rhesus	7	**86**
Blood flow to the GI tract	78±30	same	Rhesus	7	**86**
Blood flow to the total splanchnic bed	134±32	same	Rhesus	7	**86**
Blood flow to the liver	41±37	same	Rhesus	7	**86**
Blood flow to the bronchial circulation (lung tissue)	34±31	same	Rhesus	7	**86**
Blood flow to the adrenals	267±104	same	Rhesus	7	**86**
Blood flow to the chest wall	28±9	same	Rhesus	7	**86**

References

1. Glantz, S.A., *Primer of Biostatistics*, McGraw-Hill Book Co., San Francisco, 1981
2. Humphrey, S.J., Zins, G.R., The effects of indomethacin on systemic hemodynamics and blood flow in the conscious dog, *Res. Commun. Chem. Pathol. Pharma.* 39:229-240, 1983
3. Vatner, S.F., Smith, N.T., Effects of halothane on left ventricular function and distribution of regional blood flow in dogs and primates, *Circ. Res.*, 34:155-167, 1974
4. Vatner, S.F., Monroe, R.G., McRitchie, R.J., Effect of anesthesia, tachycardia and autonomic blockade on the Anrep effect in intact dogs, *Am. J. Physiol.*, 226:1450-1456, 1974
5. Manders, W.T., Vatner, S.F., Effects of sodium pentobarbital anesthesia on left ventricular function and distribution of cardiac output in dogs, with particular reference to the mechanism for tachycardia, *Circ. Res.*, 39:512-517, 1976
6. Grimditch, G.K., Barnard, R.J., Duncan, H.W., Effect of exhaustive exercise on myocardial performance, *J. Appl. Physiol.*, 51:1098-1102, 1981
7. Olsen, C.O., Tyson, G.S., Maier, G.W., Spratt, J.A., Davis, J.W., Rankin, J.S., Dynamic ventricular interaction in the conscious dog, *Circ. Res.*, 52:85-104, 1983
8. Tomoike, H., Franklin, D., McKown, D., Kemper, W.S., Guberek, M., Ross J.Jr., Regional myocardial dysfunction and hemodynamic abnormalities during strenuous exercise in dogs with limited coronary flow, *Circ. Res.*, 42:487-496, 1978
9. Osaka, G., Sasayama, S., Kawai, C., Hijakawa, A., Kemper, W.S., Franklin, D., Ross, J. Jr., The analysis of left ventricular wall thickness and shear by an ultrasound triangulation technique in the dog, *Circ. Res.*, 47:173-181, 1980
10. Schneider, R.M., Roberts, K.B., Morris, K.G., Stanfield, J.A., Cobb, F.R., Relation between radionucleide angiographic regional ejection fraction and left ventricular regional ischemia in awake dogs, *Am. J. Cardiol.*, 53:294-301, 1984
11. Bacchus, A.N., Ely, S.W., Knabb, R.M., Rubio, R., Berne, R.M., Adenosine and coronary blood flow in conscious dogs during normal physiological stimuli, *Am. J. Physiol.*, 243:H628-H633, 1982
12. Liard, J.F., Deriaz, O., Schelling, P., Thibonnier, M., Cardiac output distribution during vasopressin infusion or dehydration in conscious dogs, *Am. J. Physiol.*, 243:H663-H669, 1982
13. Barron, K.W., Bishop, V.S., Reflex cardiovascular changes with veratridine in the conscious dog, *Am. J. Physiol.*, 242:H810-H817, 1982
14. Hill, R.C., Kleinman, L.H., Tiller, W.H.Jr., Chitwood, W.R.Jr., Rembert, J.C., Greenfield, J.C.Jr., Wechsler, A.S., Myocardial blood flow and function during gradual coronary occlusion in awake dogs, *Am. J. Physiol.*, 244:H60-H67, 1983

15. Theroux, P., Ross, J.Jr., Franklin, D., Kemper, W.W., Sasayama, S., Coronary arterial reperfusion. III. Early and late effects on regional myocardial function and dimensions in conscious dogs, *Am. J. Cardiol.*, 38:599-606, 1976

16. Lin, Y.C., Carlson, E.L., McCutcheon, E.P., Sandler, H., Cardiovascular functions during voluntary apnea in dogs, *Am. J. Physiol.*, 245:R143-R150, 1983

17. Macho, P., Hintze, T.H., Vatner, S.F., Effects of α-adrenergic receptor blockade on coronary circulation in conscious dogs, *Am. J. Physiol.*, 243:H94-H98, 1982

18. McKensie, J.E., Steffen, R.P., Haddy, F.J., Relationships between adenosine and coronary resistance in conscious exercising dogs, *Am. J. Physiol.*, 242:H24-H29, 1982

19. Walgenbach, S.C., Donald, D.E., Cardiopulmonary reflexes and arterial pressure during rest and exercise in dogs, *Am. J. Physiol.*, 244:H362-H369, 1983

20. Dumont, L., Lamoureaux, C., Lelorier, J., Stanley, P., Chartrand, C., Intravenous infusion of nitroprusside: effects upon cardiovascular dynamics and regional blood flow distribution in conscious dogs, *Arch. Int. Pharmacodyn. Ther.*, 261:109-121, 1983

21. Liang, I.Y.S., Stone, H.L., Effect of exercise conditioning on coronary resistance, *J. Appl. Physiol.*, 53:631-636, 1982

22. Sit, S.P., Morita, H., Vatner, S.R., Responses of renal hemodynamics and function to acute volume expansion in the conscious dog, *Circ. Res.*, 54:185-195, 1984

23. Brazzamano, S., Mays, A.E., Rembert, J.C., Greenfield, J.C.Jr., Increase in collateral blood flow following repeated coronary artery occlusion and nitroglycerin administration, *Circ. Res.*, 54:204-207, 1984

24. Hitze, T.H., Vatner, S.F., Cardiac dynamics during hemorrhage relative unimportance of adrenergic inotropic responses, *Circ. Res.*, 50:705-713, 1982

25. Schwartz, G.G., McHale, P.A., Greenfield, J.C.Jr., Coronary vasodilation after a single ventricular extra-activation in the conscious dog, *Circ. Res.*, 50:38-46, 1982

26. Vatner, S.F., Hintze, T.H., Macho, P., Regulation of large coronary arteries by β-adrenergic mechanisms in the conscious dog, *Circ. Res.*, 51:56-66, 1982

27. Hintze, T.H., Vatner, S.F., Dipyridamole dilates large coronary arteries in conscious dogs, *Circulation*, 68:1321-1327, 1983

28. Macho, P., Vatner, S.F., Effects of prazosin on coronary and left ventricular dynamics in conscious dogs, *Circulation*, 65:1186-1192, 1982

29. Vatner, S.F., Hintze, T.H., Effects of a calcium-channel antagonist on large and small coronary arteries in conscious dogs, *Circulation*, 66:579-588, 1982

30. Fennell, W.H., Taylor, A.A., Young, J.B., Brandon, T.A., Ginos, J.Z., Goldberg, L.I., Mitchess, J.R., Propylbutyldopamine: hemodynamic effects in conscious dogs, normal human volunteers and patients with heart failure, *Circulation*, 67:829-836, 1983

31. Bishop, V.S., Peterson, D.F., Pathways regulating cardiovascular changes during volume loading in awake dogs, *Am. J. Physiol.*, 231:854-859, 1976

32. Sundet, W.D., Wang, B.C., Hakumaki, M.O., Goetz, K.L., Cardiovascular and renin responses to vanadate in the conscious dog: attenuation after calcium channel blockade, *Proc. Soc. Exp. Biol. Med.*, 175:185-190, 1984

33. Yeo, C.J., Jaffe, B.M., Zinner, M.J., The effects of intravenous substance P infusion on hemodynamics and regional blood flow in conscious dogs, *Surgery*, 95:175-182, 1984

34. Knight, D.R., SJtone, H.L., Alteration of ischemic cardiac function in normal heart by daily exercise, *J. Appl. Physiol.*, 55(1 Pt 1):52-60, 1983

35. Dumont, L., Lamoureux, C., Lelorier, J., Stanley, P., Chartrand, C., Intravenous infusion of phentolamine: effects on cardiovascular dynamics and regional blood flow distribution in conscious dogs, *J. Cardiovasc. Pharmacol.*, 4:1055-1061, 1982

36. Kanuscky, J.T., Hall, S.M., Strawn, W.B., Levitsky, M.C., Effects of expiratory positive airway pressure vs. continuous positive airway pressure in conscious, spontaneously breathing dogs, *Proc. Soc. Exp. Biol. Med.*, 169:47-53, 1982

37. Zinner, M.J., Kasher, F., Jaffe, B.M., The hemodynamic effects of intravenous infusions of serotonin in conscious dogs, *J. Surg. Res.*, 34:171-178, 1983

38. Cox, D.A., Hintze, T.H., Vatner, S.F., Effects of acetylcholine on large and small coronary arteries in conscious dogs, *J. Pharmacol. Exp. Ther.*, 225:764-769, 1983

39.   Driscoll, D.J., Fukushige, J., Lewis, R.M., Hartley, C.J., Entman, M.J., The comparative hemodynamic effects of propranolol in chronically instrumented puppies and adult dogs, *Biol. Neonate.*, 41:8-15, 1982

40.   Hastings, A.B., White, F.C., Sanders, T.M., Bloor, C.M., Comparative physiological responses to exercise stress, *J. Appl. Physiol.*, 52:1077-1083, 1982

41.   Bagshaw, R.J., Cox, R.H., Pulmonary vascular response to carotid sinus hypotension in the awake and anaesthetized dog, *Acta Anaesthesiol. Scand.*, 27:323-327, 1983

42.   Liang, C., Doherty, J.U., Faillace, R., Maekawa, K., Arnold, S., Gavras, H., Hood, W.B.Jr., Insulin infusion in conscious dogs. Effects on systemic and coronary hemodynamics, regional blood flows and plasma catecholamines, *J. Clin. Invest.*, 69:1321-1336, 1982

43.   Domenech, R.J., Hoffman, J.I.E., Noble, M.I.M., Saunders, K.B., Henson, J.R., Subijanto, S., Total and regional coronary blood flow measured by radioactive microspheres in conscious and anesthetized dogs, *Circ. Res.*, 25:581-596, 1969

44.   Spencer, F.C., Merrill, D.L., Powers, S.R., Bing, R.J., Coronary blood flow and cardiac oxygen consumption in unanesthetized dogs, *Am. J. Physiol.*, 160-149-155, 1950

45.   Friedman, H.S., Lowery, R., Shaughnessy, E., Scorza, J., The effects of ethanol on pancreatic blood flow in awake and anesthetized dogs, *Proc. Soc. Exp. Biol. Med.*, 174:377-382, 1983

46.   Tyson, G.S.Jr., Maier, G.W., Olsen, C.O., Davis, J.W., Rankin, J.S., Pericardial influences on ventricular filling in the conscious dog. Analysis based on pericardial pressure, *Circ. Res.*, 54:173-184, 1984

47.   Diepstra, G., Gonyea, W., Mitchell, J.H., Distribution of cardiac output during static exercise in the conscious cats, *J. Appl. Physiol.*, 52:642-646, 1982

48.   Arvidsson, S., Falk, A., Haglind, E., Haglund, U., The role of 5-hydroxytryptamine in the feline response to intravenous infusion of live E. coli. *Br. J. Pharmacol.* 79:711-718, 1983

49.   Wicker, P., Tarazi, R.C., Coronary blood flow measurements with left atrial injection of microspheres in conscious rats, *Cardiovasc. Res.*, 16:580-586, 1982

50.   Takahashi, H., Takeda, K., Ashizawa, H., Inoue, A., Yoneda, S., Yoshimura, M, Ijichi, H., Centrally induced cardiovascular and sympathetic responses to hydrocortisone in rats, *Am. J. Physiol.*, 245:H1013-H1018, 1993

51.   Lappe, R.W., Brody, M.J., Mechanisms of the central pressor action of angiotensin II in conscious rats, *Am. J. Physiol.*, 246 (1 Pt 2):R56-R62, 1984

52.   Zicha, J., Karen, P., Krpata, V., Dlouha, H., Krecek, J., Hemodynamics of conscious Brattleboro rats, *Ann. NY Acad. Sci.*, 394-413, 1982

53.   Bealer, S.L., Hemodynamic mechanisms in CNS-induced natriuresis in the conscious rat, *Am. J. Physiol.*, 244:F376-F382, 1983

54.   Feuerstein, G., Zerbe, R.L., Faden, A.I., Central cardiovascular effects of vasotocin, oxytocin and vasopressin in conscious rats, *J. Pharmacol. Exp. Ther.*, 228:348-353, 1984

55.   Ishii, M., Goto, A., Kimura, K., Hirata, Y., Yamakado, M., Takeda, T., Murao, S., Effects of chronic administration of captopril on blood pressure and the renin-angiotensin-aldosterone system in normotensive rats, *Jpn. Heart J.*, 24:623-631, 1983

56.   Flaim, S.F., Zelis, R., Effects of diltiazem on total cardiac output distribution in conscious rats, *J. Pharmacol. Exp. Ther.*, 222:359-366, 1982

57.   Flaim, S.F., Annibali, J.A., Newman, E.D., Zelis, R., Effects of diltiazem on the cardiocirculatory response to exercise in conscious rat, *J. Pharmacol. Exp. Ther.*, 223:624-630, 1982

58.   Malik, A.B., Kaplan, J.E., Saba, T.M., Reference sample method of cardiac output and regional blood flow determinations in the rat, *J. Appl. Physiol.*, 40:472-475, 1976

59.   Van Boom, M.P., Saxena, P.R., Tissue blood flow changes induced by propranolol infusion in conscious normotensive and renal hypertensive rabbits, *Arch. Int. Pharmacodyn. Ther.*, 264:96-109, 1983

60.   Undesser, K.P., Lynn, M.P., Bishop, V.S., Rapid resetting of aortic nerves in conscious rabbits, *Am. J. Physiol.*, 246:H302-H305, 1984

61.   Banks, R.A., Beilin, L.J., Duration of action of meclofenamate on haemodynamics in conscious rabbits, *Clin. Exp. Pharmacol. Physiol.*, 9:621-629, 1982

62.   Banks, R.A., Beilin, L.J., Soltys, J., Dose-dependent effects of meclofenamate on peripheral vasculature on peripheral vasculature of conscious rabbits, *Clin. Sci.*, 64:471-474, 1983

63.   Blombery, P.A., Korner, P.I., Role of aortic and carotid sinus baroreceptors on Valsalva-like vasoconstrictor and heart rate reflexes in the conscious rabbit, *J. Auton. Nerv. Syst.*, 5:303-315, 1982

64. Blake, D.W., Blombery, P.A., Korner, P.I., Effect of ketamine, althesin, and thiopentone on the Valsalva-constrictor and heart rate reflexes of the rabbit, *J. Auton. Nerv. Syst.*, 5:291-301, 1982

65. John, E., McDevitt, M., Cassady, G., Cardiac output and organ blood flow in young rabbits during intermittent positive-pressure ventilation, *Biol. Neonate*, 44:58-64, 1983

66. Dhasmana, K.M., Prakash, O., Saxena, P.R., Effects of fentanyl, and the antagonism by naloxone, on regional blood flow and biochemical variables in conscious rabbits, *Arch. Int. Pharmacodyn. Ther.*, 260:115-129, 1982

67. Archie, J.P., Fixler, D.E., Ullyot, D.J., Buckberg, G.D., Hoffman, J.I.E., Regional myocardial blood flow in lambs with concentric right ventricular hypertrophy, *Circ. Res.*, 34:143-154, 1974

68. Kubo, K., Kobayashi, T., Yoshimura, K., Fukushima, M., Handa, K., Kusama, S., Sakai, A., Ueda, G., Hemodynamic responses to prostacyclin (PGI$_2$) in the conscious sheep, *Jpn. Circ. J.*, 46:1292-1304, 1982

69. Breuhaus, B.A., Chimoskey, J.E., PGE$_2$ does not act at carotid sinus to raise arterial pressure in conscious sheep, *Am. J. Physiol.*, 245:H1007-H1012, 1983

70. Button, C., Mulders, M.S., Responses of unanaesthetized and pentobarbitone-anaesthetized sheep to a lethal does of succinyldicholine, *J. S. Afr. Vet. Assoc.*, 54:63-64, 1983

71. Kotelko, D.M., Schnider, S.M., Dailey, P.A., Brizgys, R.V., Levinson, G., Shapiro, W.A., Koike, M., Rosen, M.A., Bupivacaine-induced cardiac arrhythmias in sheep, *Anesthes.*, 60:10-18, 1984

72. Nesarajah, M.S., Matalon, S., Krasney, J.A., Farhi, L.E., Cardiac output and regional oxygen transport in the acutely hypoxic conscious sheep, *Respir. Physiol.*, 53:161-172, 1983

73. Matalon, S., Nesarajah, M.S., Farhi, L.E., Pulmonary and circulatory changes in conscious sheep exposed to 100% O$_2$ and 1 ATA, *J. Appl. Physiol.*, 53:110-116, 1982

74. Newman, J.H., Loyd, J.E., English, D.K., Ogletree, M.L., Fulkerson, W.J., Brigham, K.L., Effects of 100% oxygen on lung vascular function in awake sheep, *J. Appl. Physiol.*, 54:1379-1386, 1983

75. Matalon, S., Nesarajah, M.S., Krasney, J.A., Farhi, L.E., Effects of acute hypercapnia on the central and peripheral circulation of conscious sheep., *J. Appl. Physiol.*, 54:803-808, 1983

76. Gross, D.R., Dodd, K.T., Williams, J.D., Adams, H.R., Adverse cardiovascular effects of oxytetracycline preparations and vehicles in intact, awake calves, *Am. J. Vet. Res.*, 42:1371-1377, 1981

77. Gross, D.R., Kitzman, J.V., Adams, H.R., Cardiovascular effects of intravenous administration of propylene glycol and of oxytetracycline in propylene glycol in calves, *Am. J. Vet. Res.*, 40:783-791, 1979

78. Manohar, M., Thurmon, J.C., Tranquilli, W.J., Devous, M.D., Theodorakis, M.C., Shawley, R.V., Feller, D.L., Benson, J.G., Regional myocardial blood flow and coronary vascular reserve in unanesthetized young calves with severe concentric right ventricular hypertrophy, *Circ. Res.*, 48:785-796, 1981

79. Manohar, M., Thurmon, J.C., Devous, M.D., Tranquilli, W.J., Shawley, R.V., Benson, G.J., Regional coronary blood flow and coronary vascular reserve in unanesthetized calves at rest and during pharmacologic stress, *J. Surg. Res.*, 30:96-109, 1981

80. Manohar, M., Parks, C.M., Busch, M.A., Tranquilli, W.J., Bisgard, G.E., McPherron, T.A., Theodorakis, M.C., Regional myocardial blood flow and coronary vascular reserve in unanesthetized young calves exposed to a simulated altitude of 3500 m for 8-10 weeks, *Circ. Res.*, 50:714-726, 1982

81. Guth, B.D., White, F.C., Gallagher, K.P., Bloor, C.M., Decreased systolic wall thickening in myocardium adjacent to ischemic zones in conscious swine during brief coronary artery occlusion, *Am. Heart J.*, 107:458-464, 1984

82. Tranquilli, W.J., Parks, C.M., Thurmon, J.C., Benson, G.J., Koritz, G.D., Manohar, M., Theodorakis, M.C., Organ blood flow and distribution of cardiac output in nonanesthetized swine, *Am. J. Vet. Res.*, 43:895-897, 1982

83. Manohar, M., Bisgard, G.E., Bullard, V., Rankin, J.H.G., Blood flow in the hypertrophied right ventricular myocardium of unanesthetized ponies, *Am. J. Physiol.*, 240:H881-H888, 1981

84. Button, C., Gross, D.R., Johnston, J.T., Yahatan, G.J., Digoxin pharmacokinetics, bioavailability, efficacy and dosage regimens in the horse, *Am. J. Vet. Res.*, 41:1388-1395, 1980

85. Busija, D., Orr, J.A., Rankin, J.H.G., Liang, H.K., Wagerle, L.C., Cerebral blood flow during normocapnic hyperoxia in the unanesthetized pony, *J. Appl. Physiol.*, 48:10-15, 1980

86. Amory, D.W., Steffenson, M.C., Forsyth, R.P., Systemic and regional blood flow changes during halothane anesthesia in the rhesus monkey, *Anesth.*, 35:81-89, 1971

87.   Byrd, L.D., Gonzalez, F.A., Time-course effects of adrenergic and cholinergic antagonists on systemic arterial blood pressure, heart rate and temperature in conscious squirrel monkeys, *J. Med. Primatol.* 10:81-92, 1981

88.   Reutlinger, R.A., Karl, A.A., Vinal, S.I., Nieser, M.J., Effects of ketamine HCl-xylazine HCl combination on cardiovascular and pulmonary values of the rhesus macaque (Macaca mulatta), *Am. J. Vet. Res.*, 41:1453-1457, 1980

89.   Cornish, K.G., Gilmore, J.P., Increased left atrial pressure does not alter renal function in the conscious primate, *Am. J. Physiol.*, 243:R119-R124, 1982

90.   Peterson, T.V., Felts, F.T., Chase, N.L., Intravascular receptors and renal responses of monkey to volume expansion, *Am. J. Physiol.*, 244:H55-H59, 1983

91.   Peterson, T.V., Jones, C.E., Renal responses of the cardiac-denervated nonhuman primate to blood volume expansion, *Circ. Res.*, 53:24-32, 1983

92.   Drazen, J.M., Herd, J.A., Cardiac output at rest in the squirrel monkey, role of β-adrenergic activity, *Am. J. Physiol.*, 222:988-993, 1972

93.   Lavallee, M., Vatner, S.F., Regional myocardial blood flow and necrosis in primates following coronary occlusion, *Am. J. Physiol.*, 246:H635-H639, 1984

94.   Hayashi, S., Nehls, D.G., Kleck, C.F., Vielma, J., DeGirolami, U., Crowell, R.M., Beneficial effects of induced hypertension on experimental stroke in awake monkeys, *J. Neurosurg.*, 60:151-153, 1984

95.   Shelub, I., van Grondelle, A., McCullough, R., Hofmeister, S., Reeves, J.T., A model of embolic chronic pulmonary hypertension in the dog, *J. Appl. Physiol.*, 56:810-815, 1984

96.   Crozatier, B., Caillet, D., Bical, O., Left ventricular adaptation to sustained pressure overload in the conscious dog, *Circ. Res.*, 54:21-29, 1984

97.   Su-Fan, Q., Brun, J.M., Kaye, M.P., Bove, A.A., A new technique for producing aortic stenosis in animals, *Am. J. Physiol.*, 246:H296-H301, 1984

98.   Pagel, P.S., Kampine, J.P., Schmeling, W.T., Warltier, D.C., Effects of nitrous oxide on myocardial contractility as evaluated by the preload recruitable stroke work relationship in chronically instrumented dogs, *Anesthes.*, 73:1148-1157, 1990

99.   Pagel, P.S., Kampine, J.P., Schmeling, W.T., Warltier, D.C., Comparison of end-systolic pressure-length relations and preload recruitable stroke work as indices of myocardial contractility in the conscious and anesthetized, chronically instrumented dog, *Anesthes.*, 73:278-290, 1990

100.   Haskins, S.C., Farver, T.B., Patz, J.D., Cardiovascular changes in dogs given diazepam and diazepam-ketamine, *Am. J. Vet. Res.*, 47:795-798, 1986

101.   Hill, D.C., Chelly, J.E., Dlewati, A., Abernethy, D.R., Doursout, M.F., Merin, R.G., Cardiovascular effects of and interaction between calcium blocking drugs and anesthetics in chronically instrumented dogs, VI. Verapamil and fentanyl-pancuronium, *Anesthes.*, 68:874-879, 1988

102.   Schmeling, W.T., Kampine, J.P., Warltier, D.C., Negative chronotropic actions of sufentanil and vecuronium in chronically instrumented dogs pretreated with propranolol and/or diltiazem, *Anesth. Analg.*, 69:4-14, 1989

103.   Farver, T.B., Haskins, S.C., Patz, J.D., Cardiopulmonary effects of acepromzaine and of the subsequent administration of ketamine in the dog, *Am. J. Vet. Res.*, 47:631-635, 1986

104.   Cheng, C.P., Igarashi, Y., Little, W.C., Mechanisms of augmented rate of left ventricular filling during exercise, *Circ. Res.*, 70:9-19, 1992

105.   Pagel, P.S., Kampine, J.P., Schmeling, W.T., Warltier, D.C., Evaluation of myocardial contractility in the chronically instrumented dog with intact autonomic nervous system function: effects of desflurane and isoflurane, *Acta Anaesthesiol. Scand.*, 37:203-210, 1993

106.   Haidet, G.C., Parsons, D., Reduced exercise capacity in senescent beagles: an evaluation of the periphery, *Am. J. Physiol.*, 260:H173-H182, 1991

107.   Reimer, K.A., Jennings, R.B., Cobb, F.R., Murdock, R.H., Greenfield, J.C.Jr., Becker, L.C., Bulkeley, B.H., Hutchins, G.M., Schwartz, R.P., Bailey, K.R., Passamani, E.R., Animal models for protecting ischemic myocardium: Results of the NHLBI cooperative study, comparison of unconscious and conscious dog models, *Circ. Res.*, 56:651-665, 1985

108.   Bassenge, E., Mulsch, A., Anti-ischemic actions of molsidomine by venous and large coronary dilatation in combination with antiplatelet effects, *J. Cardiovasc. Pharmacol.*, 14(Suppl. 11):523-528, 1989

109.   Kremser, P.C., Gewertz, B.L., Effect of pentobarbital and hemorrhage on renal autoregulation, *Am. J. Physiol.*, 249:F356-F360, 1985

110. Benson, G.J., Thurmon, J.C., Tranquilli, W.J., Smith, C.W., Cardiopulmonary effects of an intravenous infusion of guaifenesin, ketamine and xylazine in dogs, *Am. J. Vet. Res.*, 46:1896-1898, 1985

111. Ilkiw, J.E., Pascoe, P.J., Haskins, S.C., Patz, J.D., Cardiovascular and respiratory effects of propofol administration in hypovolemic dogs, *Am. J. Vet. Res.*, 53:2323-2327, 1992

112. Pagel, P.S., Kampine, J.P., Schmeling, W.T., Warltier, D.C., Alteration of left ventricular diastolic function by desflurane, isoflurane, and halothane in the chronically instrumented dog with autonomic nervous system blockade, *Anesthes.*, 74:1103-1114, 1991

113. Kenny D., Proctor, L.T., Schmeling, W.T., Kampine, J.P., Warltier, D.C., Isoflurane causes only minimal increases in coronary blood flow independent of oxygen demand, *Anesthes.*, 75:640-649, 1991

114. Chen, B.B., Nyhan, D.P., Fehr, D.M., Goll, H.M., Murray, P.A., Halothane anesthesia causes active flow-independent pulmonary vasoconstriction, *Am. J. Physiol.*, 259:H74-H83, 1990

115. Merin, R.G., Bernard, J.-M., Doursout, M.-F., Cohen, M., Chelly, J.E., Comparison of the effects of isoflurane and desflurane on cardiovascular dynamics and regional blood flow in the chronically instrumented dog, *Anesthes.*, 74:568-574, 1991

116. Pagel, P.S., Kampine, J.P., Schmeling, W.T., Warltier, D.C., Influence of volatile anesthetic on myocardial contractility *in vivo*: desflurane versus isoflurane, *Anesthes.*, 74:900-907, 1991

117. Pagel, P.S., Kampine, J.P., Schmeling, W.T., Warltier, D.C., Comparison of the systemic and coronary hemodynamic actions of desflurane, isoflurane, halothane and enflurane in the chronically instrumented dog, *Anesthes.*, 74:539-551, 1991

118. Hartman, J.C., Kampine, J.P., Schmeling, W.T., Warltier, D.C., Alterations in collateral blood flow produced by isoflurane in a chronically instrumented canine model of multivessel coronary artery disease, *Anesthes.*, 74:120-133, 1991

119. Ilkiw, J.E., Pascoe, P.J., Haskins, S.C., Patz, J.D., Cardiovascular and respiratory effects of propofol administration in hypovolemic dogs, *Am. J. Vet. Res.*, 53:2323-2327, 1992

120. Benson, G.J., Thurmon, J.C., Tranquilli, W.J., Smith, C.W., Cardiopulmonary effects of an intravenous infusion of guaifenesin, ketamine, and xylazine in dogs, *Am. J. Vet. Res.*, 46:1896-1898, 1985

121. Pagel, P.S., Kampine, J.P., Schmeling, W.T., Warltier, D.C., Ketamine depresses myocardial contractility as evaluated by the preload recruitable stroke work relationship in chronically instrumented dogs with autonomic nervous system blockade, *Anesthes.*, 76:564-572, 1992

122. Haskins, S.C., Patz, J.D., Farver, T.B., Xylazine and xylazine-ketamine in dogs, *Am. J. Vet. Res.*, 47:636-641, 1986

123. Kolata, R.J., Rawlings, C.A., Cardiopulmonary effects of intravenous xylazine, ketamine and atropine in the dog, *Am. J. Vet. Res.*, 43:2196-2198, 1982

124. Poterack, K.A., Kampine, J.P., Schmeling, W.T., Effects of isoflurane, midazolam, and etomidate on cardiovascular responses to stimulation of central nervous system pressor sites in chronically instrumented cats, *Anesth. Analg.*, 73:64-75, 1991

125. Wang, Y.X., Zhou, T., Chua, T.C., Pang, C.C., Effects of inhalation and intravenous anesthetic agents on pressor response to NG-nitro-L-arginine, *Eur. J. Pharmacol.*, 198:183-188, 1991

126. Kuwahina, I., Gonzalez, N.C., Heisler, N., Piiper, J., Regional blood flow in conscious resting rats determined by microsphere distribution, *J. Appl. Physiol.*, 74:203-210, 1993

127. Malik, A.B., Kaplan, J.E., Saba, T.M., Reference sample method for cardiac output and regional blood flow determinations in the rat, *J. Appl. Physiol.*, 40:472-475, 1976

128. Armstrong, R.B., Laughlin, M.H., Exercise blood flow patterns within and among rat muscles after training, *Am. J. Physiol.*, 246:H59-H68, 1984

129. Ishise, S., Pegram, B.L., Yamamoto, J., Kitamura, Y., Frohlich, E.D., Reference sample microsphere method: cardiac output and blood flows in conscious rat, *Am. J. Physiol.*, 239:H443-H449, 1980

130. Laughlin, M.H., Armstrong, R.B., Muscular blood flow distribution patterns as a function of running speed in rats, *Am. J. Physiol.*, 243:H296-H306, 1982

131. Laughlin, M.H., Armstrong, R.B., Rat muscle blood flows as a function of time during prolonged slow treadmill exercise, *Am. J. Physiol.*, 244:H814-H824, 1983

132. Seyde, W.C., McGowan, L., Lund, N., Duling, B., Longnecker, D.E., Effects of anesthetics on regional hemodynamics in normovolemic and hemorrhaged rats, *Am. J. Physiol.*, 249:H164-H173, 1985

133. Flaim, S.F., Minteer, W.J., Clark, D.P., Zelis, R., Cardiovascular response to acute aquatic and treadmill exercise in the untrained rat, *J. Appl. Physiol.*, 46:302-308, 1979

134. Tsuchiya, M., Ferrone, R.A., Walsh, G.M., Frohlich, E.D., Regional blood flows measured in conscious rats by combined Fick and microsphere methods, *Am. J. Physiol.*, 235:H357-H360, 1978

135. Nishiyama, K., Nishiyama, A., Frolich, E.D., Regional blood flows in normotensive and spontaneously hypertensive rats, *Am. J. Physiol.*, 230:691-698, 1976

136. Ohsumi, H., Sakamoto, M., Yamazaki, T., Okumura, F., Effects of fentanyl on carotid sinus baroreflex control of circulation in rabbits, *Am. J. Physiol.*, 256:R625-R631, 1989

137. Lagutchik, M.S., Januszkiewicz, A.J., Dodd, K.T., Martin, D.G., Cardiopulmonary effects of a tiletamine-zolazepam combination in sheep, *Am. J. Vet. Res.*, 52:1441-1447, 1991

138. Iwamoto, J., Yang, S.-P., Yoshinaga, M., Krasney, E., Drasney, J., N^3-nitro-L-arginine influences cerebral metabolism in awake sheep, *J. Appl. Physiol.*, 73:2233-2240, 1992

139. Aoyagi, T., Mirsky, I., Flanagan, M.F., Currier, J.J., Colan, S.D., Fujii, A.M., Myocardial function in immature and mature sheep with pressure-overload hypertrophy, *Am. J. Physiol.*, 262:H1036-H1048, 1992

140. Fahey, J.T., Lister, G., A simple method for reducing cardiac output in the conscious lamb, *Am. J. Physiol.* 249:H188-H192, 1985

141. Woods, J.R.Jr., Nuwayhid, D.B., Brinkman, C.R. III, Assali, N.S., Cardiovascular reactivity of neonatal and adult sheep to autonomic stimuli during adrenergic depletion, *Biol. Neonate.*, 34:112-120, 1978

142. Gratama, J.W.C., Meuzelaar, J.J., Dalinghaus, M., Koers, J.H., Werre, A.J., Zijlstra, W.G., Kuipers, J.R.G., Maximal exercise capacity and oxygen consumption of lambs with an aortopulmonary left-to-right shunt, *J. Appl. Physiol.*, 69:1479-1485, 1990

143. Lin, H.C., Thurmon, J.C., Tranquilli, W.J., Benson, G.J., Olson, W.A., Hemodynamic response of calves to tiletamine-zolazepam-xylazine anesthesia, *Am. J. Vet. Res.*, 52:1606-1610, 1991

144. McKirnan, M.D., Gray, C.G., White, F.C., Effects of feeding on muscle blood flow during prolonged exercise in miniature swine, *J. Appl. Physiol.*, 70:1097-1104, 1991

145. Manohar, M., Right heart pressures and blood-gas tensions in ponies during exercise and laryngeal hemiplegia, *Am. J. Physiol.*, 251:H121-H126, 1986

146. Williams, D.O., Boatwright, R.B., Rugh, K.S., Garner, H.E., Griggs, D.M.Jr., Myocardial blood flow, metabolism, and function with repeated brief coronary occlusions in conscious ponies, *Am. J. Physiol.*, 260:H100-H109, 1991

147. Manohar, M., Vasodilator reserve in respiratory muscles during maximal exertion in ponies, *J. Appl. Physiol.*, 60:1571-1577, 1986

148. Rutkowski, J.A., Eades, S.C., Moore, J.N., Effects of xylazine-butorphanol on cecal arterial blood flow, cecal mechanical activity, and systemic hemodynamics in horses, *Am. J. Vet. Res.*, 52:1153-1158, 1991

149. Olson, N.C., Meyer, R.E., Anderson, D.L., Effects of flunixin meglumine on cardiopulmonary responses to endotoxin in ponies, *J. Appl. Physiol.*, 59:1464-1471, 1985

150. Hubbell, J.A.E., Bednarski, R.M., Muir, W.W., Xylazine and tiletamine-zolazepam anesthesia in horses, *Am. J. Vet. Res.*, 50:737-742, 1989

10. Naturally occurring models of cardiovascular disease

Although most naturally occurring cardiovascular diseases of man have been identified in one or more species of animals as well, the utility of all of these animals as research models is not well established. Many of the so-called congenital defects are also associated with non-cardiovascular defects. These may result in infertility, impotence and other problems which preclude, in any practical sense, the breeding of these animals to obtain adequate numbers for research purposes. Some of the defects may, in fact, be a result of teratogenic insult rather than a true genetic defect. The possibility of identifying specific genes responsible for specific defects exists, along with the possibility of creating specific transgenic animal models of these defects, but no reports of the successful accomplishment of this have been found.

Congenital heart defects have been documented in most domestic species. The most practical species for a breeding colony of congenital defects is probably dogs. They are still the most commonly used animal model for cardiovascular studies and, as documented in this text, we have the most information accumulated about them. Dog breeding is well understood, facilities are more easily acquired and the opportunity to find suitable animals for breeders is greater.

A review of the records from the Veterinary Teaching Hospital at Texas A & M University, conducted in 1983, revealed the following most commonly encountered cardiac defects in dogs, in their order of incidence: Patent ductus arteriosus (PDA), pulmonic stenosis (PS), ventricular septal defects (VSD), atrial septal defects (ASD), Tetralogy of Fallot and a range of other combined defects. In their 1965 survey, Detweiler and Patterson reported on 27 congenital defects out of 4,831 dogs examined ($\approx$0.5% incidence). They found 6 PS, 5 PDA, 3 aortic stenosis (AS) (subvalvular), 3 Tetralogy of Fallot, 2 persistent right aortic arch, combined PS and PDA, 1 VSD, and 6 with incomplete diagnosis.[1] Patterson reported 238 cardiovascular anomalies in 212 dogs; 61 PDA, 47 PS, 32 AS, 18 persistent right aortic arch, 13 VSD, 9 Tetralogy of Fallot, 9 ASD, 10 venous anomalies, 4 pericardial anomalies, 3 arterial anomalies (excluding those with persistent right aortic arch), 1 mitral insufficiency, 1 Ebstein's anomaly of the tricuspid valves, 1 origin of both great vessels from the right ventricle, 1 partial anomalous pulmonary venous drainage into the right atrium, 2 conduction disturbances without gross malformation and 26 incompletely diagnosed anomalies.[2]

The range of combined defects seen in Patterson's 10 year study were also similar to those seen in humans. He found 1 case of PDA with a patent foramen ovale, 2 PDA's with PS, 3 PS with ASD, 1 PS, ASD and pericardial diaphragmatic hernia, 3 PS and AS, 1 VSD, persistent left cephalic vena cava and anomalous right subclavian artery, 1 VSD and persistent left cephalic vena cava, 7 persistent right aortic arch with persistent left cephalic vena cava, 2 persistent right aortic arch with PDA, 1 origin of both great vessels from the right ventricle with VSD and ASD, 1 Tetralogy of Fallot with PDA and 1 Tetralogy of Fallot with persistent left cephalic vena cava.

Gopal *et al.* have reported a 14 year study of congenital cardiac defects in calves. They found 78 defects in 36 calves; interventricular septal defect (11), ectopia cordia cervicalis (10), left ventricular hypoplasia (10), right ventricular hypoplasia (10), dextraposed aorta (8), valvular hematomas (7), patent ductus arteriosus (5), patent foramen ovale (5), common aortic trunk (3), endocardial fibroelastosis with calcification (3), hypoplastic aorta (2), interatrial septal defect (2), duplicated major trunks (1), and cor triloculare biatriatum (1).[19]

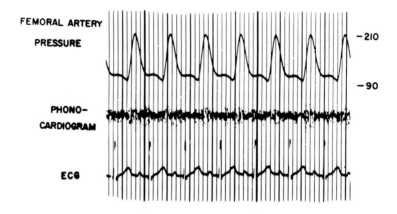

Figure 1: Recording of pressure, phonocardiogram and ECG from a dog with PDA.

The apparent predisposition of certain breeds to specific malformations suggests a genetic linkage, and chromosomal abnormalities have been reported in 2 of 15 dogs with cardiovascular malformations.[3] The existence of chromosomal abnormalities, however, does not guarantee that the specific cardiovascular defect will be genetically transmitted. Aortic stenosis seems to be most frequently reported in German Shepherds and Boxers. Poodles seem to be the breed most predisposed to PDA and German Shepherds to persistent right aortic arch. Pulmonic stenosis has been observed most frequently in English Bulldogs and Chihuahuas.[2]

Seventy-eight members of a family of Keeshonden dogs have been studied extensively. Thirteen of these dogs had a variety of congenital cardiovascular defects. Two clinically normal sisters bred to the same apparently normal male produced affected pups. A sister littermate bred to the same male had 2 affected puppies of 7 in one litter and 3 of 8 in another. A puppy with PS from one of the latter litters was bred back to her sire and produced 1 of 3 pups with a defect. A brother-sister mating from the same family of dogs produced 2 of 9 pups with congenital defects.[2]

Five poodle puppies from apparently normal parents were affected with VSD and 3 Siberian Husky puppies from clinically normal parents all had both great vessels originating from the right ventricle and a VSD. Three female pups with subvalvular AS were found in a family of Newfoundland dogs.[2] These incidents might easily be ascribed to a teratogenic agent, if complete histories during gestation were available.

Coarctation of the aorta, a relatively common malformation in humans, has apparently not been observed in dogs, whereas AS is fairly common in dogs but rare in humans. When AS does occur in humans, it is usually of the valvular type, whereas in dogs it is most commonly a subvalvular fibrous ring.[4]

Perhaps with most convincing evidence of a genetic link is provided by Patterson, Haskins and Jerzyk. Planned breedings were conducted in Poodles with PDA. Ten matings resulted in 35 offspring with an 82.9% incidence of PDA. Beagles with PS were mated 10 times, producing 35 offspring with a 25.7% incidence of the lesion. Five matings in Newfoundlands with AS produced 26 offspring with a 38.5% incidence. A 10% incidence of persistent right aortic arch resulted from 3 breedings and 30 puppies from German Shepherds with that lesion. Four matings in Keeshonden produced 11 offspring and a 90% incidence of Tetralogy of Fallot.[5]

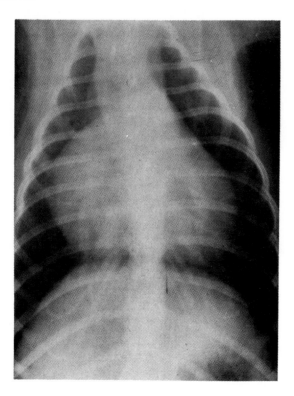

Figure 2: Dorso-ventral radiograph of a dog with PDA, note the biventricular enlargement.

Documentation of congenital cardiovascular defects is easily accomplished in dogs. Clinical catheterizations are easily performed in dogs using Innovar [fentanyl (0.04 mg/kg), droperidol (2.2 mg/kg)], intravenously, followed immediately by pentobarbital sodium (15 mg/kg), iv. An endotracheal tube is placed and the dogs are allowed to spontaneously ventilate room air. Additional pentobarbital is given, as needed, to effect during the procedure. This regimen provides normal sinus arrhythmia with normal heart rates, good baroreceptor responsiveness, normal blood gas levels (since the dogs are breathing room air), a short duration of anesthesia (20-30 min.), and relatively smooth recovery providing the dogs are kept in a dark quiet place during the recovery period.

Examples of documentation of PDA are given as Figures 1-4. Figure 1 is a recording of the lead II ECG, a phonocardiogram and femoral arterial pressure. Figures 2 and 3 are radiographs showing biventricular enlargement and Figure 4 is a contrast medium injection which demonstrates simultaneous filling of the aortic root and the pulmonary artery.

Pulmonic stenosis is frequently encountered and easily documented. Figures 5-9 demonstrate this lesion. Figure 5 shows ECG's and phono, Figure 6 is a right side contrast injection in a normal dog while Figure 7 shows a case of pulmonic

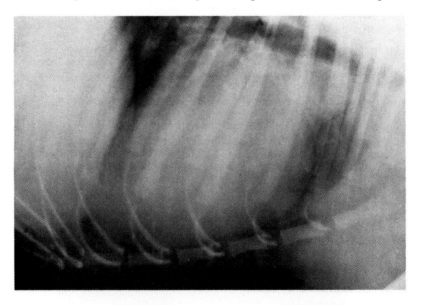

Figure 3: Lateral view radiograph of the same dog as in Figure 2, showing biventricular enlargement.

stenosis. Note the stricture at the valve and the large post-stenotic dilatation. Figure 8 is a dorso-ventral radiograph which shows the right side enlargement and the post-stenotic dilatation. Figure 9 shows pressure catheterization data of right side pullback pressures from the pulmonary artery through the right ventricle and into the right atrium along with 3 simultaneously recorded ECG leads.

An atrial septal defect usually results in right ventricular overload. The murmur associated with this lesion is very similar to the pulmonic stenosis murmur, harsh, crescendo-decrescendo. Because of the volume overload a relative pulmonic stenosis results. Figure 10 is a contrast media injection into the right atrium with simultaneous filling of both atria.

Left ventricular lesions are slightly more difficult to demonstrate since the catheter must be passed retrograde through the aortic valve. In dogs, this is easily accomplished via the carotid artery. We normally catheterize through a longitudinal incision in either the right or left jugular vein and right or left common carotid. The hole in the vessel is then repaired with 5 or 6-0 monofilament nylon. It is also feasible to cannulate using percutaneous techniques through the femoral artery and vein in dogs but this requires holding a compression pack over the femoral artery for at least 30 minutes to avoid a massive hematoma. Both techniques can be used to save the vessels for future catheterizations if necessary. Figure 11 is an example of a left ventricular contrast media injection in a normal dog. Figure 12 is a direct left ventricular injection of contrast media into a dog with a VSD. This technique is rarely used on client owned animals. Figure 13 is a dorso-ventral radiograph of a dog with an aortic stenosis. Note the greatly enlarged left ventricle and the post-stenotic dilatation of the aorta. Figure 14 is a lateral view of a dog with aortic stenosis. The stenosis and post-stenotic dilatation are very obvious.

Congenital cardiac abnormalities in dogs are not limited to structural defects. We and others have reported on the probable genetic basis of sinoatrial syncope in Miniature Schnauzer dogs (see Figure 15).[6,7] James has reported on the incidence of Jervelle and Lange-Neilsen syndrome in 9 Dalmatian dogs who were also afflicted with congenital deafness and abnormal pigmentation. This complex is characterized electrocardiographically by prolonged Q-T intervals.[8] We have observed a similar syndrome in a Harlequin Great Dane, also associated with deafness.

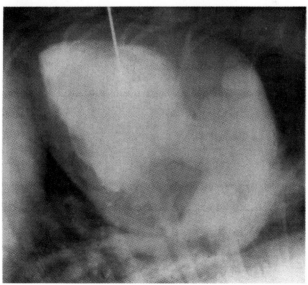

Figure 4: Left ventricular injection of radio-opaque contrast showing simultaneous filling of the aorta and pulmonary arteries, PDA.

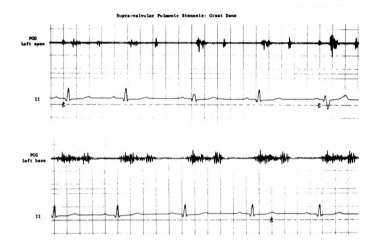

Figure 5: ECG's and phonocardiograms showing the well localized systolic murmurs characteristic of pulmonic stenosis (PS).

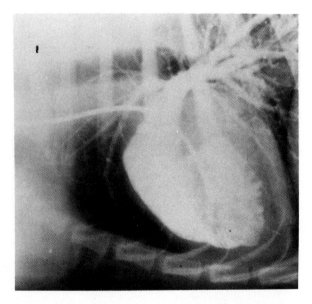

Figure 6: Radio-opaque contrast medium injection into the right ventricle of a normal dog, for reference.

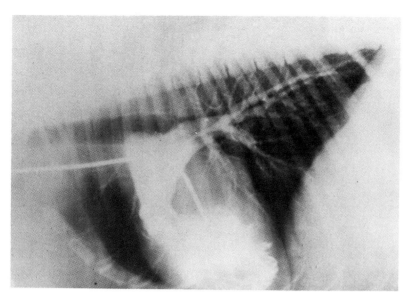

Figure 7: Radio-opaque contrast medium injection into the right ventricle of a dog with pulmonic stenosis. The valvular stricture and large post-stenotic dilatation are very apparent.

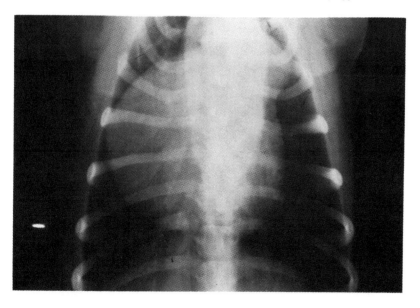

Figure 8: Dorso-ventral radiograph of a dog with PS showing right ventricular enlargement and a post-stenotic dilatation.

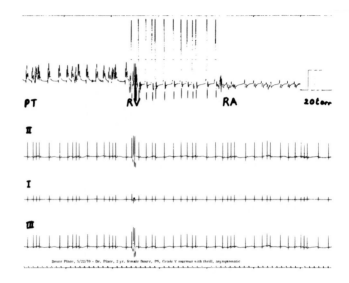

Figure 9: Catheterization pullback recording from the pulmonary trunk (PT) to the right ventricle (RV) to the right atrium (RA), a significant pressure drop across the pulmonary valve.

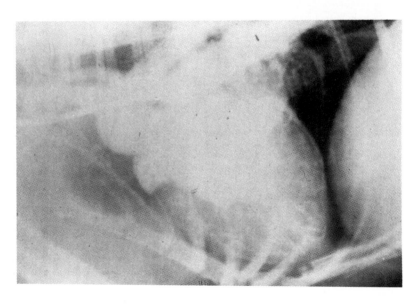

Figure 10: Radio-opaque contrast media injection into the right atrium with simultaneous filling of both atria, an atrial-septal defect.

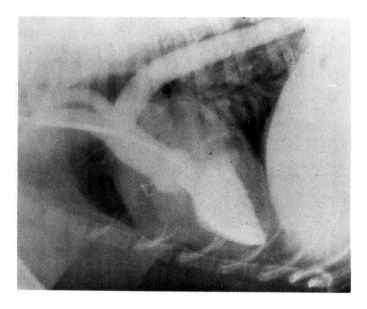

Figure 11: Normal dog, left ventricular injection of contrast media.

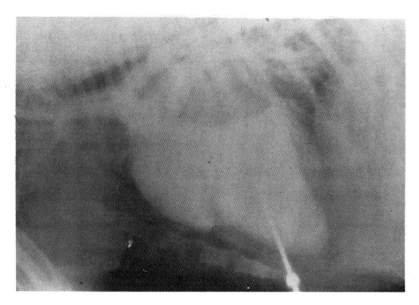

Figure 12: Dorso-ventral view of a dog with aortic stenosis (AS), the left ventricle is greatly enlarged.

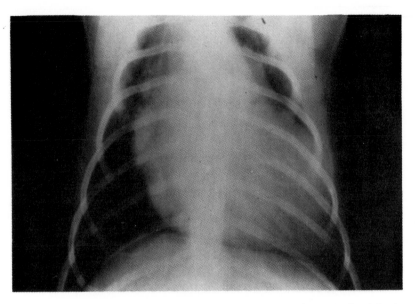

Figure 13: Dog with a ventricular septal defect (VSD), direct left ventricular injection of contrast. Both ventricles fill simultaneously.

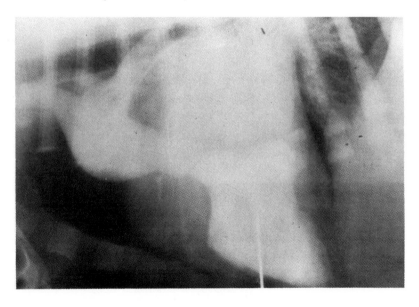

Figure 14: Aortic stenosis, contrast media injection. Compare this to Figure 11. The stenosis and post-stenotic dilatation are clearly visualized, mitral regurgitation.

Kating/6-27-71
9/15/Fs/3

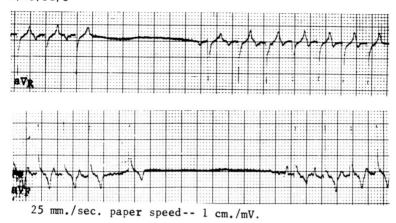

25 mm./sec. paper speed-- 1 cm./mV.

Figure 15: Sinoatrial syncope in a Miniature Schnauzer dog. Note prolonged periods of sinus arrest.

AORTIC INS.

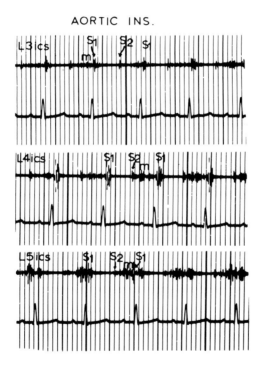

Figure 16: Recordings from a 2 year old Arabian mare with congenital aortic insufficiency, late diastolic murmur.

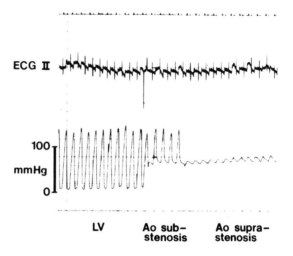

ECG II

100

mmHg

0

LV   Ao sub-   Ao supra-
            stenosis   stenosis

Figure 17: Left ventricular pressure with a pullback into the aorta. Anesthetized foal with a supravalvular aortic stenosis.

Another fairly common heart disease seen in dogs is idiopathic cardiomyopathy, also known as primary myocardial disease or myocardiopathy. Cardiomyopathy is actually a nonspecific term used to describe conditions in which lesions are located in the myocardial tissues as opposed to the other anatomic structures of the heart. It is also reserved for myocardial lesions not secondary to primary cardiac lesions involving other cardiac structures. The term encompasses a broad variety of possible etiologies. There has not been definitive work reported which fully establishes if this syndrome is congenital or acquired in dogs. It is, however, seen almost exclusively in the larger breeds. It has been reported in the following; Boxer, Bouvier des Flanders, Doberman, English Bulldog, German Shepherd, Great Dane, Irish Setter, Irish Wolfhound, Newfoundland and St. Bernard. The condition is characterized by biventricular cardiac dilatation which results in dilation of the atrioventricular valvular annuli. This leads to both mitral and tricuspid incompetence, atrial dilatation and atrial fibrillation.[9] The disease is recognized in domestic cats as well.

A cardiomyopathic strain of Syrian golden hamster has been derived from inbred lines of *Mesocricetus auratus*.[10] The BIO 14.6 strain from the Bio-Research Institute, Boston, MA, has been studied extensively. The cardiac disease develops from a genetic metabolic defect which has been established to be inherited as a recessive autosome. Viral and other infectious agents, along with Vitamin E, potassium and magnesium deficiencies have been ruled out as etiological factors in this model.[11] New strains of these animals are undergoing development and characterization. Studies have shown that, on the basis of ultrastructural analysis, the ventricular myocardium is not developmentally retarded. This seems to argue against a connection between developmental retardation and a predilection for cardiomyopathy.[12] No differences in the kinetics of Ca^{2+} exchange or on the role of Ca^{2+} in the excitation-contraction coupling process were found between normal and myopathic hamster hearts.[13]

Other species have been associated with congenital cardiovascular disease. Persistent left 4th aortic arch and VSD have been reported in chickens.[5] A variety of intracardiac anomalies have been reported in mice.[5] VSD's have been found in rats and vestigial pulmonary artery and retroesophageal right subclavian artery in rabbits.[5] Cats have been shown to have endocardial fibroelastosis and a strain of Miniature pigs has been found with hypoplastic left heart.[5] Ventricular septal defects have been found in cattle.[5] We have reported tricuspid atresia in a foal[14] and congenital aortic valvular insufficiency in a foal (Figure 16).[15] We have also seen many horses with VSD's and one foal with a supravalvular aortic stenosis (Figure 17).

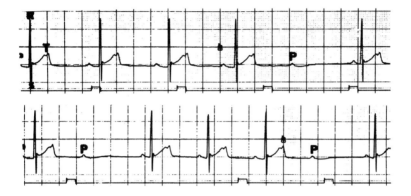

Figure 18: Second degree A-V block from a dog with no other obvious cardiovascular disease.

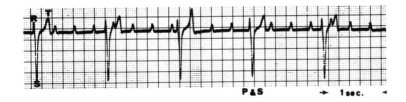

Figure 19: Complete A-V block from a dog with cardiomyopathy.

Separate from the congenital cardiovascular diseases are a host of acquired diseases. These include many responses to infectious agents and other stimuli that can result in valvular endocardiosis and myocarditis. Valvular lesions can also be acquired from tumors and migrating larval forms of parasites, particularly *Strongyle sp.* in horses. The latter is the most common cause of aortic insufficiency which is seen fairly commonly in aged horses. Heart worm disease (*Dirofilaria immitis*) of dogs is characterized by pulmonary hypertension, right ventricular hypertrophy and eventual right heart failure.

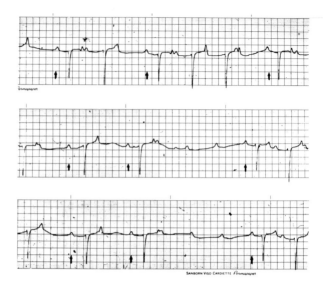

Figure 20: Second degree A-V block in a normal horse. The arrhythmia disappears with exercise and is a normal mechanism for controlling blood pressure in the very fit horse.

A host of acquired arrhythmias can be, and have been, diagnosed in animals, including partial and complete A-V block (Figures 18 and 19). The unwary investigator must take care. Figure 20 is recorded from a 6-year old, Standardbred stallion, who was completely normal. Very fit horses hold their aortic pressures and heart rates down via baroreceptor responses and high parasympathetic tone. The second degree A-V block seen in this recording is normal and, with exercise, it will disappear, but will return when the horse is resting. The correlation between pressure and the second degree block is seen in Figure 21.

Premature ventricular contractions are commonly seen from all species when the ventricular myocardium is excited from any of a host of insults. Figure 22 is from a Great Dane with cardiomyopathy. Figure 23 is from a mixed breed dog with septicemia and myocarditis.

Certain species may show an inheritable predilection to develop specific

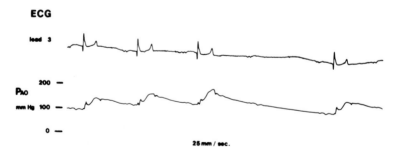

Figure 21: Second degree A-V block in a normal horse. Blockade coincides with the increase in aortic pressure (Pao).

cardiovascular diseases. A prime example of this is the so-called "high altitude" or "brisket" disease of cattle. Increased pulmonary arterial pressures in these animals lead to congestive right heart failure and the marked subcutaneous edema characteristic of the disease (Figure 24).[16,17,18]

Conrad *et al.* have found both clinical and pathological changes suggestive of heart failure in some, but not all, aged spontaneously hypertensive rats they examined. They were able to demonstrate marked left ventricular papillary muscle dysfunction in those rats between 18-24 months of age which had clinical evidence of heart failure. They concluded that impairment of intrinsic myocardial function could precede the development of heart failure.[20]

Recent breakthroughs have made it possible to experimentally target gene expression to specific tissues in both adult and developing mice. The role of extra-renal renin and angiotensin have been the subject of many transgenic experiments which have established some features of the tissue-specific regulation of mouse renin genes. A hypertensive phenotype has been created in mice by the introduction of the rat angiotensinogen gene. The transgene which expressed at a

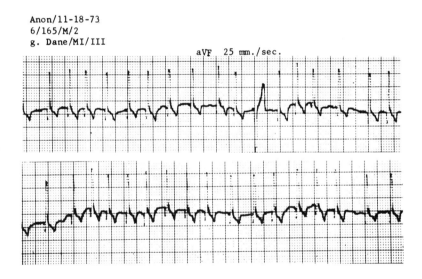

Anon/11-18-73
6/165/M/2
g. Dane/MI/III

aVF   25 mm./sec.

Figure 22: Premature ventricular contraction in a dog with idiopathic cardiomyopathy.

high level in the liver and brain and at lower levels in the heart, kidneys and testis developed mild hypertension.[21] It is not yet clear if there is a specific model available to study the importance of endothelium-derived angiotensin in hypertension and heart failure.

Considerable effort has been made to map the signalling pathways that co-ordinate the responses leading to inappropriate cardiac hypertrophy. Various stimuli capable of inducing hypertrophy have been shown to induce a transient expression of *c-myc* before the development of hypertrophy. This type of response, however, appears to be very general and is present in many physiological systems.[21]

Rubin *et al.* have constructed a transgenic mouse model that over-expresses human apo A-1 and this seems to be protective against formation of fatty lesions in the aortas of these animals despite higher total cholesterol levels (attributed to higher HDL levels) and triglyceride levels the same as in control animals fed a high fat diet.[22]   Others have introduced human apo A-1 genes into mice as well as human cholesterol ester transfer protein, apo E and apo B-100.[21]   The role of plasminogen activator inhibitors on *in vivo* thrombosis has also been studied using transgenic models.

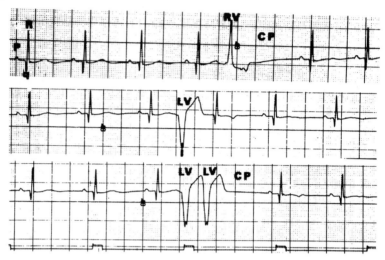

Figure 23: Multifocal premature ventricular contractions from a dog with myocarditis.

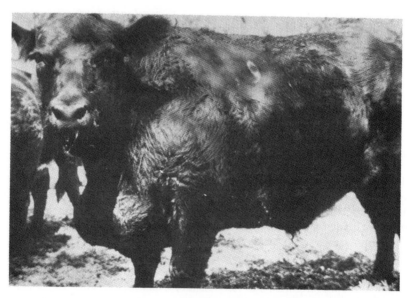

Figure 24: Marked subcutaneous ventral edema typical of "Brisket Disease" in a steer with classical signs of right heart failure.

Acknowledgements

Many of the figures presented in this chapter are courtesy of my Mentor, Professor R.L. Hamlin of The Ohio State University. He graciously allowed me to make copies from his extensive files.

References

1.   Detweiler, D.K., Patterson, D.F., The prevalence and types of cardiovascular disease in dogs, *Annals New York Academy of Sciences*, Vol. 127:481-516, 1965

2.   Patterson, D.F., Congenital heart disease in the dog, *Annals New York Academy of Sciences*, Vol.127:541-569, 1956

3.   Patterson, D.F., Hare, W.C., Shive, R.J., Luginbuhl, H.R., Congenital malformations of the cardiovascular system associated with chromosomal abnormalities. A report of the clinical, pathologic and cytogenetic findings in 2 dogs, *Zentralbl-Veterinarermed* (A), 13:669-686, 1966

4.   Fontana, R.S., Edwards, J.E., Congenital cardiac disease: A review of 357 cases studied pathologically, Saunders, Philadelphia, 1962

5.   Patterson, D.F., Haskins, M.E., Jezyk, P.F., Models of human genetic disease in domestic animals, *Adv Hum Genet*, 12:263-339, 1982

6.   Clark, D.R., Knauer, K.W., Hobson, H.P., Gross, D.R., Humphries, J., Artificial pacemaker implantation for control of sinoatrial syncope in a Miniature Schnauzer, *Southwestern Vet*, 28:101-107, 1975

7.   Hamlin, R.L., Smetzer, D.L., Breznock, E.M., Sino-atrial syncope in Miniature Schnauzers, *J AVMA*, 161:1022-1028, 1972

8.   James, T.N., Congenital deafness and cardiac arrhythmias, *Am J Cardiol*, 19:627-643, 1967

9.   Ettinger, S.J., Suter, P.F., Canine Cardiology, W.B. Saunders Co, Philadelphia, 1970

10.   Homburger, F., Baker, J.R., Nixon, C.W., Whitney, R., Primary generalized polymyopathy and cardiac necrosis in an inbred line of Syrian hamsters, *Med Exp*, 6:339, 1962

11.   Gertz, E.W., Cardiomyopathic Syrian hamster: A possible model of human disease, *Progr Exp Tumor Res*, 16:242-260, 1972

12.   Kidd, P.M., Jones, A.L., Lemanski, L.F., Rudolph, A., Allen, L., Histological and electron microscopic stereological study of the myocardium of newborn genetically cardiomyopathic hamsters, *J Ultrastruc Res*, 76:107-119, 1981

13.   Ma, T.S., Bailey, L.E., Excitation-contraction coupling in normal and myopathic hamster hearts. I: Identification of a calcium pool involved in contraction, *Cardiovasc Res*, 13:487-498, 1979

14.   Button, C., Gross, D.R., Allert, J.A., Kitzman, J.V., Tricuspid atresia in a foal, *J AVMA*, 172:825-830, 1978

15.   Gross, D.R., Clark, D.R., McDonald, D.R., McCrady, J.D., Allert, J.A., Congestive heart failure associated with congenital aortic valvular insufficiency in a horse, *Southwestern Vet*, 30:27-34, 1977

16.   Alexander, A.F., Jenson, R., Pulmonary vascular pathology of high altitude induced pulmonary hypertension in cattle, *Am J Vet Res*, 24:1112-1122, 1963

17.   Hecht, H.H., Kuida, H., Lange, R.L. Thorne, J.L., Brown, A.M., Brisket disease II, Clinical and hemodynamic observations in altitude dependent right heart failure of cattle, *Am J Med*, 32:171-182, 1961

18.   Will, D.H., Alexander, A.F., Reeves, J.T., Grover, R.F., High altitude induces pulmonary hypertension in normal cattle, *Circ Res*, 10:172-177, 1961

19.   Gopal, T., Leipold, H.W., Dennis, S.M., Congenital cardiac defects in calves, *Am J Vet Res*, 47:1120-1121, 1986

20.   Conrad, C.H., Brooks, W.W., Robinson, K.G., Bing, O.H.L., Impaired myocardial function in spontaneously hypertensive rats with heart failure, *Am J Physiol, 260 (Heart Circ Physiol, 29)*:H136-H145, 1991

21.   Barrett, G., Mullins, J.J., Transgenic models of cardiovascular disease, *Current Opinion in Biotechnology*, 3:637-640, 1992

22.   Rubin, E.M., Spangler, E.A., Versturyft, J.G., Clift, S.M., Inhibition of early atherogenesis in transgenic mice by human apolipoprotein A 1, *Nature*, 353:265-267, 1991

11. Iatrogenic models for studying heart disease

Heart failure models

Research associated with heart failure has, over the years, been aimed at three general areas: 1) The identification, characterization and quantification of injured tissue, including the so-called "border zone controversy". 2) The testing and evaluation of a large variety of interventions of potential therapeutic value. The latter include both pharmacologic and mechanical interventions. 3) Studies designed to evaluate the dynamics and mechanisms of heart failure per se. The common requirement of all studies of this nature is an adequate and appropriate model of heart failure. A wide variety of models have been used, each of which generates a characteristic type or a specific phase of failure.

Heart failure is, by definition, the inability of the heart to supply adequate tissue blood flow (left heart failure) or pulmonary alveolar blood flow (right heart failure) to meet the metabolic demands of the body. In man chronic heart failure also involves complex reflex changes in several physiological systems. Sympathetic system changes occur along with changes in the renin-angiotensin system and changes in adrenal steroid secretions. These changes result in vasoconstriction and retention of salt and water. Heart failure also is associated with subcellular abnormalities in both the directly affected and the residual, still viable, myocardium. These abnormalities may include, but not be limited to, depletion of intracellular calcium ion stores, changes in myosin and in a variety of subcellular enzymes. There is a reduction in the number and functional sensitivity of myocardial β-adrenergic receptors.

The majority of patients with heart failure have coronary artery disease, almost always associated with atherosclerosis. Under these circumstances the primary lesion is ischemia induced but excessive work load or volume overloading may produce additive effects. From a practical standpoint it is very difficult to control the degree and severity of heart failure with any of the commonly used models and the use of a model combining ischemia with pressure or volume overloading becomes even more difficult to manage.

Hypertrophy/heart failure models

Increasing the ventricular workload is a very common technique for inducing heart failure. Thus is generally accomplished by; 1) pressure overloading, 2) volume overloading, or 3) creating a valvular insufficiency. Each of these techniques pose their own particular difficulties, shortcomings and limitations. The techniques described have been used most frequently in dogs and cats but also is pigs, sheep, ponies, rabbits, guinea pigs, rats and baboons. Hearts exposed to increases in ventricular workload compensate by dilation and/or hypertrophy but do not always terminate in heart failure. Dilation and/or hypertrophy seem to be a normal compensatory mechanism to compensate for the higher workload. When the compensation is no longer able to meet the demand the system fails. All of the methods to be described produce some degree of dilation and/or hypertrophy but, for the most part, the final level of failure and its rate of progression are beyond the control of the experimenter. Human pathological states which these models are designed to mimic are primarily congenital in nature and actually represent a small percentage of the total cases of heart failure seen clinically in man.

Table 11.1 summarizes several different techniques for producing ventricular pressure overload. Not included in this table are a variety of techniques for inducing reno-vascular hypertension. These techniques are described in detail in Chapter 13. All of these models can also be used for left ventricular hypertrophy/failure models. Table 11.2 summarizes some models of volume overload and cardiac valvular insufficiencies and stenoses. The most common technique for accomplishing the latter is the creation of an aorto-caval or femoral artery-vein shunt. Frequently pressure overload alone or volume overload alone is not sufficient to result in heart failure within a short enough time frame to be useful for the experiment to be conducted. In these instances a combination model is often used. Overload failure has been produced by surgical creation of mitral insufficiency followed by a subsequent surgery to produce an arterio-venous shunt.[2] Right atrioventricular valvectomy and pulmonary arterial stenosis have been combined to produce right heart failure.[39]

Table 11.1 Techniques for producing ventricular pressure overload induced heart failure.

Technique	Results	Comments	Ref
Peri-arterial hydraulic occluder on the pulmonary artery	Spectrum of lesions from right ventricular dilation alone to dilation with severe stenosis and hypertrophy	Some control over the amount of dilation and hypertrophy by varying the degree of occlusion	1,2
Pulmonary stenosis by a constricting nylon band	Right ventricular hypertrophy and failure	Difficult to control the degree of occlusion, the amount of dilation and the rate to failure development	3
Banding of pulmonary artery	Hypertrophy caused by a sudden pressure overload	Histopathological and biochemical differences exist between this model and naturally occurring disease	4,109-118,134, 135

Technique	Results	Comments	Ref
Band around pulmonary artery in cats, 2 different sizes used to obtain either 80% or 90% constriction	Right congestive failure obvious in 20 of 26 cats prepared in this manner	Short time course of development	5
Acute banding of pulmonary artery	Response of right and left ventricles to acute pressure overload	Experimental data used to develop and verify a mathematical model of the response of both right and left ventricles	6
Banding of pulmonary artery in kittens 7-9 weeks of age, 6 months later reoperated and bands removed	Chronic progressive pressure overload, reversible	Compared banded to sham operated siblings, sham group reoperated after 6 months as well. Produces persistent, ongoing abnormalities of contractile, energetic and biochemical function *in vitro* and *in vivo*. Pump function appeared to be normal. Was fully reversible by operative removal of the band	**Ref** 7
Partial clamping of the ascending aorta with a Satinsky clamp	Acute pressure overload	Open chest, acute effects	8
Ligature around ascending aorta in guinea pigs, size 0 braided silk	Congestive heart failure	Closed to approximately 67% of the original size, i.e. approximately 33% patent	9
Woven dacron tube wrapped around intact ascending aorta, inflatable cuff placed around graft and injection bulb implanted subcutaneously	Dacron prevents aortic rupture from pressure necrosis, causes afterload increases	Jacobson hydraulic cuff, inflated after animal recovered from the surgery. Available from Davol Rubber Co.	10

Technique	Results	Comments	Ref
Banding of ascending aorta, usually done in young, they are allowed to grow during which time the degree of stenosis continuously increases	Chronic congestive left heart failure	When banded young often results in aortic rupture, even when protected by a Dacron or other material patch or graft. Because the stenosis is distal to the coronary ostia the coronary vasculature "sees" a high pressure, in humans aortic stenosis is almost always valvular and the coronary vessels therefore "see" normal pressures	**11,12,13, 14,15, 117,119- 125,133**
So called "subcoronary" or "supravalvular" banding of the aorta	Chronic congestive left heart failure with the left common coronary exposed to "normal" pressures	The ligature is applied so it passes under the left main coronary. The right coronary still "sees" the high pressure and may contribute to more of the left ventricular supply than it does under normal circumstances	**16,17, 126,127**
Inflatable cuff around the ascending aorta, not inflated until the dog has recovered from the surgery (7-14 days)	Cuff inflated to produce an approximately 60% increase in peak systolic left ventricular pressure	Response of the conscious dog. Is difficult to adjust the amount of constriction required to maintain the pressure increase constant over any prolonged period of time	**18**
Balloon cuff around the ascending aorta, 2 weeks later created a side-to-side, infrarenal, aorto-caval anastomosis, 11-16 mm long and 5-7 mm diameter	No change in ventricular contractility with hypertrophy even though there was obvious failure with fluid retention	Animals studied 29-49 days after aorto-caval anastomosis. Combination model of volume and pressure overload	**19**
Aortic constriction with a nylon band	Left ventricular hypertrophy and failure	Aortic rupture can be a problem and required exercise to produce failure	**20**

Technique	Results	Comments	Ref
Ameroid clip on ascending aorta	Gradual swelling of hydroscopic Ameroid causes gradual occlusion and pressure overload	Most of occlusion occurs rapidly *in vivo*, difficult to control amount of constriction achieved, models tend to have large variability	21
Banding the aorta in puppies and allowing them to gradually stenose as they grow	Stable left ventricular hypertrophy, usually does not progress to failure unless the dogs are exercised excessively	Stenosis is supravalvular and myocardial function is usually normal even though the heart muscle is hypertrophied	22
Stenosis or lesioning of the aortic valve	Left ventricular hypertrophy and failure	Extremely difficult to cause the same degree of aortic valvular stenosis in every animal and the degree of pressure overload therefore varies considerably	114,128-132

Table 11.2   Techniques for the production of ventricular volume overload induced hypertrophy/heart failure including valvular insufficiencies (and stenoses).

Technique	Results	Comments	Ref
Volume overloading accomplished by infusion of 10% dextran in 0.9% NaCl at 50 ml/kg in 5-10 min. The dogs were paced from the right atrium at approx. 40 bpm greater than their control rate to match the tachycardia associated with acute volume loading	Signs of acute heart failure	If pacing could not be achieved because of a compensatory heart block the dogs were given atropine (0.2-0.4 mg, iv). The dogs were sedated with morphine sulfate (30 mg, im) 30 min prior to the experiment then given Diazepam (5 mg).	22
Aorto-caval shunt	Congestive failure	Difficult to control the rate of development or the degree of failure produced	23
Aorto-caval shunts in rats, designed to equal about 50% of the total cardiac output	High output failure, significant bilateral ventricular hypertrophy	Two months of post surgical recovery allowed before used	24

Technique	Results	Comments	Ref
Aorto-caval shunts in rats, large volume defects	High output failure, significant bilateral ventricular hypertrophy, increased myocyte size	Five months following surgery	**136-138**
Aorto-caval fistula in rats	Volume overload, high output failure	Model exhibits: 1) chronically increased ventricular filling pressure, 2) increased skeletal and aortic smooth muscle catecholamine content, 3) decreased myocyte catecholamine stores, 4) increased systemic vascular resistance, 5) decreased blood flow to vascular beds under primary sympathetic control and 6) a substantial increase in total cardiac output	**25**
Bilateral femoral artery-vein shunts	Left ventricular overload, hypertrophy and failure	Works the same as aorto-caval shunts, high output failure	**2**
Modified Blalock-Taussig shunt (left subclavian artery to pulmonary artery GoreTex conduit graft)	Chronic volume overload with left ventricular dilation and hypertrophy	Same type of left ventricular responses as documented for aorto-caval shunts	**139**
Simulated mitral regurgitation in the dog. Thoracotomy, shunt from the base of the left ventricular freewall to the left atrium. Used a stainless steel cannula with a Teflon sewing ring and a portion of a Dacron prosthetic graft	Produced left ventricular overload, hypertrophy and failure	Hard to control left atrial pressure, passive congestion of the lungs and pulmonary edema prior to heart failure in a percentage of cases	**26**

Technique	Results	Comments	Ref
Mitral insufficiency, cut 1 or more chordae tendinea of the freewall cusp using a special instrument inserted through the left ventricular apex. Guided the instrument by finger through the left atrium. In this way they were able to palpate the mitral valve cusp and the chordae to be cut	Mitral regurgitation, left ventricular hypertrophy and failure	Can be done with caval occlusion, difficult to control the amount of regurgitation, produces uneven models	27
Perforated aortic valves in rabbits	Aortic insufficiency and chronic heart failure	Took 8-12 months post-op to achieve total heart failure. Difficult to produce equal amount of insufficiency in each case	28
Same as above	Same as above	Similar technique as above but produced failure in 4-7 weeks	29
Direct suturing or clipping of the aortic leaflets to cause aortic stenosis	Frequently results in valvular insufficiency because of tearing of the valve leaflet at the high stress areas where the sutures or clips are applied	Want pressure overload failure and end up with regurgitant, volume overload failure instead. Difficult to control the amount of stenosis produced, even if successful	30,31
Plication of the non-coronary cusp of the aortic valve	Trying to produce pressure overload by causing aortic stenosis	Often results in small valve gradients and valvular incompetence	32,33,34, 35
Aortic valvular stenosis, Teflon felt rolled into a 4-5 mm diameter, 8-9 mm length cylinder, covered with autologous pericardium and sutured into the sinuses of valsalva below the coronary orifices	Produces a true valvular stenosis and pressure overload failure	Requires by-pass surgery, care must be taken not to injure the aortic and mitral valve leaflets or get insufficiency as well	36
Pulmonary and/or aortic valve cusps cauterized with silver nitrate sticks	Pulmonic and aortic stenosis with subsequent pressure overload hypertrophy and eventual failure	Requires by-pass surgery, very difficult to control the amount of stenosis produced	37

Technique	Results	Comments	Ref
Acute tricuspid regurgitation produced by introducing a wire coiled into a spiral through the tricuspid valve via a puncture incision in the right atrium. Wire was advanced by screwing in as with a cork screw	Regurgitation produced by preventing complete apposition of the valve leaflets while permitting retrograde flow to occur through the spiral lumen and between the windings of the wire	So far only reported for acute intervention. Probably could be modified to be used in chronic preparations	**140**

Ischemic disease is the single most prevalent condition resulting in heart failure in humans. In this instance, ventricular dilation, hypertrophy, biochemical alterations, and eventual edema formation are all a result of the poor pumping capacity of the damaged myocardium. There are many experimental models available for the study of myocardial ischemia and tissue protection and, during the last 25 years there have been thousands of experimental and clinical studies conducted using a wide variety of these models.[40] Two very different types of ischemia have been studied; global ischemia, associated with cardiac arrest and regional ischemia, associated with a localized myocardial infarction. These two types of ischemia differ widely in their biochemical and electrophysiological characteristics and deservedly need to be studied as separate conditions.

Global ischemia, under surgically induced circumstances, i.e. the use of aortic cross-clamping and cardioplegia, is characterized by a fixed, relatively short duration and is readily reversible by reperfusion. Protective agents can be administered at the moment of, or prior to, the induction of ischemia. In the clinical situation the infarction lesion is nonfinite, it may or may not be reversible, the exact time of onset is frequently unknown, and it is rarely possible to administer any kind of protective agent prior to the actual onset of injury.

It is essential that pump function be maintained during infarction. A major effort in cardiovascular research has been, and still is, directed at the development of physical and/or pharmacological interventions to reduce infarct size, to assist the viable tissue in maintaining a normal level of contractile ability and to speed recovery of the damaged area. To accomplish these aims it is essential that the model used should mimic, as closely as possible, the clinical situation. Most experiments which have been conducted to evaluate tissue salvage and/or reduction of infarct size have assumed that, within an area of regional ischemia, tissue injury is heterogeneous with the most severely ischemic tissue in the core of the area affected. A "border zone" of intermediately injured tissue is presumed to exist around the severely injured core. This border zone is the target of most interventions. It appears that in most experimental models, particularly the acute infarction models in dogs and pigs, no such border zone exists. There is a sharp, but irregular transition from normal to ischemic myocardium.[40] The absence of an area of intermediate injury is different from that seen in slowly progressing coronary artery disease in man and adds a question to the utility of these acute models in evaluating beneficial interventions. The same is true when these models are used in studies of ischemia-reperfusion injury.

Overwhelmingly, the animal model most commonly used for coronary circulation studies has been the dog. There seems to be little doubt that the pig coronary vascular system is more similar to that of man than the dog coronary distribution.[41] The left circumflex coronary artery and left anterior descending coronary artery each supply about 40% of the myocardium and the right coronary artery about 15% in the dog. In pigs the right coronary and left anterior descending are about equal and the left circumflex plays a relatively minor role, more similar to the situation in man.[39] There are also similarities between man and pigs in intramural coronary artery branching patterns, coronary supply to papillary muscles and to nodal conduction tissue.[42,43] The dog seems to have a most extensive and recruitable collateral system. They usually have 3-4 relatively large subepicardial collateral vessel anastomoses. Pigs have some small endocardial anastomoses between the right and left coronaries. Man seems to fall somewhere between these two extremes, perhaps tending more toward the situation in pigs. There is considerable evidence that a gradual narrowing of the coronary arteries is the greatest stimulus for the formation of the collateral vessels.[41] When the blood supply to one of the major arteries is interrupted acutely in pigs the anastomoses are generally not adequate to prevent necrosis and/or fatal ventricular arrhythmias but in dogs a high survivor rate is common following acute constriction.[41]

Baboons have a coronary circulation very similar to that in man, although the diagonal branches are grouped into a single "third primary" coronary. Acute coronary ligation in baboons results in a very well circumscribed lesion with a clearly defined edge and marked tissue changes. There is no apparent "border zone".[44] Diffuse myocardial necrosis and, on occasion, infarct-like lesions have been recorded in captured baboons, in the absence of coronary artery disease. These lesions are presumed to be endocrine/ neurogenic from the stress and massive catecholamine discharge experienced during the capture process.[45]

The dog compensates for changes in venous return and afterload chiefly by changes in vagal tone. The baboon seems to respond to these perturbations by changes in sympathetic tone and man responds somewhere between these two extremes.[46] There is some evidence that the pig is even more of a sympathetic responder than the baboon.[44] Table 11.3 summarizes some of the published techniques for causing heart failure as a result of ischemic disease.

Table 11.3 Techniques for producing coronary ischemic disease.

Technique	Results	Comments	Ref
Two-stage ligation of left anterior descending coronary approximately 2 cm distal to its origin, in dogs	Reduced both *in vivo* and *in vitro* left ventricular compliance curves	Acute, open thorax preparation	**47**
Tourniquet around the left anterior descending coronary, open chest acute and closed chest acute and chronic, primates	Amount of reaction dependent upon length of time of occlusion	Tourniquet left in place for 1 hr, 2 hr, 4 hr, 6 hr or chronically	**48**

Technique	Results	Comments	Ref
Acute ligation of coronary arteries in dogs	Acute infarction model	Limitations and criteria for this type of thrombosis model are discussed in detail in ref # 52	**49,50, 51**
Acute ligation in swine	Same as above	Closed thorax model	**52**
Stepwise occlusion of the coronaries using a constrictor device with a U-shaped base which fits around the vessels, a plate and a screw inside a threaded portion. The screw is turned down pushing the plate and giving more control to the amount of stenosis caused, dogs	The vessel is squeezed between the plate and the base resulting in an asymmetrical constriction	There is fair control over the amount of constriction but no control over the geometry of the constriction. This is still an acute ligation model	**53**
Stepwise twisting of a copper wire placed around the vessel, dogs	Some control over the amount of constriction	Another acute ligation model but it could also be used chronically	**54**
Constriction and/or occlusion produced by compressing the vessel between a hook-shaped stainless steel plate and a silicone rubber covered chromel plunger bent to fit the pressure plate. To provide the flexibility needed for coronary arteries on the beating heart, the hook-shaped plate is silver soldered to a piece of 17 gauge thin wall stainless steel tubing approx. 12 inches long. The upper end of the tubing is silver soldered into a collar rigidly fixed into a lucite mounting block with a set screw. The chromel plunger is freely movable within the thin wall tubing and is silver soldered to a second, spring-loaded metal collar. The latter maintains constant pressure against the spindle of the micrometer	This device creates a linear compression of the cross-sectional area of the vessel at the level of the stenosis	There is also a direct drive lever that, when manually depressed, fully occludes the vessel. The advantage of this device is precision, ease of application and manipulation and reproducibility of a specific stenosis	**55**

Technique	Results	Comments	Ref
Two 0 nylon suture is looped through a very small ring and held at each end by 2 blocks of plastic. The 2 plastic blocks are mounted on a pair of metal rods, one of which is moveable and alters the loop diameter	The distance between the blocks can be accurately measured with a Vernier caliper and the relationship between that distance and the radius of the loop is linear	Reproducible stenosis, accurately measurable	56
2-3 mm wide band of umbilical tape passed around the artery, then through a stiff tubing and attached to a machinist's micrometer	Investigators were able to close the snare by small, precise amounts	Reproducible stenosis, good accuracy	57
Acute coronary occlusion in dogs	3 major periods of ventricular arrhythmias produced: 1) Malignant within min. 2) Release of acute occlusion 3) 15-24 hours, subacute period of spontaneous arrhythmias, lasts up to 72 hours	1) Persist for about 30 min, often lead to fibrillation, there is some evidence that the mechanism is due to slow conduction and re-entry within the ischemic myocardium 2) Also associated with malignant arrhythmias 3) Rarely results in fibrillation, dominant rhythm disturbance seems to be due to enhanced automaticity in the Purkinje system	58,147
Use of hydraulic occluders, chronic in awake dogs after prior instrumentation surgery	1/4 of volume needed to occlude at original surgery injected into the occluder every 15 min until occlusion complete	Dogs protected by morphine (1 mg/kg),and lidocaine (1 mg/kg, iv and 2-3 mg/min in a continuous iv drip	59
Hydraulic occluder	Design described in paper	This is the same device sold by In Vivo Metric Systems, Healdsburg, CA	60,61, 62,149
Another type of hydraulic occluder	Indirect pressure of balloon against the vessel inside a rigid plastic ring	Design is well described	63

Technique	Results	Comments	Ref
Still another type of hydraulic occluder made from a # 5 French polyvinyl feeding tube	Creates a balloon pressure around most of the vessel circumference	Simple, inexpensive, but difficult to get consistent levels of occlusion from the injection of the same amount of fluid in different occluders	64
Balloon cuff type occluder filled with Mercury	At the time of the experiment more Mercury is added to the cuff until the measured flow is reduced a predetermined amount	More control of the amount of occlusion, less likely to leak and loose the constriction with time. Some danger associated with handling the Hg	65
Another hydraulic occluder similar in design to those described above	Occlusion from the hydraulic cuff	Commercially available from Rhodes Medical Inst., Woodland Hills, CA. Very difficult to control the amount of occlusion from animal to animal with this particular devise	66,67
Use of Ameroid constrictors. Ameroid is a hydroscopic casein plastic material	In saline at 38 °C the ring narrowed from 3 to 1.5 mm id in 24 days, to 1.3 mm in 40 days and from 3-1.98 mm in 4 days	The Ameroid casein material was obtainable in 6 mm and 12 mm diameter rods from American Plastics Corp., Bainbridge, NY (1957 ref)	68
Ameroid constrictors	Most investigators agree that this technique lacks predictability and reliability to produce a functional stenosis. The degree of stenosis cannot be adjusted nor predicted	Ameroid cylinder is eccentrically placed. With this method it is not necessary to use a rigid encasement as is usually described. The thicker portion of the cylinder is at the side of the slot. The constrictor can be held in position with 3 or 4 stainless steel wires in grooves made in the material. Expansion is greater on the thicker side, so the slot will occlude more rapidly than the lumen	69,70

Technique	Results	Comments	Ref
Ameroid constrictors	30% of total constriction within the first 48 hours after application	Difficult to have a post-operative period for baseline control measurements. Some skill is needed to fit the devices properly	**71,149 150**
Coronary embolization done in closed chest dogs, coronary catheterization. Injection of 0.1 ml glass beads, 400-600 μm diameter, dispersed in 0.4 ml contrast media and injected under fluoroscopic observation to make sure there was no reflux into the aortic root	To prevent acute fibrillation the dogs were given lidocaine (1 mg/min, iv) started 15 min prior to embolization and continued for 1 hr post-embolization, still lost 9 or 20 dogs	Damage is acute, indiscriminate and widespread. A very small amount of embolization is required to cause terminal failure	**75**
Coronary embolization using a variety of modifications of the basic technique described above. Most recent modification is to do multiple coronary catheterizations (7-10 or more) at 2 week intervals and inject small numbers of 50-100 μm microspheres each time	Difficult to control the amount and location of the damage. Onset is slow but still have a rather large risk of acute ventricular arrhythmias after 6 or 7 embolizations	Maintaining femoral arteries patent and healthy for repeated percutaneous catheterizations is difficult and tedious. Hematomas are frequently a problem. In our experience there is still a rather high acute mortality during the last embolizations	**73,74, 141**
Internal (intravascular) plugs, 2 different types; 1) streamlined entrance, 2) blunt, step up entrance. A variety of plug lumen diameters of known geometry can be used	Polycarbonate plugs, outside diameter of plug matched to within 0.25 mm of the inside diameter of the vessel, fluid mechanics can be well defined	Requires surgical implantation, which can be difficult in the beating heart	**75**
Internal occlusion with helically-shaped copper wire, anesthetized, closed thorax dogs	Able to selectively release a wire into a coronary vessel by delivering with a double catheter system using fluoroscopic visualization	Difficult to reproduce the same degree of constriction consistently	**76,77**

Technique	Results	Comments	Ref
Electrical injury to the coronary endothelium producing an injury site and thrombus formation. Anodal current of 50-200 μA is delivered using a DC source. Described in both open and closed chest dogs. The injury induces platelet adhesion and aggregation at the damaged site. The process is followed by further platelet aggregation and consolidation with the growing thrombus entrapping red blood cells	Current can be delivered acutely at higher doses or slowly at lower doses. The latter results in more slowly developing obstructive lesions. Used primarily to evaluate various thrombolytic therapies	Cannot control the amount of constriction or occlusion developed but it is a reasonably realistic model	**78,142 - 144, 148**
Thrombin-induced clot formation. The vessel is deendothelialized by external trauma using a forceps. Snare occluders are then placed proximal and distal to the injury site and 10 units of thrombin are injected into the isolated segment of vessel, usually in a small volume via a side branch into the isolated segment. Autologous blood (0.3-0.4 ml), mixed with $CaCl_2$ (0.05 M) is also injected into the isolated segment producing a stasis-type red clot superimposed on an injured blood vessel. The snares are released after 2-5 min.	Total occlusion usually occurs and can be used to evaluate thrombolytic therapies	Realistic but causes acute and complete occlusion	**145, 146**
Radiolucent, physiologically inert plastic (Lexan) cylinders, 3 mm long with varying internal diameters, placed around the outside of the vessels to create a stenosis	Noted time changes in the amount of obstruction with a constant aortic pressure and flow. Considered to be due to platelet aggregation and disaggregation	Something was obviously happening inside the stenosis and the flow changes could be blocked with aspirin	**79**

Technique	Results	Comments	Ref
Essentially the same as above except plastic cylinder was 2.5 mm long. The diameter was designed to produce a 60-80% narrowing of the vessel.	On average it was found that a 72% stenosis was necessary to abolish the reactive hyperemic response. When the obstructive cylinder is in place the phasic flow downstream is largely abolished but the mean flow is in the same range as before the cylinder is applied. Causes cyclical reductions in flow, caused by intravascular platelet aggregation and temporary thrombosis	Aspirin abolished the cyclic flow changes seen in the presence of constant aortic pressure and flow. The cyclic changes were not influenced by heparin administration, i.e. not fibrin deposition. Not all dogs showed the cyclic reductions in flow but those that did all had greater ADP-induced platelet aggregation reactions	**80**
A 0.95 mm thick thermosonde is introduced into the coronary artery via catheterization. The tip of the thermosonde is heated to 45-65°C for 1-2 min, then the catheter is removed, in sheep	When tip is heated an acute infarction occurs	Provides acute injury, reproducible, advantage is that it is a closed chest procedure	**108**
Acute left coronary, ligation 2-3 mm from the origin of the left coronary between the pulmonary artery conus and the left atrium, in rats	The ligations are done using sterile technique and the rats used for a variety of studies from 3 to 85 days later. Well defined infarcted areas are produced but incidence of severe ventricular arrhythmias is low	Rat hearts seem to accommodate to this injury rather well and the true relevance of this model to the human ischemic infarct is not clear	**151-155**
Acute, 2 stage coronary ligation in dogs	Ligature first tied with a 20 gauge needle laid longitudinally on the coronary artery. After the ligature is tied the needle is removed. After some period of time (typically 40-60 min) another ligature is tied to occlude the vessel	This is a type of ischemic preconditioning and alters the metabolic and functional responses to the ischemic insult	**156**

Technique	Results	Comments	Ref
Acute coronary ligation, in pigs	Ligatures tied acutely around the coronary arteries result in clearly demarcated ischemic zones	Can result in serious ventricular arrhythmias. Not clear how this model relates to human disease	**157, 158**
Direct myocardial damage with ultrasound, dogs	Thermal injury induced by high power, high frequency, ultrasonic irradiation	Can direct the ultrasound beam at specific myocardial locations. Acute lesions produced have questionable relation to human lesions except for acute injury type lesions	**159**

Cardiomyopathy is a general term applied to a variety of diseases which result in myocardial lesions not related to disease states initiated in other cardiac structures. The term therefore encompasses a wide variety of conditions initiated by a wide variety of etiologies. In humans this condition is an important cause of myocardial failure which often leads to severe functional abnormalities and death. Cardiomyopathy has been reported in rabbits associated with high stress levels attributed to overcrowding. At necropsy these animals show normal heart weights but biventricular dilation. Histologically these rabbits demonstrate myocardial edema, myocytolysis and myofibrillar coagulative necrosis. Multifocal areas of necrosis are replaced with fibrous connective tissue in longer term survivors along with basophilic mucinous degeneration. Animals surviving for more than one month had a thickened endocardium localized at the ventricular apexes. The thickening was due to excessive accumulation of collagen and elastic fibers.[160] Table 11.4 summarizes a wide variety of techniques which have been used to create cardiomyopathic models of heart failure. Perhaps most recent, and most popular is the rapid supraventricular pacing model. This has clearly been shown to produce a dilated cardiomyopathy characterized by increased left ventricular (LV) chamber dimensions, elevated end-diastolic pressure, reduced wall thickness and increased LV wall stress.[164-166,168-171] This model has several advantages but, perhaps, the most important is the ease with which it can be created and the uniformity of the lesions produced. Another, perhaps related model derived from observations on patients with pheochromocytoma related cardiomyopathy which indicate that excess circulating catecholamines are responsible for the cardiomyopathy.[179]

Table 11.4 Techniques for the induction of cardiomyopathic heart failure.

Technique	Results	Comments	Ref
Right ventricular pacing at 260 bpm for 10 days, compared sham operated controls to paced dogs	Congestive heart failure characterized by: decreased cardiac output and stroke volume, increased total peripheral vascular resistance, right atrial pressure and pulmonary arterial mean pressure	Was used to evaluate usefulness of an atrial natriuretic peptide fragment (ANP-95-126) in the treatment of congestive heart failure	**161**
Right ventricular pacing in previously instrumented dogs, 140 bpm for 24±4 days, compared the same 8 dogs before and after pacing	Congestive heart failure characterized by: increases in LV end-diastolic pressure, heart rate, LV end-diastolic diameter, LV end-systolic diameter, end-systolic long-axis diameter, LV end-systolic stress, LV end-diastolic stress, LV end-diastolic volume, LV end- systolic volume and plasma volume; decreases in LV end-systolic wall thickness, LV long-short axis, LV wall thickness (short axis), LV +dP/dt, LV -dP/dt, LV mean velocity of circumferential fiber shortening, LV ejection fraction and LV stroke work	Demonstrated that this degree of rapid ventricular pacing resulted in dilated congestive cardiomyopathy in conscious dogs characterized by globally depressed myocardial systolic function and changes in LV shape	**162**
Atrial pacing, 3 weeks at 240 bpm, compared unpaced controls to paced pigs	Cardiomyopathy characterized by: decreased LV fractional shortening and capillary luminal diameter; increased left atrial pressures, myocardial blood flow, coronary vascular resistance and capillary-myocyte distance; capillary density did not change	Supraventricular pacing also causes a tachycardia induced cardiomyopathy	**163**

Technique	Results	Comments	Ref
Unipolar electrode advanced to the right ventricular apex via the jugular vein, paced at 250 bpm until the end point was achieved in each of 17 dogs. End point defined as development of severe congestive heart failure defined as radiographic pulmonary edema, a >25% increase in planimetered chest X ray cardiac area and/or a >10% increase in body weight. Comparisons made to a sham operated control group monitored for 4 weeks	Congestive heart failure with marked LV remodelling. The extent of ventricular dilation correlated with the time required for the development of signs of severe heart failure. Mitral regurgitation was found as an epiphenomenon and was most likely caused by the increase in LV cross sectional area	Attempt to create a more consistent model but continued pacing until well defined end-points were achieved	167
A left thoracotomy was used to suture a shielded stimulating electrode to the left atrium, supraventricular pacing at 240 bpm for 3 weeks, treated vs sham operated pigs	There was a significant reduction of LV fractional shortening, increased end-diastolic dimensions and lengthening of isolated myocytes. Myocyte attachment to laminin was significantly decreased with similar reductions in myocyte attachment to fibronectin and collagen IV. There were focal disruptions of the basement membrane-sarcolemmal interface and a reduced number of sarcolemmal festoons	The observed structural changes may play a significant role in the progression of ventricular dysfunction	172

Technique	Results	Comments	Ref
Same as above, also in pigs, paced vs sham controls. LV function evaluated by echocardiography and catheterization. Isolated myocyte function was studied using computer-assisted video microscopy with cells examined in the unloaded, unattached state and after attachment to a basement membrane substrate	LV fractional shortening and peak +dP/dt significantly decreased. Isolated myocyte % shortening and normalized peak velocity of shortening of myocytes adherent to a basement membrane were significantly lower. Extent and velocity of shortening reduced over 50% in SVT vs control. For both attached and unattached SVT myocytes responsiveness to increases in extracellular Ca^{2+} were significantly blunted vs controls. % vol of myofibrils within isolated myocytes was reduced in SVT vs controls	SVT cardiomyopathy probably due to a primary defect in isolated myocyte contractile performance. Reduced contractile function of SVT cardiomyopathic myocytes was associated with abnormalities in cytoarchitecture and Ca^{2+} responsiveness	**173**

Technique	Results	Comments	Ref
36 paced vs 36 control mongrel dogs, bipolar pacing electrode introduced under aseptic conditions into the right ventricular apex. Paced at 250 bpm until overt heart failure observed, i.e. ascites, fatigue, shortness of breath, anorexia and >9% weight gain	Decreased; β-adrenergic receptor-mediated stimulation of adenylate cyclase, basal adenylate cyclase activity, the V_{max} of 5'-guanylylimidodiphosphate and forskolin stimulation of adenylate cyclase activity. Pertussis toxin-mediated ADP-ribosylation of membranes revealed a significant decrease in the inhibitory guanine nucleotide binding protein content with adenylate cyclase activity remaining depressed in the failing heart after pertussis toxin treatment. Mechanical studies on isolated papillary muscles and trabeculae revealed a decrease in baseline total tension, and maximal tension and dT/dt was significantly lower in the presence of isoproterenol	Seems that a decrease in adenylate cyclase reactivity contributes to the blunted β-adrenergic response to catecholamine stimulation in this model. The β-adrenergic signal transduction pathway abnormalities were accompanied by a decrease in activity of membrane-bound Na^+,K^+-ATPase. The defects may be a reflection of more widespread dysfunction of sarcolemmal-bound enzymes and may play a role in the decrease in contractility and the development of heart failure in this model.	**174**

Technique	Results	Comments	Ref
Treatment vs control groups of dogs compared, right ventricular apex pacing @ 250 bpm for 26.3±2.9 days. Studies performed on isolated, metabolically supported hearts coupled to a computer-controlled left ventricular loading system. Pressure-volume relations and myocardial oxygen consumption (MVO_2) measured to assess chamber systolic and diastolic function	Systolic function reduced in failed hearts vs controls, i.e. slope of end-systolic pressure-volume relation and lowered end-systolic stiffness at matched stress. Diastolic chamber and myocardial stiffness were unaltered in failure hearts but unstressed diastolic-arrested volume was significantly larger. Inotropic response to increased heart rate and exogenous β-adrenergic stimulation was significantly impaired in the failure hearts which also had a lowered slope of the MVO_2-PVA relation (indicating increased efficiency of chemomechanical energy conversion)	Reduced chamber and myocardial contractility, dilatation without alteration of passive myocardial properties, impaired contractile reserve and novel alterations in cardiac efficiency found in this model	**175**
Rabbits paced at 400 bpm for 29.4±10.6 days, paced vs control group. Two stainless-steel-tipped pacing wires pushed into left ventricular myocardium then sutured to the epicardium to hold in place. Measured passive and active length-tension relations and postrest contraction behavior in right ventricular papillary muscles	Active tension reduced at muscle lengths of 0.95 x L_{max} and above. Both control and paced groups sowed increased force development when the concentration of Ca^{2+} in the buffer was increased. No differences between the groups in the passive-length-tension relations	Sustained tachycardia will lead to myocardial depression in rabbits as in other species	**176**

Technique	Results	Comments	Ref
Mongrel dogs, control vs paced, anesthetized and a unipolar pacemaker lead placed in the right ventricular apex via the right external jugular vein. Paced at 250 bpm until severe heart failure achieved as judged by >25% increase in heart size accompanied by pulmonary edema and/or a >10% increase in body weight (4-6 weeks)	The myocardium had a significantly lower energy charge in the failed hearts due to lower concentrations of ATP, ADP and AMP, however the total adenine nucleotide pool was not different between the two groups. Myocardial lactate concentration was also unchanged. Glycogen was significantly lower. Adenine nucleotides were similar among the endo-, mid- and epicardium. Enalapril (angiotensin-converting enzyme inhibitor) administration decreased vascular resistance but had no effect on myocardial energy status	Findings suggest that the lower energy charge in the failed hearts is not the result of subendocardial ischemia, endogenous glycogen depletion or increased lactate concentrations. The energy status of the myocardium in rapid ventricular pacing failed hearts is different than that seen in ischemia-induced heart failure	**177**

Technique	Results	Comments	Ref
Mongrel dogs, unipolar active fixation pacing lead positioned in the right ventricular apex with fluoroscopic control. Paced at 250 bpm. Right heart hemodynamics evaluated along with plasma renin activity, arginine vasopressin, atrial natriuretic factor, and noradrenalin assays done during the development of failure	Onset of rapid pacing accompanied by a fall in cardiac output and a rise in pulmonary arterial, pulmonary capillary wedge and right atrial pressures. Noradrenaline and atrial natriuretic factor increased. Plasma renin activity showed an initial fall followed by a rise. Arginine vasopressin was unchanged in first 8 hr. After 35 days of rapid pacing clinical signs of fluid retention appeared by day 28, with further decreases in cardiac output and increases in right side pressures. Atrial natriuretic factor peaked at around 14 days whereas plasma renin activity, arginine vasopressin and noradrenalin tended to reach a plateau at about day 20 and then to show further increases as clinical signs of fluid retention appeared, plasma renin activity showed the most marked increase	These findings suggest a major role for renin, vasopressin and/or noradrenaline in the pathophysiology of the fluid retention of heart failure induced using this technique	**178**
Rats with pheochromocytomas	Investigated effects of chronic exposure to high concentrations of catecholamines on desensitization of α- & β-adrenergic receptor-mediated responses	Was found to be a useful model	**180**

Technique	Results	Comments	Ref
New England Deaconess Hospital rats implanted with pheochromocytoma, control vs treated with captopril	Captopril treated did not develop hypertension. Plasma norepinephrine levels increased in both captopril treated and untreated implanted rats vs control (no pheochromocytoma implantation). Plasma renin activities slightly lower in pheochromocytoma rats vs unimplanted controls. Captopril markedly attenuated pheochromocytoma induced cardiomyopathy	Captopril will block the development of hypertension and cardiomyopathy in rats implanted with pheochromocytoma tumor cells	**181**
Measured inotropic reactivity and β-adrenoceptor density of right ventricular myocardial strips from rats treated for 1 month with isoproterenol	Hyperresponsiveness to inotropic effects of the calcium channel activator Bay K 8644, subsensitivity to isoproterenol and decreased β-adrenoceptor density	A form of cardiomyopathy is developed with chronic treatment with the β-adrenergic agonist isoproterenol	**182**
Isoprenaline administered subcutaneously (0.25 mg/kg/day, single dose) for 10 days in adult rats	Developed both right and left ventricular hypertrophy and functional reserve of the left ventricle decreased, collagen concentration increased	Developed both functional and structural differences than hypertrophy induced by thyroxine treatment	**183**
Thyroxine administered subcutaneously (0.30 mg/kg/day, single dose) for 10 days in adult rats	Developed both right and left ventricular hypertrophy, functional reserve of the left ventricle increased significantly while collagen concentration was unchanged	Opposite functional and structural differences than hypertrophy induced by isoprenaline treatment	**183**

Technique	Results	Comments	Ref
Limipramine, a tricyclic antidepressive agent, administered as a continuous infusion (7.5 mg/kg/hr for 30 min) in dogs.	LV dP/dt_{max} decreased, LV end-diastolic pressure increased, LV peak pressure, ejection fraction decreased. No ECG changes or supraventricular /ventricular arrhythmias were seen. Function partially recovered after cessation of infusion. Able to repeat the treatment during a 2 week interval with same results	Reversible heart failure, may be useful for testing the efficiency of supportive interventions	184
Rabbits given Adriamycin (1 mg/kg, iv) twice per week for 8 weeks, then allowed to recover for 2 weeks. (Adriamycin is an anthracycline antibiotic widely used for chemotherapy)	Long lasting decrease in cardiac output and other measures of cardiac function	Useful model of cardiomyopathy	185
Same as above	Cardiac myocytes enzymatically isolated showed a decrease in contraction amplitude, velocity and oxygen consumption compared to controls. Myosin content was decreased, no decrease in β-adrenoceptor sensitivity	Intrinsic changes in cardiac myocyte structure and performance are probable cause of reduced cardiac function in this model	186

Technique	Results	Comments	Ref
Wistar rats injected with streptozotocin (90 mg/kg, intraperitoneal at 2 days of age)	Produces a marked glucose intolerance but plasma fasting and non-fasting glucose values were at or near normal values for 12 months of the study. Hearts exhibited a progressive cardiomyopathy with both contractile and metabolic abnormalities. There were decreases in cardiac output, ventricular pressure, cardiac work and glucose utilization. Abnormalities not corrected by acute exposure to insulin or changes in work load	In the rat a progressive cardiomyopathy results from persistent glucose intolerance in the absence of fasting hyperglycemia. The cardiomyopathy is reminiscent of that described in human noninsulin-dependent diabetes	**187**
Male Fischer 344 rats, 4 mos of age, given 30% ethanol in their drinking water every day for 8 mos.	Body and cardiac growth depressed, LV weight reduced by 14%, no difference in RV weight. Arterial pressures and peak LV pressures decreased with no change in heart rates. Myocardial contractility depressed, LV end-diastolic pressure increased 5.2-fold and RV 2.9-fold. LV diastolic chamber volume increased while thickness decreased. The volume % of myocardial lesions increased 342% in the wall of the LV	Chronic consumption of moderate amounts of alcohol results in ventricular dysfunction that is precipitated by myocardial damage and ventricular wall remodeling	**188**

Technique	Results	Comments	Ref
Pregnant guinea pigs were given 2.5% ethanol in drinking water from day 30 to the end of pregnancy. At delivery ethanol intake was stopped and litter size and perinatal mortality recorded.	Maternal deaths, litter size, number of stillborn, newborn body weight and heart weight were not different in ethanol treated vs control guinea pigs and their offspring. Calcium ion uptake, binding and calcium ion stimulated ATPase activity in isolated sarcoplasmic reticulum were all reduced in 1-3 day old offspring from ethanol treated mothers.	Moderate ethanol exposure in utero produced functional cardiac alterations in the newborn which were slowly reversible with abstinence from ethanol	**189**

Other heart failure models

Pulmonary embolism is a technique that has been employed by many investigators who have injected substances of various sizes, shapes, weights and composition into the pulmonary vasculature. These have included pumice powder, lycopodium spores, starch granules, glass beads, fat emboli, endotoxin, balloons, collagen suspensions, buckshot, birdshot, etc. These various products may activate different mechanisms, i.e. glass beads result in intravascular coagulation, balloons do not. Intravascular coagulation has also been stimulated with thrombin. This causes the release of clots formed elsewhere in peripheral veins. Another technique involves the intravenous injection of preformed autologous blood clots. With this technique it is difficult to control the size of the vessels obstructed. Air emboli have been used, but they generally distribute to upper lung regions whereas glass beads and gunshot distribute to dependent regions.[81] Awake rabbits have been subjected to intermittent micro-embolization with particles of aggregated human albumin (10-40 μm in diameter). Using a catheter in the right atrium 13.5 mg/kg of albumin suspended in Ringer's solution was infused during the first 3 hours followed by an additional 4 mg/kg at 6-8, 12-14 and 18-20 hours. The technique resulted in approximately 80% of the pulmonary microvessels being occluded.[82] Microspheres of Sephadex have been repeatedly injected until chronic pulmonary hypertension was well established, a procedure which took 16-30 weeks and eventually resulted in right heart failure.[83]

Production of heart block and severe arrhythmias is another technique for the creation of heart failure. With dogs on total by-pass an encircling endocardial ventriculotomy has been described which produces ventricular tachyarryhthmias.[84] Weir et al. summarize and evaluate several techniques for producing complete A-V block.[85] Following thoracotomy, atriotomy and venous inflow occlusion, the A-V nodal area can be mechanically destroyed by; 1) sectioning or crushing of the A-V node or His bundle or 2) ligature of the A-V node or His bundle. Chemical necrosis of the area can be produced by formalin, alcohol or other noxious agents. Electrocautery has been used as has the local application of cold. Other procedures are done using a thoracotomy, but blindly through a purse-string suture in the atrium or via a needle puncture.[86] Injury to the area is accomplished as previously described by mechanical, chemical, electrocautery or cold insult. Temporary A-V block has been produced, after a thoracotomy, by ligation of the coronary artery branches to the A-V nodal area and by injection of pharmacological agents into the coronary branches to the area. A-V block has also been produced in closed chest subjects using a catheter with a needle on the end. After guiding the catheter to the A-V nodal area fluoroscopically a chemical necrosis is produced, usually with formalin. Similar techniques have been described using a fluoroscopically guided catheter and electrocautery.[85] After production of complete A-V block most animals will develop right and left side failure, either spontaneously or after several weeks of daily exercise.[87]

Cardiac tamponade has been produced as another method of causing heart failure. Animals were previously instrumented, including a catheter into the pericardium. Tamponade was produced by continuous infusion of 0.9% saline at 37°C into the pericardial space at 10 ml/min. The procedure resulted in right ventricular diastolic collapse and resulting failure.[88]

Radiation-induced myocardial damage has been employed with some success to produce progressive heart failure. Stone, Bishop and Guyton used ^{60}Co irradiation of intact dogs.[89,90] The results were not highly reproducible and the mechanism of failure was not defined. The insult also produced widespread damage to other tissues, i.e. the chest wall, lungs and pericardium. These lesions led to complications, including pericarditis and cardiac tamponade.

Repetitive direct current has been used by Carlyle and his colleagues to produce myocardial damage and subsequent failure.[91,92] A premeasured soft metallic guide wire was passed, via a catheter, into the left ventricle. The wire was positioned, using fluoroscopy, just below the aortic valve and against the intraventricular septum. An electrode was then placed on the left chest wall over the point of maximal intensity of the apex beat and a second electrode was attached to the guide wire. The dogs were given repetitive dc shocks of 75-80 joules every 10 seconds at the rate of 1 shock/kg body weight. The dogs usually had A-V block by the second shock and most stayed in that rhythm throughout the study. Two dogs spontaneously reverted to sinus rhythm, but after several more shocks they also converted to complete A-V block.[91] Two of 14 dogs died from the procedure acutely and a third died 3 weeks after the insult. All dogs developed signs of left ventricular failure, the amount of pump dysfunction seemed to be related to the area of necrosis which resulted.[92]

Neurogenic stress in adrenalectomized animals will result in heart failure. Two different type of reactions to adrenal insufficiency have been described: The first type of failure takes days and is characterized by a slow debilitation with associated electrolyte and circulating volume changes. The second is a short, cataclysmic cardiovascular failure without frank alterations in electrolytes or circulating volume. The latter occurs within hours after excessive sympathetic excitation.[93]

Pure right ventricular failure has been produced by creating a right ventricular freewall infarct, double ventriculotomy and tricuspid insufficiency and pulmonary arterial banding in dogs. These lesions had an effect on the total hemodynamic state of the dogs but were not a direct cause of death in these animals if the pulmonary band was removed prior to circulatory collapse.[190]

Ventricular fibrillation is obviously an acute model of heart failure which has been used in many different species. It has been reported as being very useful in a sheep model to test the efficacy of a percutaneously introduced large bore venous drainage catheter.[191]

Vena cava constriction is an old and well defined model of low cardiac output congestive heart failure.[192] This model was recently used in dogs by placing a band around the thoracic inferior vena cava and causing an approximately 50% reduction in diameter. The model was used to study the roles of endothelin-1 and atrial natriuretic factor in this form of heart failure.[193] A similar technique was used to produce low cardiac output failure in lambs. In this case a balloon catheter was introduced into the right atrium via a jugular vein. By inflating the balloon the investigators we able to reduce cardiac output to as low as 20% of the baseline resting cardiac output and to maintain the preparation in a stable condition.[194]

Pharmacological infarction has been created in rabbits using abrupt withdrawal of chronic nitroglycerin pretreatment.[195] A similar model was described in which rabbits were pretreated with nitroglycerin paste (2%) applied as a 2-inch strip of paste three times daily for 42 days to a shaved interscapular region. Forty hours after the last dose of nitroglycerin the rabbits were challenged with either ergonovine (0.2 mg/kg, i.v.) or indomethacin (25 mg/kg, i.v.). Following either of the challenges the rabbits developed ECG changes such as single ventricular premature beats, nonsustained ventricular tachycardia and ST segment deviations all indicative of localized myocardial ischemia.[196]

Portal hypertension models

There are many different methods of producing portal hypertension and these have been reviewed by Halvarsen and Myking.[95] Dogs and monkeys rarely get chronically elevated portal vein pressures as a result of these procedures. It seems that enough collateral circulation either exists or develops in those species to rapidly decompress the portal vein. Rats, however, have proven to be good models for this syndrome. Total occlusion of the portal vein using Ameroid constrictors has resulted in sustained increases in portal vein pressure.

Isolated heart preparations

The use of an isolated heart preparation permits studies under highly controlled conditions in which the various aspects of cardiac function can be evaluated. The classic Langendorff preparation, i.e. retrograde perfusion of the coronary vasculature using a balanced buffered crystalloid solution saturated with a 95/5% mixture of O_2 and CO_2 has been used and modified by many investigators but the basic elements have been retained.[96,97,98] This preparation is most commonly used in mice and rats but is also useful in rabbits. Similar designs have been used in larger species, including dogs, but in our experience hearts from any animal larger than a 4 or 5 kg rabbit require some circulating blood cells in the preparation to increase oxygen carrying capacity. Without this capability the heart is, at minimum, borderline ischemic and will function poorly if the workload is increased. The advantages of the Langendorff type preparation are that the heart is perfused through its own coronary distribution, it is beating at a relatively normal heart rate and the temperature can be adjusted and controlled to normal body temperatures. The method is particularly useful for studies of myocardial metabolism since it is very easy to measure total coronary flow and oxygen consumption. Modifications of this preparation include the use of a support animal in which case the isolated heart is blood perfused and the support animal not only acts as an oxygenator and CO_2 extractor it also acts as a pH buffer and supplies all metabolic requirements as well as providing liver and kidneys for metabolic waste disposal.[99] If an intraventricular balloon is positioned properly and the isolated heart is beating isovolumetrically the mechanical function of the heart can be evaluated. However with the balloon in place there is some possibility that subendocardial ischemia is present. This could effect the metabolism of the preparation.[97] The same author has also pointed out that, in the classic Langendorff preparation, pressure, volume and internal cardiac work can all vary independently. Changes in metabolic function may occur which are secondary to altered mechanical function or to a primary adaptation in the metabolic pathway and special techniques are necessary to separate the two.[97]

Elzinga and Westerhof used an isolated cat heart preparation in a climate controlled box in which the heart is made to pump through a hydraulic loop.[100] This "working heart" preparation has been used by many investigators including ourselves to study the effects of changes in afterload on the efficiency of the heart as a pump. With this system, or a variety of modifications of it, it is possible to vary both preload and afterload, independently. The left ventricle ejects into a hydraulic model of the input impedance of the animal's systemic arterial tree, characterized by 2 resistances and 1 capacitance (the three-element Windkessel model). These systems usually involve some method of direct retrograde perfusion until the harvested heart recovers and is beating well. At that point there is usually some method of switching so that the heart is preloaded and starts to eject, supplying its own aortic root with blood under sufficient pressure to allow coronary perfusion. Although these, and similar preparations (i.e. isolated heart-lung preparations) both *in situ* and isolated, offer considerable control over the variables involved in cardiac function they cannot serve to answer all questions concerning cardiovascular mechanisms. They are denervated and separated from both nervous and endocrine influences. The heart must respond to various perturbations in any way that it can. A perfect demonstration of this is the Frank-Starling mechanism which is the major way in which the isolated heart copes with increases in preload. *In vivo* responses to preload changes are almost entirely compensated for by changes in heart rate. These preparations to serve a useful role as a "bridge" between highly controlled isolated papillary muscle type preparations and much less controlled *in vivo* studies.

Spontaneously beating mouse hearts have been maintained in organ culture media. These preparations are not perfused, per se, but have proven very useful for biochemical studies.[105,106]

Microvascular studies

Some of the classical preparations for microvascular studies include hamster cheek pouches, rat cremaster muscle, cat, mouse and rat mesenteric preparations, bat wings, frog toe-web, human cuticle and other similar experimental setups. Many of these preparations were developed almost concurrently with the light microscope. A more recent development has been described by Greenblatt and his associates from a technique first detailed by Gilmore and Zipes.[101] This preparation allows *in vivo* studies of the coronary microcirculation as well as electrophysiological studies. Functioning hamster neonatal cardiac tissue is transplanted to the adult hamster cheek pouch. Cubes of 1-2 mm of transmural right atrial and left ventricular endocardial sections have been used for this purpose.[101,102,103,104]

Chilian et al. developed a unique and ingenious system for measuring epicardial coronary microvessel diameters and pressures in a beating, *in situ* cat heart.[197] This system uses high frequency jet ventilation to minimize artifact produced by lung inflation/deflation. The left ventricle is partially restrained to eliminate the up-and-down movement associated with ventricular contraction. This enables the spatial relationship between the epicardial surface and the objective lens of the intravital microscope to be maintained. The epicardium is illuminated with a xenon arc stroboscopic light source. The strobe light is triggered by a computer programmed to synchronize the light with a predetermine gate off a left ventricular pressure pulse signal. Vascular diameters are measured by capturing a video image at different times during the cardiac cycle with the strobe light and analyzing the freeze-frame images. Small vessel intravascular pressures are measured using a micropipette system in which the micropipette is mounted in an electromechanical micromanipulator, termed the "Wobbler". This device consists of electromagnets arranged so that their field strengths are perpendicular to each other in a 3-dimensional array. The system moves in the X,Y and Z axes and is synchronized to the movement of a particular epicardial microvessel on the myocardium. The vessel appears stationary because the strobe is flashed once per cardiac cycle at the same temporal point during each cardiac cycle. The operator uses a joy stick to track the microvessel. The computer program replicates the exact position of the micropipette for a certain point in the cardiac cycle. Once the operator tracks the vessel over a few composite cardiac cycles the computer program correctly replicates the full cycle of movement by using the Wobbler to move the micropipette. The micropipette was then advanced into the microvessel and the pressure can be measured using standard servonull microvascular techniques. Chilian and DeFily recently reviewed a variety of methodological approaches for the study of the coronary microcirculation *in situ*.[198] Chilian also describes techniques for studying the subendocardial microcirculation.[199]

Experimental endocarditis/carditis

Beagles iatrogenically infected with an opossum-derived strain of *Trypanosoma cruzi* demonstrate features of early and chronic chagasic cardiomyopathy, i.e. increases in PR interval, A-V block, premature ventricular contractions, ventricular tachycardia and decreased LV ejection fraction. Infection with a canine strain of the same organism did not result in these signs. The opossum-derived strain was found to produce the typical signs via depression of β-adrenergic adenylate cyclase activity as a result of changes in the G_s protein complex, most likely resulting in an uncoupling of the β-adrenergic receptor from the G_s protein.[200]

Round heart disease, a viral myocarditis of turkeys, produces left atrial and left ventricular dilatation, reduced LV shortening fraction, systemic hypotension, low cardiac output, relative subendocardial underperfusion and an increase in ventricular mass. It is said to be a useful model for congestive cardiomyopathy.[201]

When certain genetic strains of rabbits are given repeated infections, by intradermal injection of group A streptococci, a few of the rabbits will develop focal cardiac lesions characterized by acute and chronic inflammation. It is not certain, from the work that has been done on this model, that the group A streptococcus is solely responsible for the lesions seen. Cardiac lesions resembling those associated with rheumatic fever have also been produced using viridans streptococci, various streptococcal culture filtrates, crystalline streptococcal proteinase, sonicated streptococci and various group A streptococcal constituents, including cell wall components. Mice, rabbits, and monkeys infected with group A streptococci by the pharyngeal route have been shown to develop scattered myocardial inflammatory reactions but they only slightly resemble the classical Aschoff bodies. Rheumatic-like lesions have also been produced in rabbits and rats using a variety of immunological procedures including the use of; duck anti-rabbit heart sera, injecting nephrectomized rabbits with massive doses of gamma globulin, mixtures of rat heart extract and dead hemolytic streptococci, rabbit heart extract emulsified with paraffin, and isologous heart homogenates. Serum sickness will also cause rheumatic-like lesions. No reproducible *in vivo* or *in vitro* model systems using cross-reacting antibody have been found as of this writing. There are some indications, but a lack of experimental evidence, the viral or other infectious agents are also involved in the etiology of rheumatic fever. There is also circumstantial evidence that genetic susceptibility may be involved.[107]

Polyethylene catheters with their tips at the entrance to or within the right side of the heart have been shown to produce sterile marantic endocarditis and tricuspid valvulitis. Introducing as few at 100 microorganisms within the catheter predictably produces staphylococcal endocarditis. It is suggested that this model is suitable for the study of the bacteriological, pathological, and immunologic aspects of bacterial endocarditis and reproduces some of the complications of indwelling venous catheters in humans.[202]

References

1. Higgins, C.B., Panalec, R., Vatner, S.F., Modified technique for production of experimental right-sided congestive heart failure, *Cardiovasc. Res.*, 7:860-878, 1973

2. Conway, G., Heazlitt, R.A., Montag, J., Mattingly, S.F., The ATPase activity of cardiac myosin from failing and hypertrophied hearts, *J. Mol. Cell. Cardiol.*, 7:817-822, 1975

3. Braunwald, E., Mechanics and energetics of the normal and failing heart, *Trans. Assoc. Am. Phys.*, 84:63-72, 1971

4. Bishop, S.P., Melsen, L.R., Myocardial necrosis, fibrosis and DNA synthesis in experimental cardiac hypertrophy induced by sudden pressure overload, *Circ. Res.*, 39:238-241, 1976

5. Spann, J.F. Jr., Buccino, R.A., Sonnenblick, E.H., Production of right ventricular hypertrophy with and without congestive heart failure in the cat, *Proc. Soc. Exp. Biol. Med.*, 125:522-524, 1967

6. Mirsky, I., Laks, M.M., Time course of changes in the mechanical properties of the canine right and left ventricles during hypertrophy caused by pressure overload., *Circ. Res.*, 46:530-542, 1980

7. Cooper, G., Marino, T.A., Complete reversibility of cat right ventricular chronic progressive pressure overload, *Circ. Res.*, 54:323-331, 1984

8. Pirzada, F.A., Ekong, E.A., Vokonas, P.S., Apstein, C.S., Hood, W.B.Jr., Experimental myocardial infarction. XIII. Sequential changes in left ventricular pressure-length relationships in the acute phase, *Circ.*, 53:970-975, 1976

9. Gestler, M.M., Production of experimental congestive heart failure in the guinea pig, *Proc. Soc. Exp. Biol. Med.*, 102:396-397, 1959

10. Sasayama, S., Ross, J.Jr., Franklin, D., Bloor, C.M., Bishop, S.P., Dilley, R.B., Adaptations of the left ventricle to chronic pressure overload, *Circ. Res.*, 38:172-178, 1976

11. Gaertner, R.A., Blalock, A., Experimental coarctation of the ascending aorta, *Surgery*, 40:712-717, 1956

12. McLaughlin, J.S., Morrow, A.G., Buckley, M.J., The experimental production of hypertrophic subaortic stenosis, *J. Thorac. Cardiovasc. Surg.*, 48:695-703, 1964

13. O'Kane, H.O., Geha, A.S., Kleiger, R.E., Abe, T., Salaymeh, M.T., Malik, A.B., Stable left ventricular hypertrophy in the dog, *J. Thorac. Cardiovasc. Surg.*, 65:264-271, 1973

14. Rodger, W.A., Bishop, S.P., Hamlin, R.L., Experimental production of supravalvular aortic stenosis in the dog, *J. Appl. Physiol.*, 30:917-920, 1971

15. Taylor, D.E.M., Whamond, J.S., A method of producing graded stenosis of the aortic and mitral valves in sheep for fluid dynamic studies, *J. Physiol. (London)*, 244:16-17, 1975

16. Griggs, D.M.Jr., Chen, C.C., Tchokaer, V.V., Subendocardial anaerobic metabolism in experimental aortic stenosis, *Am. J. Physiol.*, 224:607-612, 1973

17. Iyengor, S.R.R., Charrettee, E.J.P., Iyengor, C.K.S., An experimental model with left ventricular hypertrophy caused by subcoronary aortic stenosis in dogs, *J. Thorac. Cardiovasc. Surg.*, 66:823-827, 1973

18. Crozatier, B., Caillet, D., Bical, O., Left ventricular adaptation to sustained pressure overload in the conscious dog, *Circ. Res.*, 54:21-29, 1984

19. Taylor, R.R., Covell, J.W., Boss, J.Jr., Left ventricular function in experimental aorta-caval fistula with circulatory congestion and fluid retention, *J. Clin. Invest.*, 47:1333-1342, 1968

20. Wollenberger, A., Responses of the heart mitochondria to chronic cardiac overload and physical exercise, *Rec. Adv. Stud. Cardiol. Metab.*, 1:213-220, 1972

21. Schwartz, A., Biochemical studies concerning etiology of hypertrophy, heart failure and cardiomyopathy, *Rec. Adv. Stud. Cardiol. Metab.*, 2:501-509, 1973

22. Crawford, M.H., Badke, F.R., Amon, K.W., Effect of the undisturbed pericardium on left ventricular size and performance during acute volume loading, *Am. Heart J.*, 105:267-272, 1983

23. Porter, C.B., Walsh, R.A., Badke, F.R., O'Rourke, R.A., Differential effects of dilitiazem and nitroprusside on left ventricular function in experimental chronic volume overload, *Circ.*, 68:685-692, 1983

24. Flaim, S.F., Minteer, W.J., Nellis, S.H., Clark, D.P., Chronic arteriovenous shunt: evaluation of a model for heart failure in rat, *Am. J. Physiol.*, 236:H698-H704, 1979

25. Flaim, S.F., Peripheral vascular effects of nitroglycerin in a conscious rat model of heart failure, *Am. J. Physiol.*, 243:H974-H981, 1982

26. Spratt, J.A., Olsen, C.O., Tyson, G.S.Jr., Glower, D.D.Jr., Davis, J.W., Rankin, J.S., Experimental mitral regurgitation. Physiological effects of correction on left ventricular dynamics, *J. Thorac. Cardiovasc. Surg.*, 86:479-489, 1983

27. Morais, D.J., Richart, T.S., Fritz, A.J., Acree, P.W., Davila, J.C., Glover, R.P., The production of chronic experimental mitral insufficiency, *Ann. Surg.*, 145:500-508, 1957

28. Fizelona, A., Figel, A., Myocardial metabolic changes in cardiac hypertrophy and heart failure, *Rec. Adv. Stud. Cardiol. Struc. Metab.*, 1:200-210, 1972

29. Ito, J., Suko, J., Chidsey, C.A., Intracellular calcium and myocardial contractility. V. Calcium uptake of sarcoplasmic reticulum fractions in hypertrophied and failing rabbit hearts, *J. Mol. Cell. Cardiol.*, 6:237-243, 1974

30. Copeland, J.G., Marm, B.J., Luka, N.L., Ferrans, V.J., Michaelis, L.L., Experimental production of aortic valvular stenosis: short-term and long-term studies in dogs, *J. Thorac. Cardiovasc. Surg.*, 67:361-379, 1974

31. Salerno, R.A., The experimental production of valvular aortic stenosis, *Ann. Surg.*, 149:368-373, 1959

32.   Allard, J.R., O'Neill, M.J.Jr., Hoffman, J.I.E., Valvular subcoronary aortic stenosis in dogs, *Am. J. Physiol.*, 236:H780-H784, 1979

33.   Attarian, D.E., Jones, R.N., Currie, W.D., Hill, R.C., Sink, J.D., Olsen, C.O., Chitwood, W.R.Jr., Wechsler, A.S., Characteristics of chronic left ventricular hypertrophy induced by subcoronary valvular aortic stenosis, *J. Thorac. Cardiovasc. Surg.*, 81:382-388, 1981

34.   Roper, K.O., Levitsky, O.S., Vorachek, M.A., Wright, R.N., Eckner, F.A.O., Feinberg, H., Development of a new model of subcoronary valvular aortic stenosis to create ventricular hypertrophy, *J. Surg. Res.*, 24:302-306, 1979

35.   Sink, J.D., Attarian, D.E., Chitwood, W.R.Jr., Hill, R.C., Pellom, G.L., Wechsler, A.S., An improved technique for producing ventricular hypertrophy with a subcoronary valvular aortic stenosis model, *Ann. Thorac. Surg.*, 30:285-290, 1980

36.   Su-Fan, Q., Brum, J.M., Kaye, M.P., Bove, A.A., A new technique for producing aortic stenosis in animals, *Am. J. Physiol.*, 246:H296-H301, 1984

37.   Raju, S., Cibulski, A., Hendrix, M.B., Experimental induction of intrinsic valve stenosis, *Am. Surg.*, 46:485-493, 1980

38.   Button, C., Gross, D.R., Allert, J.A., Applications of individualized digoxin dosage regimens to canine therapeutic digitalization, *Am. J. Vet. Res.*, 41:1238-1242, 1980

39.   Schapes, W., The collateral circulation of the heart, Elsevier/North-Holland, Amsterdam, 1979

40.   Hearse, D.J., Models and problems in the study of myocardial ischemia and tissue protection, *Eur. Heart J.*, C:43-48, 1983

41.   Verdouw, P.D., Wolffenbuttel, B.H., van der Glessen, W.J., Domestic pigs in the study of myocardial ischemia, *Eur. Heart J.*, C-61-67, 1983

42.   Eckstein, R.W., Coronary interarterial anastomoses in young pigs and mongrel dogs, *Circ. Res.*, 11:460-465, 1954

43.   Brooks, H., Al-Sadir, J.,Schwartz, J., Rich, B., Harper, P., Resnekor, L., Biventricular dynamics during quantitated anteroseptal infarction in the porcine heart, *Am. J. Cardiol.*, 36:765-774, 1975

44.   Opie, L.H., Bruyneel, K.J., Lube, W.F., What has the baboon to offer as a model of experimental ischemia?, *Eur. Heart J.*, C:55-60, 1983

45.   Groover, M.E., Seljeskog, E.L., Haglin, J.J., Hitchcock, C.R., The relationship of coronary disease to myocardial infarction in the baboon. In Vagtbord, H., ed. The baboon in medical research, Southwest Foundation for Research and Education, University of Texas Press: 543-556, 1965

46.   Scher, A.M., Ohm, W.W., Burngarner, K., Boynton, R., Young, A.C., Sympathetic and parasympathetic control of heart rate in the dog, baboon and man, *Fed. Proc.*, 31:1219-1225, 1972

47.   Hood, W.B.Jr., Bianco, J.A., Kumar, R., Experimental myocardial infarction IV. Reduction of left ventricular compliance in the healing phase, *J. Clin. Invest.*, 49:1316-1328, 1967

48.   Smith, G.T., Soeter, J.R., Haston, H.H., McNamara, J.J., Coronary reperfusion in primates. Serial electrocardiographic and histologic assessment, *J. Clin. Invest.*, 54:1420-1427, 1974

49.   Opie, L.H., Owen, P., Glycolysis in acute experimental myocardial infarction: pathways of metabolism and preliminary results, *Rec. Adv. Stud. Card. Struc. Metab.*, 2:567-579, 1973

50.   Gross, D.R., Animal Models in Cardiovascular Research, Chp 1 in Quantitative Cardiovascular Studies, ed. Hwang, Gross, Patel, University Park Press, Baltimore, 1979

51.   Wilde, J., Sedlarik, K., Eger, H., Renniman, G., Limitations of and criteria for a coronary thrombosis model, *Z. Exp. Chir.*, 9:296-301, 1976

52.   Sedlarik, K., Eger, H., Wilde, J., Vollmar, F., Reimann, G., Schilling B., Seelig, G., Fiehring, H., Experimental model of coronary thrombosis in the closed thorax in swine, Z. Exp. Chir., 9:302-315, 1976

53.   Elzinga, W.E., Skinner, D.B., Hemodynamic characteristics of critical stenosis in canine coronary arteries, *J. Thorac. Cardiovasc. Surg.*, 69:217-222, 1975

54.   van der Meer, J.J., Reneman, R.S., An improved technique to induce a standardized functional stenosis of a coronary artery, *Eur. Surg. Res.*, 4:407-418, 1972

55.   Hosko, M.J., Gross, G.J., Warltier, D.C., Technique for precise, graded arterial stenosis and occlusion, *Bas. Res. Cardiol.*, 72:651-659, 1977

56.   Berguer, R., Hwang, N.H.C., Critical arterial stenosis: a theoretical and experimental solution, *Ann. Surg.*, 180:39-45, 1974

57.   Gould, K.L., Lipscomb, K., Calvert, C., Compensatory changes of the distal coronary vascular bed during progressive coronary constriction, *Circ.*, 51:1085-1094, 1975

58.   Spear, J.F., Michelson, E.L., Moore, E.N., The use of animal models in the study of the electrophysiology of sudden coronary deaths, *Ann. NY Acad. Sci.*, 382:78-89, 1982

59. Patterson, R.E., Jones-Collins, B.A., Aamodt, R., Impaired collateral blood flow reserve early after nontransmural myocardial infarction in conscious dogs, *Am. J. Cardiol.*, 50:1133-1140, 1982

60. Khouri, E.M., Gregg, D.E., An inflatable cuff for zero determination in blood flow studies, *J. Appl. Physiol.*, 23:395-397, 1967

61. Murdock, R.H.Jr., Harlan, D.M., Morris, J.J., Pryor, W.W.Jr., Cobb, F.R., Transitional blood flow zones between ischemic and nonischemic myocardium in the awake dog. Analysis based on distribution of the intramural vasculature, *Circ. Res.*, 52:451-459, 1983

62. Huddleston, C.B., Lupinetti, F.M., Laws, K.H., Collins, J.C., Clanton, J.A., Hawiger, J.J., Oates, J.A., Hammon, J.W.Jr., The effects of Ro-29-4679, a thromboxane synthetase inhibitor, on ventricular fibrillation induced by coronary artery occlusion in conscious dogs, *Circ. Res.*, 52:608-613, 1983

63. Jacobsen, E.D., Swan, K.G., Hydraulic occluder for chronic electromagnetic blood flow determinations, *J. Appl. Physiol.*, 21:1400-1402, 1966

64. Debley, V.G., Miniature hydraulic occluder for zero blood flow determination, *J. Appl. Physiol.*, 31, 138-139, 1971

65. Neill, W.A., Oxendine, J., Phelps, N., Anderson, R.P., Subendocardial ischemia provoked by tachycardia in conscious dogs with coronary stenosis, *Am. J. Cardiol.*, 35:30-36, 1976

66. Hirsch, L.J., Rone, A.S., Mesenteric blood flow response to dopamine infusion during myocardial infarction in the awake dog, *Circ. Shock*, 10:173-178, 1983

67. Grunwald, A.M., Watson, D.D., Holzgrefe, H.H.Jr., Irving, J.F., Beller, G.A., Myocardial [201]thallium kinetics in normal and ischemic myocardium, *Circ.* 64:610-618, 1981

68. Litvak, J., Siderides, L.E., Vinoberg, A.M., The experimental production of coronary artery insufficiency and occlusion, *Am. Heart J.*, 53:505-518, 1957

69. Berman, J.K., Fields, D.C., Judy, H., Mori, V., Parker, R.J., Gradual vascular occlusion, *Surgery*, 39:399-410, 1956

70. Bredee, J.J., Blickman, J.R., Homan van der Heide, J.N., Kootstra, G.J., Zeelenberg, H.J., Zijlstra, W.G., Standardized induction of myocardial ischemia in the dog, *Eur. Surg. Res.*, 17:269-286, 1975

71. Elliot, E.C., Jones, E.L., Bloor, C.M., Lean, A.S., Gregg, D.E., Day-to-day changes in coronary hemodynamics secondary to constriction of circumflex branch of left coronary artery in conscious dog, *Circ. Res.*, 22:237-242, 1968

72. Franciosa, J.A., Hechel, R., Limas, C., Chon, J.N., Progressive myocardial dysfunction associated with increased vascular resistance, *Am. J. Physiol.*, 239:H477-H482, 1980

73. Stone, H.L., Bishop, V.S., Guyton, A.C., Cardiac function after embolization of coronaries with microspheres, *Am. J. Physiol.*, 204:16-27, 1963

74. Marcus, E., Katz, L.N., Pick, R., Stamler, J., The production of myocardial infarction, chronic coronary insufficiency and chronic coronary heart disease in the dog, *Acta. Cardiol.*, 13:190-198, 1958

75. Young, D.F., Cholrin, N.R., Roth, A.C., Pressure drop across artificially induced stenosis in the femoral arteries of dogs, *Circ. Res.*, 36:735-743, 1975

76. Kordenat, R.K., Electrocardiogram during experimental coronary thrombolysis, *J. Electrocardiol.*, 9:41-46, 1976

77. Kordenat, R.K., Kezdi, P., Stanley, F.L., A new catheter technique for producing experimental coronary thrombosis and selective coronary visualization, *Am. Heart J.*, 83:360-367, 1972

78. Romson, J.L., Bush, L.R., Haack, D.W., Lucchesi, B.R., The beneficial effects of oral ibuprofen on coronary artery thrombosis and myocardial ischemia in the conscious dog, *J. Pharmacol. Exp. Ther.*, 215:271-278, 1980

79. Gallagher, K.P., Folts, J.D., Rowe, G.G., Comparison of coronary arteriograms with direct measurements of stenosed coronary arteries in dogs, *Am. Heart J.*, 95:338-347, 1978

80. Folts, J.D., Crowell, E.B., Rowe, G.G., Platelet aggregation in partially obstructed vessels and its elimination with aspirin, *Circ.*, 54:365-370, 1976

81. Malik, A.B., Pulmonary microembolism, *Physiol. Rev.*, 63:1114-1207, 1983

82. Wolf, H.R., Seeger, H.W., Experimental and clinical results in shock lung treatment with vitamin E., *Ann. NY Acad. Sci.*, 393:392-410, 1982

83. Shelub, I., van Grondelle, A., McCullough, R., Hofmeister, S., Reeves, J.T., A model of embolic chronic pulmonary hypertension in the dog, *J. Appl. Physiol.*, 56:810-815, 1984

84.   Ungerleider, R.M., Holman, W.L., Stanley, T.E., Lofland, G.K., Williams, J.M., Smith, P.K., Quick, G., Cox, J.L., Encircling endocardial ventriculotomy for refractory ischemic ventricular tachycardia. II. Effects on regional myocardial blood flow, *J. Thorac. Cardiovasc. Surg.*, 83:850-856, 1982

85.   Weir, E.K., McMustry, I.F., Grover, R.F., Experimental models of complete heart block, *Basic Res. Cardiol.*, 70:446-455, 1975

86.   Leininger, B.J., Raghunath, T.K., Neville, J.A., A simplified method of producing experimental heart block, *Ann. Thorac. Surg.*, 10:560-562, 1970

87.   Starzl, T.E., Gaertner, R., Chronic heart block in dogs. A method for producing experimental heart failure, *Circ.*, 12:259-270, 1955

88.   Leimgruber, P.P., Klopfenstein, H.S., Wann, L.S., Brooks, H.L., The hemodynamic derangement associated with right ventricular diastolic collapse in cardiac tamponade: an experimental echocardiographic study, *Circ.*, 68:612-620, 1983

89.   Stone, H.L., Bishop, V.S., Guyton, A.C., Progressive changes in cardiovascular function after unilateral heart irradiation, *Am. J. Physiol.*, 206:289-294, 1964

90.   Stone, H.L., Bishop, V.S., Guyton, A.C., Ventricular function following radiation damage of the right ventricle, *Am. J. Physiol.*, 211:1209-1213, 1966

91.   Carlyle, P.F., Cohn, J.N., A nonsurgical canine model of chronic left ventricular myocardial dysfunction, *Am. J. Physiol.*, 244:H769-H774, 1983

92.   Mehta, J., Runge, W., Cohn, J.N., Carlyle, P., Myocardial damage after repetitive direct current shock in the dog: correlation between left ventricular end-diastolic pressure and extent of myocardial necrosis, *J. Lab. Clin. Med.*, 91:272-279, 1978

93.   Cleghorn, R.A., Cardiovascular failure in experimental adrenal insufficiency: a historical revival, *Perspect. Biol. Med.*, 27:135-155, 1983

94.   Bonilla, C.A., DiClementi, D., MacCarter, D.J., Hemodynamic effects of slow and rapid defibrination with defibrizyme, the thrombin-like enzyme from venom of the timber rattlesnake, *Am. Heart J.*, 90:43-49, 1975

95.   Halvarsen, J.F., Myking, A.O., Prehepatic portal hypertension in the rat. Immediate and long-term effects on portal vein and aortic pressure of a graded portal vein stenosis, followed by occlusion of the portal vein and spleno-renal collaterals, *Eur. Surg. Res.*, 11:89-98, 1979

96.   Hearse, D.J., Chain, E.B., The role of glucose in the survival and recovery of the anoxic isolated perfused rat heart, *Biochem. J.*, 128:1125-1133, 1972

97.   Scheuer, J., The advantages and disadvantages of the isolated perfused working rat heart, *Med. Sci. Sports*, 9:231-238, 1977

98.   Okamatsu, S., Lefer, A.M., The protective effects of nifedipine in the isolated cat heart, *J. Surg. Res.*, 35:35-40, 1983

99.   Serur, J.R., Galyean, J.R., Urschel, C.W., Sonnenblick, E.H., Experimental myocardial ischemia: dynamic alterations in ventricular contractility and relaxation with dissociation of speed and force in the isovolumic dog heart, *Circ. Res.*, 39:602-607, 1976

100.   Elzinga, G., Westerhof, N., Pump function of the feline left heart: changes with heart rate and its bearing on the energy balance, *Cardiovasc. Res.*, 14:81-92, 1980

101.   Gilmour, R.F.Jr., Zipes, D.P., Electrophysiological response of vascularized hamster cardiac transplants to ischemia, *Circ. Res.*, 50:599-609, 1982

102.   Greenblatt, M., Choudari, K.U.R., Sanders, A.G., Subik, P., Mammalian microcirculation in the living animal: methodologic considerations, *Microvasc. Res.*, 1:420-432, 1969

103.   Greenblatt, M., Kaufman, J., Choudari, K.U.R., Functioning heart homografts in hamsters, *Transplantation*, 11:50-55, 1971

104.   Cornish, K.G., Joyner, W.L., Gilmore, J.P., Evidence for the conversion of angiotensin I to angiotensin II by the coronary microcirculation, *Blood Vessels*, 16:241-246, 1979

105.   Ingwall, J.S., Roeske, W.R., Wildenthal, K., The fetal mouse heart in organ culture: Maintenance of the differential state. *in* Methods in Cell Biology, ed. by Harris, C.C., Trump, B.F., Stoner, G.D., New York, Academic Press Inc.: 167-185, 1980

106.   Wildenthal, K., Longterm maintenance of spontaneously beating mouse hearts in organ culture, *J. Appl. Physiol.*, 30:153-157, 1971

107.   Unny, S.K., Middlebrooks, B.L., Streptococcal rheumatic carditis, *Microbiol. Rev.*, 47:97-120, 1983

108.   Helnius, G., Myocardial infarction without coronary occlusion. A study with a new experimental model in sheep, *J. Med. Sci.* (Suppl.), 29:1-28, 1980

109. Spann, J.F., Buccino, R.A., Sonnenblick, E.H., Braunwald, E., Contractile state of cardiac muscle obtained from cats with experimentally produced ventricular hypertrophy and heart failure, *Circ. Res.*, 21:341-354, 1967

110. Anderson, P.A.W., Manring, A., Arentzen, C.E., Rankin, J.S., Johnson, E.A., Pressure-induced hypertrophy of cat right ventricle, *Circ. Res.*, 41:582-588, 1977

111. Bassett, A.L., Gelband, H., Chronic partial occlusion of the pulmonary artery in cats, *Circ. Res.*, 32:15-26, 1973

112. Holman, E.F., Hemicardiac hypertrophy due to increased peripheral resistance: a study of pulmonic and aortic stenosis experimentally produced, *J. Thorac. Surg.*, 9:262-273, 1940

113. Gerbode, F., Selzer, A., Experimental cardiac hypertrophy: the acute effect of pulmonic and aortic stenosis, *Surgery*, 24:505-511, 1948

114. Laks, M.M., Morady, F., Garner, D., Swann, H.J.S., Relation of ventricular volume, compliance, and mass in the normal and pulmonary arterial banded heart, *Cardiovasc. Res.*, 6:187-198, 1972

115. Wyse, R.K.H., Welham, K.C., Jones, M., Silove, E.E., de Leval, M.R., Haemodynamics, regional myocardial blood flow and sarcoplasmic reticulum calcium uptake in right ventricular hypertrophy and failure, *Adv. Myocardial.*, 4:97-105, 1983

116. Welham, K.C., Silove, E.D., Wyse, R.K.H., Experimental right ventricular hypertrophy and failure in swine, *Cardiovasc. Res.*, 12:61-65, 1978

117. Burrington, J.D., Response to experimental coarctation of aorta and pulmonic stenosis in fetal lamb, *J. Thorac. Cardiovasc. Surg.*, 75:819-826, 1978

118. Manohar, M., Bisgard, G.E., Bullard, V., Rankin, J.H.G., Blood flow in the hypertrophied right ventricular myocardium of unanaesthetized ponies, *Am. J. Physiol.*, 240:H881-H888, 1981

119. Dhalla, N.S., Das, P.K., Sharma, G.P., Subcellular basis of cardiac contractile failure, *J. Mol. Cell. Cardiol.*, 10:363-385, 1978

120. Mercadier, J.J., Lompre, A.M., Wisnewski, C., Samuel, J.L., Bercovici, J., Swynghedauw, B., Schwartz, K., Myosin isoenzyme changes in several models of rat cardiac hypertrophy, *Circ. Res.*, 49:525-532, 1981

121. Alexander, N., Hinshaw, L.B., Drury, D.R., Mechanism of congestive heart failure following aorta constriction in rabbits, *Circ. Res.*, 5:375-381, 1957

122. Sordahl, L.A., Wood, W.G., Schwartz, A., Production of cardiac hypertrophy and failure in rabbits with ameroid clips, *J. Mol. Cell. Cardiol.*, 1:341-344, 1970

123. Gaertner, R.A., Blalock, A., Experimental coarctation of the ascending aorta, *Surgery*, 40:712-717, 1956

124. Kleinmann, L.H., Wichsler, A.S., Rembert, J.C., Fedor, J.M., Greenfield, J.C., A reproducible model of moderate to severe concentric left ventricular hypertrophy, *Am. J. Physiol.*, 234:H515-H519, 1978

125. Womble, J.R., Haddox, M.K., Russell, D.H., Epinephrine elevation in plasma parallels canine cardiac hypertrophy, *Life Sci.*, 23:1951-1957, 1979

126. Rogers, W.A., Bishop, S.P., Hamlin, R.L., Experimental production of supravalvular aortic stenosis in the dog, *J. Appl. Physiol.*, 30:917-920, 1971

127. Iyengar, S.R.K., Charnette, E.J.P., Iyendor, C.K.S., Lynn, R.B., An experimental model with left ventricular hypertrophy caused by subcoronary aortic stenosis in dogs, *J. Thorac. Cardiovasc. Surg.*, 66:823-827, 1973

128. Leclercq, J.F., Sebag, C., Swynghedauw, B., Experimental cardiac hypertrophy in rabbits after aortic stenosis or incompetence or both, *Biomedicine*, 28:180-184, 1978

129. Copeland, J.G., Maron, B.J., Luka, N.L., Ferrans, V.J., Michaelis, L.L., Experimental production of aortic valvular stenosis: short-term and long-term studies in dogs, *J. Thorac. Cardiovasc. Surg.*, 67:371-379, 1974

130. Allard, J.R., O'Neill, M.J., Hoffman, J.I.E., Valvular subcoronary aortic stenosis in dogs, *Am. J. Physiol.*, 236:H780-H784, 1979

131. Carabello, B.A., Mee, R., Collins, J.J., Kloner, R.A., Levin, D., Grossman, W., Contractile function in chronic gradually developing subcoronary aortic stenosis, *Am. J. Physiol.*, 240:H80-H86, 1981

132. Barger, A.C., Roe, B.B., Richardson, G.S., Relation of valvular lesions and of exercise to auricular pressure, work tolerance, and to the development of chronic, congestive failure in dogs, *Am. J. Physiol.*, 169:384-399, 1952

133. Ishihara, K., Zile, M.R., Tomita, M., Tanaka, R., Kanazawa, S., Carabello, B.A., Left ventricular hypertrophy in a canine model of reversible pressure overload, *Cardiovasc. Res.*, 26:580-585, 1992

134. Buccino, R.A., Harris, E., Spann, J.F., Sonnenblick, E.H., Response of myocardial connective tissue to development of experimental hypertrophy, *Am. J. Physiol.*, 216:425-428, 1969

135. Olivetti, G., Lagrasta, C., Ricci, R., Sonnenblick, E.H., Capasso, J.M., Anversa, P., Long-term pressure-induced cardiac hypertrophy: capillary and mast cell proliferation, *Am. J. Physiol.*, 257:H1766-H1772, 1989

136. Liu, Z., Hilbelink, D.R., Crockett, W.B., Gerdes, A.M., Regional changes in hemodynamics and cardiac myocyte size in rats with aortocaval fistulas, 1. Developing and established hypertrophy, *Circ. Res.*, 69:52-58, 1991

137. Liu, Z., Hilbelink, D.R., Gerdes, A.M., Regional changes in hemodynamics and cardiac myocyte size in rats with aortocaval fistulas, 2. Long-term effects, *Circ. Res.*, 69:59-65, 1991

138. Garcia, R., Lachance, D., Thibault, G., Atrial natriuretic factor release and natriuresis in rats with high-output heart failure, *Am. J. Physiol.*, 259:H1374-H1379, 1990

139. Gewillig, M., Daenen, W., Aubert, A., van der Hauwaert, L., Abolishment of chronic volume overload: implications for diastolic function of the systemic ventricle immediately after Fontan repair, *Circ. (Suppl. II)*, 86:II-93-II-99, 1992

140. Kinney, T.E., Olinger, G.N., Sagar, K.B., Boerboom, L.E., Acute, reversible tricuspid insufficiency: creation in a canine model., *Am. J. Physiol.*, 260:H638-H641, 1991

141. Sabbah, H.N., Stein, P.D., Kono, T., Gheorghiade, M., Levine, T.B., Jafri, S., Hawkins, E.T., Goldstein, S., A canine model of chronic heart failure produced by multiple sequential coronary microembolizations, *Am. J. Physiol.*, 260:H1379-H1384, 1991

142. Salazar, A.E., Experimental myocardial infarction, induction of coronary thrombosis in the intact closed-chest dog, *Circ. Res.*, 9:135-136, 1961

143. Schumacher, W.A., Lee, E.C., Lucchesi, B.R., Augmentation of streptokinase-induced thrombolysis by heparin and prostacyclin, *J. Cardiovasc. Pharmacol.*, 7:739-746, 1985

144. Benedict, C.R., Matthew, B., Rex, K.A., Cartwright, J.Jr., Sordahl, L.A., Correlation of plasma serotonin changes with platelet aggregation in an in vivo dog model of spontaneous occlusive coronary thrombus formation, *Circ. Res.*, 58:58-67, 1988

145. Collen, D., Stassen, J.M., Verstraete, M., Thrombolysis with human extrinsic (tissue-type) plasminogen activator in rabbits with experimental jugular vein thrombosis, *J. Clin. Invest.*, 71:368-376, 1983

146. Gold, H.K., Fallon, J.T., Yasuda, T., Leinbach, R.C., Khaw, B.A., Newell, J.B., Guerrero, J.L., Vislosky, F.M., Hoyng, C.F., Grossbard, E., Collen, D., Coronary thrombolysis with recombinant human tissue-type plasminogen activator, *Circ.*, 70:700-707, 1984

147. Reimer, K.A., Jennings, R.B., Cobb, F.R., Murdock, R.H., Greenfield, J.C.Jr., Becker, L.C., Bulkley, B.H., Hutchins, G.M., Schwartz, R.P.Jr., Bailey, K.R., Passamani, E.R., Animal models for protecting ischemic myocardium: results of the NHLBI cooperative study: comparison of unconscious and conscious dog models, *Circ. Res.*, 56:651-665, 1985

148. Kitzen, J.M., McCallum, J.D., Harvey, C., Morin, M.E., Antithrombotic activity of the phosphodiesterase III inhibitor pelrinone in a canine model of coronary artery thrombosis: enhancement of efficacy with concurrent α_2-adrenergic antagonism, *J. Cardiovasc. Pharmacol.*, 18:777-790, 1991

149. Hartman, J.C., Kampine, J.P., Schmeling, W.T., Warltier, D.C., Actions of isoflurane on myocardial perfusion in chronically instrumented dogs with poor, moderate, or well-developed coronary collaterals, *J. Cardiothorac. Anesth.*, 4:715-725, 1990

150. Hartman, J.C., Kampine, J.P., Schmeling, W.T., Warltier, D.C., Alterations in collateral blood flow produced by isoflurane in a chronically instrumented canine model of multivessel coronary artery disease, *Anesth.*, 74:120-133, 1991

151. Nishikimi, T., Uchino, K., Frohlich, E.D., Effects of α_1-adrenergic blockade on intrarenal hemodynamics in heart failure rats, *Am. J. Physiol.*, 262:R198-R203, 1992

152. Anversa, P., Loud, A.V., Levicky, V., Guideri, G., Left ventricular failure induced by myocardial infarction. I. Myocyte hypertrophy, *Am. J. Physiol.*, 248:H876-H882, 1985

153. Anversa, P., Loud, A.V., Levicky, V., Guideri, G., Left ventricular failure induced by myocardial infarction. II. Tissue morphometry, *Am. J. Physiol.*, 248:H883-H889, 1985

154. Hirsch, A.T., Talsness, C.E., Schunkert, H., Paul, M., Dzau, V.J., Tissue-specific activation of cardiac angiotensin converting enzyme in experimental heart failure, *Circ. Res.*, 69:475-482, 1991

155. Mill, J.G., Stefanon, I., Leite, C.M., Vassallo, D.V., Changes in performance of the surviving myocardium after left ventricular infarction in rats, *Cardiovasc. Res.*, 24:748-753, 1990

156. Kedem, J., Zurovski, Y., Miller, H., Battler, A., Effect of reserpine upon the haemodynamic course of recovery following experimental myocardial infarction, *Arch. Internat. Physiol. Bioch.*, 88:427-436, 1980

157. van Woerkens, L.J., van der Giessen, W.J., Verdouw, P.D., Cardiovascular effects of dopamine and dobutamine in conscious pigs with chronic heart failure, *Critical Care Med.*, 21:420-424, 1993

158. Sakai, K., Watanabe, K., Millard, R.W., Defining the mechanical border zone: a study in the pig heart, *Am. J. Physiol.*, 249:H88-H94, 1985

159. Gillebert, T.C., de Hert, S.G., Andries, L.J., Jageneau, A.H., Brutsaert, D.L., Intracavitary ultrasound impairs left ventricular performance: presumed role of endocardial endothelium, *Am. J. Physiol.*, 263:H857-H865, 1992

160. Bishop, S.P., Sole, M.J., Tilley, L.P., Cardiomyopathies. *in* Spontaneous Animal Models of Human Diseases, ed. by Andrews, E.J., Ward, B.C., Altman, N.H., New York, Academic Press Inc., vol I., pp.59-64, 1979

161. Riegger, G.A.J., Elsner, D., Forssmann, W.-G., Kromer, E.P., Effects of ANP-(95-126) in dogs before and after induction of heart failure, *Am. J. Physiol.*, 259:H1643-H1648, 1990

162. Shannon, R.P., Komamura, K., Stambler, B.S., Bigaud, M., Manders, W.T., Vatner, S.F., Alterations in myocardial contractility in conscious dogs with dilated cardiomyopathy, *Am. J. Physiol.*, 260:H1903-H1911, 1991

163. Spinale, F.G., Zellner, J.L., Tomita, M., Tempel, G.E., Crawford, F.A., Zile, M.R., Tachycardia-induced cardiomyopathy: effects on blood flow and capillary structure, *Am. J. Physiol.*, 261:H140-H148, 1991

164. Packer, D.L., Bardy, G.H., Worley, S.J., Smith, M.S., Cobb, F.R., Coleman, R.E., Gallagher, J.J., German, L.D., Tachycardia-induced cardiomyopathy: a reversible form of left ventricular dysfunction, *Am. J. Cardiol.*, 57:563-570, 1986

165. Damiano, R.J., Tripp, H.F., Asano, T., Small, K.W., Jones, R.H., Lowe, J.E., Left ventricular dysfunction and dilatation resulting from chronic supraventricular tachycardia, *J. Thorac. Cardiovasc. Surg.*, 94:135-143, 1987

166. Wilson, J.R., Douglas, R.P., Hickey, W.F., Lanoce, V., Ferraro, N., Muhammad, A., Reichek, N., Experimental congestive heart failure produced by rapid ventricular pacing in the dog: cardiac effects, *Circ.*, 75:857-867, 1987

167. Howard, R.J., Moe, G.W., Armstrong, P.W., Sequential echocardiographic-Doppler assessment of left ventricular remodelling and mitral regurgitation during evolving experimental heart failure, *Cardiovasc. Res.*, 25:468-474, 1991

168. Coleman, III H.N., Taylor, R.R., Pool, P.E. et al., Congestive heart failure following chronic tachycardia, *Am. Heart J.*, 81:790-798, 1971

169. Armstrong, P.W., Stoops, T.P., Ford, S.E., de Bold, A.J., Rapid ventricular pacing in the dog: pathophysiologic studies of heart failure, *Circ.*, 74:1075-1084, 1986

170. Moe, G.W., Stoops, T.P., Howard, R.J., Armstrong, P.W., Early recovery from heart failure: insights into the pathogenesis of experimental chronic pacing-induced heart failure, *J. Lab. Clin. Med. Sci.*, 62:426-432, 1988

171. Riegger, A.J.G., Liebau, G., The renin-angiotensin-aldosterone system, antidiuretic hormone and sympathetic nerve activity in an experimental model of congestive heart failure in the dog, *Clin. Sci.*, 62:465-469, 1982

172. Zellner, J.L., Spinale, F.G., Eble, D.M., Hewett, K.W., Crawford, F.A.Jr., Alterations in myocyte shape and basement membrane attachment with tachycardia-induced heart failure, *Circ. Res.*, 69:590-600, 1991

173. Spinale, F.G., Fulbright, B.M., Mukherjee, R., Tanaka, R., Hu, J., Crawford, F.A., Zile, M.R., Relation between ventricular and myocyte function with tachycardia-induced cardiomyopathy, *Circ. Res.*, 71:174-187, 1992

174. Calderone, A., Bouvier, M., Li, K., Juneau, C., de Champlain, J., Rouleau, J.-L., Dysfunction of the β- and α-adrenergic systems in a model of congestive heart failure: the pacing-overdrive dog, *Circ. Res.*, 69:332-343, 1991

175. Wolff, M.R., de Tombe, P.P., Harasawa, Y., Burkhoff, D., Bier, S., Hunter, W.C., Gerstenblith, G., Kass, D.A., Alterations in left ventricular mechanics, energetics, and contractile reserve in experimental heart failure, *Circ. Res.*, 70:516-529, 1992

176. Freeman, G.L., Colston, J.T., Myocardial depression produced by sustained tachycardia in rabbits, *Am. J. Physiol.*, 262:H63-H67, 1992

177.   Montgomery, C., Hamilton, N., Ianuzzo, C.D., Energy status of the rapidly paced canine myocardium in congestive heart failure, *J. Appl. Physiol.*, 73:2363-2367, 1992

178.   Travill, I., Williams, T.D.M., Pate, P., Song, G., Chalmers, J., Lightman, S.L., Sutton, R., Noble, M.I.M., Hemodynamic and neurohumoral response in heart failure produced by rapid ventricular pacing, *Cardiovasc. Res.*, 26:783-790, 1992

179.   Wilkenfeld, C., Cohen, M., Lansman, S.L., Courtney, M. et al., Heart transplantation for end-stage cardiomyopathy caused by an occult pheochromocytoma, *J. Heart Lung Transplant.*,11(2 Pt 1):363-366, 1992

180.   Hoffman, B.B., Adrenergic pharmacology in rats harboring pheochromocytoma, *Hypertension*, 18(5 Suppl):III35-III39, 1991

181.   Hu, Z.W., Billingham, M., Tuck, M., Hoffman, B.B., Captopril improves hypertension and cardiomyopathy in rats with pheochromocytoma, *Hypertension*, 15:210-215, 1990

182.   Gunasekaran, S., Young, J.A., Tenner, T.E.Jr., Pharmacological study of isoproterenol and diabetic cardiomyopathies in rat right ventricular strips, *Pharmacology*, 46:101-108, 1993

183.   Cihak, R., Kolar, F., Pelouch, V., Prochazka, J., Ostadal, B., Widimsky, J., Functional changes in the right and left ventricle during development of cardiac hypertrophy and after its regression, *Cardiovasc. Res.*, 26:845-850, 1992

184.   Lucas, C.M., Cheriex, E.C., van der Veen, F.H., Habets, J., van der Nagel, T., Penn, O.C., Wellens, H.J., Imipramine induced heart failure in the dog: a model to study the effect of cardiac assist devices, *Cardiovasc. Res.*, 26:804-809, 1992

185.   Wanless, R.B., Anand, I.S., Poole-Wilson, P.A., Harris, P., An experimental model of chronic cardiac failure using adriamycin in the rabbit: central haemodynamics and regional blood flow, *Cardiovasc. Res.*, 21:7-13, 1987

186.   Jones, S.M., Kirby, M.S., Harding, S.E., Vescova, G., Wanless, R.B., Libera, L.D., Poole-Wilson, P.A., Adriamycin cardiomyopathy in the rabbit: alterations in contractile proteins and myocyte function, *Cardiovasc. Res.*, 24:834-842, 1990

187.   Schaffer, S.W., Tan, B.H., Wilson, G.L., Development of a cardiomyopathy in a model of noninsulin-dependent diabetes, *Am. J. Physiol.*, 248:H179-H185, 1985

188.   Capasso, J.M., Li, P., Guideri, G., Anversa, P., Left ventricular dysfunction induced by chronic alcohol ingestion in rats, *Am. J. Physiol.*, 261:H212-H219, 1991

189.   Staley, N.A., Tobin, J.D.Jr., Reversible effects of ethanol in utero on cardiac sarcoplasmic reticulum of guinea pig offspring, *Cardiovasc. Res.*, 25:27-30, 1991

190.   Fantidis, P., Castejon, R., Fernandez, R.A., Madero-Jarabo, R., et al., Does a critical hemodynamic situation develop from right ventriculotomy and free wall infarct or from small changes in dysfunctional right ventricle afterload?, *J. Cardiovasc. Surg. (Torino)*, 33:229-234, 1992

191.   Rossi, F., Kolobow, T., Foti, G., Borelli, M., Mandava, S., Long-term cardiopulmonary bypass by peripheral cannulation in a model of total heart failure, *J. Thorac. Cardiovasc. Surg.*, 100:914-920, 1990

192.   Davis, J., Howell, D., Mechanisms of fluid and electrolyte retention in experimental preparations in dogs. II. With thoracic inferior vena cava constriction, *Circ. Res.*, 1:171-178, 1953

193.   Underwood, R.D., Aarhus, L.L., Heublein, D.M., Burnett, J.C.Jr., Endothelin in thoracic inferior vena caval constriction model of heart failure, *Am. J. Physiol.*, 263:H951-H955, 1992

194.   Fahey, J.T., Lister, G., A simple method for reducing cardiac output in the conscious lamb, *Am. J. Physiol.*, 249:H188-H192, 1985

195.   Reeves, W.C., Cook, L., Wood, M.A., Whitesell, L., Coronary artery spasm after abrupt withdrawal of nitroglycerin in rabbits, *Am. J. Cardiol.*, 55:1066-1070, 1985

196.   Booth, D.C., Cunningham, M.R., Rountree, R.M., Elion, J., Nissen, S.E., Gillespie, M.N., Coronary arteriography in the intact rabbit: Demonstration of coronary vasomotor and electrocardiographic effects of ergonovine and indomethacin in rabbits after abrupt cessation of prolonged nitroglycerin treatment, *Am. Heart J.*, 114:343-349, 1987

197.   Chilian, W.M., Eastham, C.L., Marcus, M.L., Microvascular distribution of coronary vascular resistance in beating left ventricle, *Am. J. Physiol.*, 251:H779-H788, 1986

198.   Chilian, W.M., DeFily, D.V., Methodological approaches used for the study of the coronary microcirculation in situ, *Blood Vessels*, 28:236-244, 1991

199.   Chilian, W.M., Microvascular pressures and resistances in the left ventricular subepicardium and subendocardium, *Circ. Res.*, 69:561-570, 1991

200.   Morris, S.A., Barr, S., Weiss, L., Tanowitz, H., Wittner, M., Bilezikian, J.P., Myocardial β-adrenergic adenylate cyclase complex in a canine model of Chagasic cardiomyopathy, *Circ. Res.*, 69:185-195, 1991

201. Einzig, S., Staley, N.A., Mettler, E., Nicoloff, D.M., Noren, G.R., Regional myocardial blood flow and cardiac function in a naturally occurring congestive cardiomyopathy of turkeys, *Cardiovasc. Res.*, 14:396-407, 1980

202. Garrison, P.K., Freedman, L.R., Experimental endocarditis. I. Staphylococcal endocarditis in rabbits resulting from placement of a polyethylene catheter in the right side of the heart, *Yale J. Biol. Med.*, 42:394-409, 1970

12. Animal models of atherosclerosis

Atherosclerosis is a pathological process which primarily occurs in large conduit arteries. There are focal accumulations of; cells within the intima of the artery, both intra- and extra-cellular lipids, fibrous connective tissue, complex proteoglycans, minerals, blood and blood products. As the disease progresses necrosis often occurs, especially at the base of the lesion, along with damage to the media of the vessel, ulceration and eventually thrombosis.[1] The disease is thought to occur when the influx and deposition of cholesterol into the wall exceeds the elimination from the wall, i.e. the process is continuous and dynamic. The cholesterol that is deposited seems to be derived from specific types of plasma lipoproteins. The mechanism(s) of deposition probably involve oxysterol metabolism as well. Other types of plasma lipoproteins may be able to participate in the elimination processes which mobilize cholesterol from the arterial cells and transport it to the liver for elimination.[2]

The use of animal models in atherosclerosis research dates from as early as 1908.[21] Vesselinovitch has listed the following requirements for the ideal animal model to be used in atherosclerosis research:

1. Available and inexpensive
2. Easy to maintain and manipulate
3. Proper size
4. Available as genetically pure-bred lines
5. Reproduce easily in captivity
6. Develop lesions with relative ease
    a. Nutritional manipulation conducive to development of advanced plaques
    b. Practical length of time for the development of severe disease
7. Low incidence of spontaneously developed disease
8. Similar to human anatomy, physiology, and biochemistry
9. Similar to human atherosclerosis regarding
    a. Serum lipoprotein and lipid metabolism (lack of loading of reticuloendothelial system)
    b. Pathogenesis of lesions (eg. hypercholesterolemia and hypertension)
    c. Topography of lesions (sparing of small arteries)
    d. Lesion components
    e. Clinical complications (eg. ischemia, myocardial infarction, thrombosis and gangrene).[22]

The search for the ideal animal model for any particular study has led investigators to use high fat diet feeding, alone and in combination with injury to the endothelium produced by direct physical injury, chemical injury, and immunologic injury, or a variety of combinations of these insults.[22] However it is rare to find a single animal model that is suitable for all different kinds of studies. There are always some features of the disease that are different from the naturally occurring disease in humans. It is therefore necessary to make some sort of compromise and select an animal model that offers the most characteristics fitting the problem being investigated.

The use of animal models which demonstrate accelerated plaque formation has been criticized because it would appear that the pathogenesis differs from the slowly developing atherogenesis seen in humans. However examples of accelerated plaque formation do occur in humans particularly patients with familial hypercholesterolemia and in patients with organ transplants. These special cases have similarities to both the slowly developing human disease and the experimentally produced disease in certain animal models.

Quantification

A wide variety of techniques have been used to quantify both naturally occurring and experimentally induced atherosclerosis. Some of these techniques are very involved and sophisticated, others less so.[3] Most commonly the large conduit vessels are perfusion fixed at physiological pressures as a prelude to quantification. They are then opened longitudinally and usually stained with Sudan IV, or some other lipophilic dye. The extent of fatty streaks, raised plaque and/or complicated lesions are then evaluated. Techniques used have included planimetry, point-counting, percent involvement, arbitrary grading, photometry and densitometry.[4,35] A variety of biochemical analyses have also been used. The wide variety of techniques that have been described lends credence to the idea that none of them is totally satisfactory. Sudanophilia may actually decrease, especially during regression of lesions, while the cholesterol deposits persist. Cholesterol and certain cholesterol esters do not stain with Sudan IV. Progressive intimal fibrosis may actually mask deeply seated lipid deposits. Most investigators have relied on the use of the same quantification techniques between groups, within the study. They have usually used blind evaluations by more than one observer and have quantified all the animals from an experiment at the same time. This has enabled the results to be more consistent and valid for any particular experimental design but has created problems in comparing results from different experiments. There does not appear to be a universally acceptable solution to this problem at present.

Pathogenesis

There seems to be little disagreement that the pathogenesis of atherosclerosis involves a complex interaction between the cells of the arterial wall and a variety of blood components, including lipoproteins, platelets, other blood cells and a variety of chemical constituents. These interactions result in a complex series of biochemical changes within the arterial wall as the plaque develops.[1] The response to injury hypothesis has many adherents and the role of platelets is probably tied to this concept along with prostacyclin and thromboxane.[5] This is also the rationale for causing endothelial injury when creating an atherosclerotic model. The most common method of doing this is balloon injury where a balloon catheter is advanced beyond the region where plaque is desired, the balloon is inflated to some predetermined pressure and the catheter is withdrawn a predetermined distance with the balloon inflated. We did a pilot study using these techniques in miniature pigs and found no difference in location or amount of plaque between balloon injured and sham treated groups both fed the same high fat diet for 16 weeks. There is considerable indirect evidence which suggests that high shear stress at the arterial wall may cause local damage in regions that develop lesions.[3] Other workers feel that the lesions correspond to regions of low-shear in the flow field.[6] The response to injury hypothesis is also related to a pressure hypothesis,[7] the turbulence hypothesis[9] and developmental factors.[10] Nakata has shown that disturbances in the microcirculation of the vasa vasorum affected the site of atherosclerotic predilection in high cholesterol diet fed rabbits.[11]

Four major changes have been identified in animals fed high cholesterol-high fat diets: 1) There is a reduction in concentration of typical high density lipoprotein (HDL) without apo-E. 2) There is an increase in HDL with apo-E. 3) There is an increase in low density lipoprotein (LDL) in the plasma. 4) Cholesterol-rich lipoproteins which have beta-electrophoretic mobility, so called β-very low density lipoprotein (β-VLDL), appear in the plasma.[2,12] LDL and β-VLDL can transform macrophage-monocytes into foam cells. Several studies indicate that individuals with low levels of HDL have an increased risk of atherogenesis.[2] There is also support for the theory that proliferating cells of an atherosclerotic plaque all stem from one mutated cell, the monoclonal hypothesis.[10] It has also been shown that interfacial tensions at the lesion surface were significantly increased over normal endothelial surface tensions. This may reflect a change in the strength of hydrophilic interactions associated with the lesion surface, i.e. there may be physico-chemical components of the atherogenic process.[13]

Natural Occurrence

Some animals do, in fact, develop atherosclerotic-like lesions as a naturally occurring disease. Roberts and Straus[14] edited a comprehensive text which provided a review of reports of naturally occurring arterial disease in animals. The following table (Table 12.1) has been compiled from that text.

Table 12.1 Reported incidence of naturally occurring arterial disease in animals.

Animals affected	Atheroma	Medial sclerosis	Fatty streaking
Canidae (domestic)	+	+	-
Felidae	+	+	-
Ursidae (bears)	+	-	-
Rodentia (rabbits, rats, etc.)	+	+	-

Marsupialia (kangaroos, etc.)	+	+++	-
Pinnipedia (seals, sea lions, etc.)	+	-	-
Artiodactyla (swine)	++	-	-
Artiodactyla (bovine)	+	++	-
Artiodactyla (nondomestic)	++	++	-
Perissodactya (equine)	-	-	-
Aves Pelecaniformes (pelicans)	+	-	-
Aves Ciconiiformes (herons)	+	-	-
Aves Anseriformes (ducks)	++	-	-
Aves Falconiformes (falcons)	+	-	-
Aves Galliformes (domestic fowl)	++	-	++
Aves Columbiformes (pigeons)	++	-	-
Aves Psiitaciformes (parrots)	++	-	-
Aves Passeriformes (crows)	+	-	-
Aves Coaciiformes (hornbills)	+	-	-
Primates Lemuridae	+	-	-
Primates Cebidae (squirrel monkey)	+	-	-
Primates Cercopithecidae (macaque, baboon, etc.)	+	+	-
Primates Pongidae (chimpanzees, gorillas, etc.)	+	-	-

+ = reported; ++ = fairly common; +++ = common, - = not reported

Specific Animal Models

The challenge in identifying and establishing suitable animal models has been to characterize a model which develops the same type of atherosclerotic lesion, at the same locations as are seen in man. The lesions should form over a relatively short period of time (to save on costs) but with the same sequence of development as seen in the very long term lesions characteristic of the human disease. The same factors of diet, stress and heredity known to play a role in the human disease should influence the course of events in the animal model.

Rabbits: As cited previously the high cholesterol diet fed rabbit model has been around since at least 1908.[21]   Rabbits seldom develop spontaneous true atherosclerosis but do develop some unusual types of degenerative medial lesions.[15] These lesions occur primarily in the aortic arch and thoracic aorta and consist of mineralization of the media. They resemble Monckeberg's medial sclerosis of humans and it has been possible to selectively breed for the presence of these lesions.[34]   When rabbits are fed regular rabbit chow with 2% cholesterol (sheep lanolin derived) added, free choice, they will go from normal total plasma cholesterol levels of 50-75 mg/dl to >1500 mg/dl in 6-8 weeks. The cells of the reticuloendothelial system, particularly in the liver, become massively engorged with cholesterol.   The kidneys and other internal organs are also severely affected.[25] These lesions are reminiscent of a lipid storage disorder or "fat toxicosis" and the rabbits are demonstrably ill. If allowed to progress a certain percentage of these animals will die of liver and/or renal failure. The rabbits also accumulate cholesterol within the intima of the large conduit arteries under these circumstances.[1] The lesions predominate in the aortic arch and the thoracic aorta, however the content of the lesions and the sites of distribution are not the same as seen in man.[16] The amount of cholesterol and the amount and type of fat included in the diet play a direct role in the severity and composition of the lesions produced in rabbits. Microscopically rabbit lesions resemble thick fatty streaks with most of the lipid localized within foam cells.   When the duration of hypercholesterolemia is increased the lipid eventually starts to accumulate extracellularly. It is rare for lesions in rabbits to develop fibrosis, hemorrhage, ulceration, and/or thrombosis, all characteristic of lesions in humans.[1] It has been reported that hypercholesterolemia causes inhibition of arterial fibrosis in rabbits but more recently it was shown that moderate hypercholesterolemia stimulates predominantly collagenous responses.[22]   Feeding of various food fats, with or without cholesterol, results in the formation of different types of lesions, depending upon the type of fat used. Some lesions are significantly fibrocellular in composition.[26,27] In spite of the many problems listed above the rabbit is still likely to be the most widely used animal model for atherosclerosis. The probable reason for this is that rabbits are easy to feed, care for, and handle, along with being inexpensive and readily available.[15]

The Watanabe heritable hyperlipidemic (WHHL) rabbit has proven to be an excellent model for homozygous familial hypercholesterolemia in humans.[28-30] These animals develop massive hypercholesterolemia as a result of a single genetic defect which very close to the same genetic defect seen in humans with this affliction. The defect seems to reside in the gene(s) for low density lipoprotein (LDL) receptor(s) and fulminating atherosclerosis occurs even when the rabbits are fed a cholesterol-free diet. The pattern of atherosclerosis development is also the same in these rabbits as is seen in humans.[17]   A hybrid hare, heterozygous for glucose-6-phosphate dehydrogenase has been described and used to study clonal characteristics of arterial lesions in cholesterol-induced atherosclerosis.[31,32]

Birds: Both naturally occurring and diet-induced atherosclerosis occurs in birds. The bulk of the research conducted has been in chickens, pigeons and Japanese quail. Birds fed a high cholesterol diet initially accumulate foam cells in the intima and inner portion of the media of the large arteries, the extent depending upon the magnitude of the hypercholesterolemia that is present. With continued exposure fibrous tissue develops followed by extracellular lipid and cell debris in the necrotic areas of the plaque. In severe lesions there is calcification, ulceration, hemorrhage and mural thrombi. These avian lesions are therefore more similar to those found in man than are the lesions produced in rabbits. In all birds studied thus far regression occurs readily when the high cholesterol diet is stopped and the hypercholesterolemia is reduced.[1] Naturally occurring lesions in chickens are most commonly found in the abdominal aorta and are almost exclusively within the intima.   These lesions are initially cellular in nature and later become predominantly fibrous. When fed a high cholesterol diet birds frequently achieve plasma cholesterol levels >1,000 mg/dl. The lesions formed with cholesterol feeding are most common in the thoracic aorta and coronary arteries.   With additional time on the diet the abdominal aorta is increasingly affected.[1] Male chickens seem to show more lipid in the atheromatous lesions than do female chickens. Neither the male nor the female lesion is exactly comparable to that found in man, although the thoracic aortic lesion in roosters is quite close.[14] Patel et al. conducted a very interesting experiment in roosters.   They fed a high cholesterol diet to 3 groups, a control group fed a normal ration, another group which received the diet alone the other received the diet plus 0.2 mg/kg valium, b.i.d. There were no significant differences between the groups for blood pressure, cardiac output or heart rate.   Both groups fed the high fat diet exhibited hypercholesterolemia (peak of 600 mg/dl in 4-6 weeks, falling to 200-300 mg/dl by week 10), and equivalent levels of triglycerides. The birds receiving only the high fat diet developed atherosclerotic lesions, more pronounced in the abdominal than the thoracic aorta. The birds fed the high fat diet plus Valium did not develop atherosclerotic   plaque.   This   obviously   suggests   other   factors   than hypercholesterolemia being responsible for plaque deposition.[33]

The lower thoracic aorta, at the site of the celiac artery bifurcation, is a highly predictable site of atherosclerosis in susceptible breeds of pigeons, where marked breed susceptibility exists. The White Carneau breed seems to be most susceptible while the Show Racer breed is the most resistant.[1] The lesions found have been reported to be very similar, microscopically, to aortic lesions in man. However the lesions are focally distributed as opposed to the general distribution found in man. The coronaries are rarely affected in pigeons.[14]

Broad-breasted bronze or white turkeys develop posterior aortic lesions that contain consideration fibrin and very little lipid. This lesion may be associated with an, so far, undefined nutritional deficiency. The lesion is apparently different in many important aspects than lesions found in humans.[15]

Almost every species of bird that has been investigated has shown some sort of lipid-containing lesions of the aortic intima. Lesions that closely resemble those of man have been reported in an 80-year old parrot and a 106 year old cockatoo.[14]

Dogs: Dogs have been shown to develop a variety of chronic arterial lesions that increase both in prevalence and severity with age. Smooth muscle cells apparently play an important role in the development of these lesions.[15] The lesions found are sclerotic but the species seems to be resistant to lipid deposition unless a marked hypercholesterolemia is produced. To accomplish this it is usually necessary to thyroidectomize the animal. It is possible to produce lipid deposition without thyroidectomy by feeding a diet extremely high in cholesterol and saturated fat but with absolutely no unsaturated fats. Even a small amount of safflower oil added to this diet will prevent lipid deposition in dogs.[1] Obviously dogs fed a diet of this nature   can   develop   severe   diarrheas   and   chronic   enteritis.   Dogs   made hypercholesterolemic will develop severe, occlusive, lesions in the abdominal aorta, the coronaries and the cerebral arteries but the coronary lesions do not develop early in the disease.[16] Dogs do not develop the diffuse thickening of the arterial intima as seen in humans, most of the lesion develops in the media.[1,14]

Rats: Rats are generally considered to be resistant to atherogenesis, although lesions have been produced by heroic measures.[16] Naturally occurring lesions in rats are not very similar to those seen in man. Although lipid-containing lesions can be produced in rats they are generally considered to be residual lesions following an acute arteritis.[14]

Pigs: The pig is an omnivore so its normal diet is similar to man. Its cardiovascular system is similar in size and the coronary distribution and behavior is very similar to that of man. It also appears that the manner in which dietary lipids are absorbed, transported and metabolized is quite similar.[35] Since the atherosclerotic lesions that pigs develop are also similar to those found in humans this model of atherosclerosis has become quite popular. The main deterrent to the use of pigs is the expense and problems involved in maintaining these animals in a research colony. These problems are somewhat abrogated by the use of miniaturized breeds of swine but even these breeds can be difficult to work with and specialized skills must be learned to handle and use swine as a model.

Atherosclerosis is naturally occurring in older swine, i.e. breeding animals, that have been maintained on normal pig rations, especially those fed cooked garbage. They develop lesions of the aorta, coronary and cerebral arteries and in other arterial sites. The lesions are most prevalent in the abdominal aorta with a very predictable pattern in or near the renal arteries and especially at the iliac trifurcation (origin of the coccygeal artery). The early naturally occurring lesions closely resemble early lesions in man.[1] There is abundant lipid in these lesions and they start as fatty streaks early in the animal's life.[15] In normally fed pigs at 6 months of age it is possible to find accumulations of smooth muscle cells, elastic fibers and collagen within the intima at sites of predilection. These accumulations tend to progress to "elastic-hyperplastic" thickening and then to deposition of lipid.[1,36] Swine fed diets with 2-3% added cholesterol can develop plasma cholesterol levels in excess of 1,000 mg/dl very easily. When fed a cholesterol free diet plasma cholesterol levels are generally less than 100 mg/dl. After being fed a 2-3% cholesterol diet for 6-7 months 10-20% of the abdominal aorta will have raised fatty lesions.[1] Higher levels of cholesterol will produce lesions within weeks, especially if preceded by some sort intimal injury.[1,18] The lesions produced by added cholesterol feeding have spindle-shaped and round cells, both containing lipid. The atheromatous lesions are characterized by a necrotic core of lipid and cell debris covered by a fibromuscular layer with fewer lipid-filled cells than in the foam cell lesions. As the duration of cholesterol feeding increases there is an increase in the proportion of atheromatous versus cellular lesions.[1]

Certain strains of pigs have become valuable because they lack the von Willebrand factor. This has permitted the development of a syndrome closely resembling von Willebrand's disease in humans.[37,38] These pigs have prolonged bleeding times and are less susceptible to aortic atherosclerosis induced either by an atherogenic diet alone or an atherogenic diet and endothelial injury.[5] This seems to suggest a role for platelets, or at least a role for some aspect of the coagulation cascade in the atherogenic swine model.

Non-human primates: Those species that are omnivores show a progression and distribution of atherosclerotic plaque very similar to that seen in man. There seem to be some species differences in susceptibility to both spontaneous and diet-induced atherosclerosis but the lesions that develop are generally limited to small areas of intimal thickening with accumulations of smooth muscle cells and connective tissue.[15] There are only small amounts of lipid deposited initially. Most of the information available has been collected from *Macaca mulatta (rhesus)* or *Macaca fascicularis (cynomolgus)*. In those species that develop diet-induced hypercholesterolemia the lesions formed are initially fatty streaks with foam cells, then fatty and fibrous plaques increase and the fatty streaks decrease. The fibrous lesions have a variety of features similar to those found in man, i.e. necrosis, calcification, cholesterol clefts, increased amounts of collagen and elastin. They will occasionally show hemorrhage, ulceration and thrombosis. The overall severity of the lesions seen in primates, even those with diet-induced hypercholesterolemia, does not appear to be as severe as those commonly seen in humans at autopsy. The abdominal aorta has an increased prevalence of raised plaques compared to the thoracic aorta. Lesions are also seen in the proximal main (left) coronary, the carotid, iliac, subclavian and femoral arteries. Intracranial cerebral artery lesions are rare in rhesus but present in about 20% of diet-induced hypercholesterolemia cynomolgus monkeys.[1]

Non-human primates are considered to be the most important animal models of atherosclerosis because of their close phylogenetic relationship to humans, the similarities in lipid levels and metabolism and the response of these systems to excessive fat in the diet, and the distribution, composition and complications caused by plaque deposition. The rhesus monkey is most commonly used for studies relating to diet-induced atherosclerosis, particularly the effects of diet modification and/or cholesterolemic lowering drug interventions. They are also useful for studying lipoprotein profiles and metabolism, lesion topography, lesion composition and the clinical complications associated with plaque deposition.[22] Cynomolgus monkey models are particularly useful for studies relating to coronary artery lesions and their associated complications, the relationships between immune responses and atherogenesis and for the effects of sex differences and behavior factors.[22] If maintained on a low level hypercholesterolemic died (200-400 mg/dl) for more than 2 years the lesions are very similar to those found in humans with fatty streaks converted to fibrous plaques.[43]

Other macaque species have also been used in atherosclerosis research including the stump-tailed, pig-tailed and the Celebes black ape.[22] There does not seem to be any special advantage for the use of these more difficult to obtain species. Different families of Squirrel monkeys may be either hypo- or hyper-responders to an atherogenic diet and the apparently genetic differences make this species useful for genetic studies. A genetic strain of baboons has been developed that has lipoprotein phenotypes which are susceptible to atherosclerosis characterized by differences in serum low- and high-density lipoprotein.[39] Baboons are perhaps most useful for studies of whole-body cholesterol metabolism since those processes are very similar to those in humans.[39,40]

To summarize some special indications for specific non-human primate species *Macaca speciosa* are useful when a larger but docile animal is needed. *Macaca fascicularis* and *Cebus* monkeys have been shown to develop severe coronary artery disease and myocardial infarctions. *Macaca mulatta* are very valuable for studies involving diet-induced atherosclerosis and regression studies. *Saimiri sciureus* exhibit cerebral infarctions when fed a high cholesterol diet and the baboon absorbs and excretes cholesterol using similar mechanisms as are seen in humans. *Macaca nemestrina* develops lesions that are predominantly fibromuscular in nature following intra-arterial balloon injury combined with a high fat diet while *Macaca fascicularis* develops mostly concentric transmural lipid-rich proliferative lesions. *Cercopithecus aethiops* (one of the African green monkeys) apparently develops predominantly fibrous and complex atheromatous lesions when fed a high-fat, cholesterol-rich diet. *Macaca fascicularis* will develop foam cell-rich lesions when fed an atherogenic diet, but this type of lesion can also be produced in other species (i.e. swine and rabbits) with the proper diet manipulation.[22]

There are three main advantages to the non-human primate as a model of atherogenesis: **1)** Lesions can be induced in a relatively short time, from a few weeks to 1 or 2 years, depending upon the amount of cholesterol and the type of fat fed. **2)** The arterial lesions are very similar to those seen in man. **3)** The arteries are easily accessible for anatomical, physiological and biochemical observation.[19]

There are also three primary limitations of non-human primates as atherogenesis models: **1)** Data on cholesterol-fed monkeys may be applicable only to people in whom atherosclerosis is related to, or aggravated by, exogenous cholesterol. In man, it is usually associated with the amount of saturated fat as well as the cholesterol intake. **2)** The effects of the dietary intake of saturated fats on plasma cholesterol and lipoproteins, in the absence of exogenous cholesterol, particularly oxidized cholesterol, is minimal in monkeys, unlike the situation in man and pigs. **3)** The induction period is short with very high cholesterolemia in most primate models, whereas in man the naturally occurring disease is usually much more prolonged in onset.[19]

Regression studies

Following cessation of high cholesterol feeding regression of atheromatous lesions has been demonstrated in rabbits, chickens, rats, dogs, pigeons, pigs and non-human primates. In addition to the withdrawal of the high cholesterol diet regression has been associated with the ingestion of cholestyramine, alfalfa meal and alfalfa saponins in monkeys maintained on a high cholesterol diet.[4] There appear to be remarkable differences in the composition and distribution of lesions in non-human primates when the animals are fed different types of fat, i.e. corn oil vs butterfat vs peanut oil vs fish oil.[41,42] The mechanisms of regression involve; **1)** a regeneration of the endothelium, **2)** an arrest of cell proliferation, and **3)** decrease in the atheromatous mass. All of these are probably interrelated processes.[19] With the possible exception of starting the regression process when the lesions are only early fatty streaks there is no return to normal. There is a remodeling and repair of the atherosclerotic plaque, including a reduction in both intra- and extra-cellular lipid, cell proliferation and necrosis and an increase in fibrosis, calcification and repair of the endothelial surface of the plaque.[1]

Upon cessation of cholesterol feeding in rabbits the lesions in the aorta initially become more severe. They then stop progressing and finally regress. This may all be related to the time required for the hypercholesterolemia to decrease. In rabbits the intracellular lipid is probably readily depleted, either by cell death or excretion from the cell, but the liberated cellular cholesterol then accumulates in the extracellular compartment where it is mobilized very slowly.[1]

When diet-induced hypercholesterolemia is reversed in swine the atherosclerotic plaque does regress. Biochemical analysis shows that levels of DNA synthesis, cell proliferation and both free and esterified cholesterol concentrations are similar to non-diseased areas and to aortas from control animals. These parameters are all increased in lesioned areas. Following regression the amount of collagen content is increased in the previously affected areas. There is also evidence which indicates that the overall severity of the initial lesion probably plays a role in the completeness of regression.[1]

Regression also occurs in non-human primates but it is apparently necessary to lower the hypercholesterolemia to less than 200 mg/dl. When the plasma cholesterol is lowered to between 200 and 300 mg/dl there is little or no regression seen. The reduction that does occur seems to be due to a decrease in both intra- and extra-cellular lipids and necrotic debris. There is some collagen replacement in these studies.[1] Another study shows an apparent functional improvement in aortic elastic properties, i.e. compliance increased with regression.   The improvements in arterial compliance seems to follow reductions in total aortic wall cholesterol concentrations and the extent of the total atherosclerotic plaque. An increase in the collagen-elastin ratio is seen with the regression of plaque. This is correlated with a decrease in arterial stiffness.[20]

Final selection of the most appropriate animal model

The most important issue when selecting an animal model is matching the model to the experiment. When doing this it is important not to just consider the end point result. The most appropriate model also has a physiopathological pathway that is as close as possible to that in humans. In choosing an atherosclerosis model there is a wide variety of choices to be made. If hypo- or hyper-responsiveness to atherogenic stimuli are of interest one should consider either pigeons or squirrel monkeys. Genetic hyperlipidemic disorders are best studied in Watanabe rabbits. Interactions between clotting disorders and atherosclerosis can be evaluated in von Willebrand's disease swine. Interactions between atherosclerosis and hypertension can be studied in rabbits, rats, spider, squirrel and woolly monkeys. *Macaca nigra* has proven to be very valuable in studies concerning the interactions between atherosclerosis and diabetes.[22] Swine have proven to be one of the best models for studying a variety of problems in atherosclerosis as well as for the testing and evaluation of new diagnostic and therapeutic regimens.[22]   Despite many shortcomings rabbits, with suitable manipulation, will yield significant insights into specific aspects of hypercholesterolemic effects.

References

1. St. Clair, R.W.; Atherosclerosis regression in animal models: current concepts of cellular and biochemical mechanisms, *Prog Cardiovasc Dis*, 26:109-132, 1983
2. Mahley, R.W.; Development of accelerated atherosclerosis. Concepts derived from cell biology and animal model studies, *Arch Pathol Lab Med*, 107:393-399, 1983
3. Roach, M.R., Smith N.B.; Does high shear stress induced by blood flow lead to atherosclerosis?, *Perspect Biol Med*, 26:287-303, 1983
4. Malinow, M.R.; Experimental models of atherosclerosis regression, *Atherosclerosis*, 48:105-118, 1983
5. Saunders, R.N.; Evaluation of platelet-inhibiting drugs in models of atherosclerosis, *Ann Rev Pharmacol Toxicol*, 22:279-295, 1982
6. Matsuda, I., Miimi, H., Moritake, K., Okumura A, Handa, H.; The role of hemodynamic factors in arterial wall thickening in the rat, *Atherosclerosis*, 29:363-371, 1978
7. Texon, M.; A hemodynamic concept f atherosclerosis with particular reference to coronary occlusion, *AMA Arch Int Med*, 99:418-421, 1957
8. Fox, J.A., Hugh, A.E.; Localization of atheroma- a theory based on boundary layer separation, *Brit Heart J*, 28:388-393, 1966
9. Wesolowski, S.A., Fries, C.C., Sabini, A.M., Sawyer, P.N.; The significance of turbulence in hemolic systems and in the distribution of the atherosclerotic lesion, *Surg*, 57:155-161, 1965
10. Benditt, E.P.; The origin of atherosclerosis, *Sci Am*, 236:74-85, 1977
11. Nakata, Y.; Relations between disturbances in microcirculation and accumulation of lipids in the aortic wall, *Jap Circ J*, 43:734-740, 1979
12. Mahley, R.W.; Atherogenic hyperlipoproteinemia. The cellular and molecular biology of plasma lipoproteins altered by dietary fat and cholesterol, *Med Clin North Am*, 66:375-402, 1982
13. Boyce, J.F., Church, S., McIver, D.J.; Interfacial tensions in healthy and atherosclerotic rabbit aortae. Higher values and lesion surfaces, *Atherosclerosis*, 37:361-370, 1980
14. Roberts, J.C., Straus, S.R., editors; Comparative atherosclerosis: the morphology of spontaneous and induced atherosclerotic lesions in animals and its relation to human disease, Harper and Row, New York, 1965
15. Gross, D.R.; Animal models in cardiovascular research, Chp. 1 in; *Quantitative cardiovascular studies, clinical and research applications of engineering principles*, Ed by N.H.C. Hwang, D.R. Gross and D.J. Patel, University Park Press, 1979
16. Kritchevsky, D.; Laboratory models for atherosclerosis, *Adv Drug Res*, 9:41-53, 1974
17. Goldstein, J.L., Kita, T., Brown, M.S.; Defective lipoprotein receptors and atherosclerosis. Lessons from an animal counterpart of familial hypercholesterolemia, *N Eng J Med*, 309:288-296, 1983
18. van Oort, G., Gross, D.R., Spiekerman, A.M.; Effects of eight weeks of physical conditioning on atherosclerotic plaque in swine, *Am J Vet Res*, 48:51-55, 1987
19. Malinow, M.R.; The role of nonhuman primates in research on atherosclerosis regression-hypothetical mechanisms implicated in regression, *Artery*, 9:2-11, 1981
20. Farrar, D.J., Green, H.D., Wagner, W.D., Bond, M.G.; Reduction in pulse wave velocity and improvement of aortic distensibility accompanying regression of atherosclerosis in the Rhesus monkey, *Circ Res*, 47:425-432, 1980
21. Ignatowski, A.C.; Influence of animal food on the organism of rabbits, *Invest Imper Voennomed Akad St Petersburg*, 16:154-173, 1908
22. Vesselinovitch, D.; Animal models and the study of atherosclerosis, *Arch Pathol Lab Med*, 112:1011-1017, 1988
23. Alonso, D.R., Starek, P.K., Minick, C.R.; Studies on the pathogenesis of atheroarteriosclerosis induced in rabbit cardiac allografts by the synergy of graft rejection and hypercholesterolemia, *Am J Pathol*, 87:415-435, 1977
24. Wissler, R.W., Vesselinovitch, D.; The development and use of animal models in atherosclerosis research, in, *Cardiovascular Disease '86*, ed. by L. Gallo, New York, Plenum Press: 337-357, 1987
25. Besterman, E.M.M.; Experimental coronary atherosclerosis in rabbits, *Atherosclerosis*, 12:75-83, 1970

26. Kritchevsky, D., Tepper, S.A., Kim, H.K. et al.; Experimental atherosclerosis in rabbits fed cholesterol-free diets: V. Comparison of peanut, corn, butter, and coconut oils, *Exp Mol Pathol*, 24:375-391, 1976

27. Kritchevsky, D., Tepper, S.A., Scott, D.A. et al.; Cholesterol vehicle in experimental atherosclerosis: SVIII. Comparison of North American, African, and South American peanut oils, *Atherosclerosis*, 38:291-299, 1981

28. Watanabe, Y.; Serial inbreeding of rabbits with hereditary hyperlipidemia (WHHL-rabbit): Incidence and development of atherosclerosis and xanthoma, *Atherosclerosis*, 36:261-268, 1980

29. Havel, R.J., Kita, T., Kotite, L., et al.; Concentration and composition of lipoproteins in blood plasma of the WHHL rabbit: An animal model of human familial hypercholesterolemia, *Arteriosclerosis*, 2:467-474, 1982

30. Buja, L.M., Kita, T., Goldstein, J.L., et al.; Cellular pathology of progressive atherosclerosis in the WHHL rabbit: An animal model of familial hypercholesterolemia, *Arteriosclerosis*, 3:87-101, 1983

31. Lee, K.T., Thomas, W.A., Janakidevi, K., et al.; Mosaicism in female hybrid hares heterozygous for glucose-6-phosphate dehydrogenase (G-6-PD):I. General properties of a hybrid hare model with special reference to atherogenesis, *Exp Mol Pathol*, 34:191-201, 1981

32. Pearson, T.A., Dillman, J., Malmros, H., et al.; Cholesterol-induced atherosclerosis: Clonal characteristics of arterial lesions in the hybrid hare, *Arteriosclerosis*, 3:574-580, 1983

33. Patel, D.J., Wong, H.Y.C., Newman, H.A.I., Nightingale, T.E., Frasinel, C., Johnson, F.B., Patel, S., Coleman, B.; Effect of valium (Diazepam) on experimental atherosclerosis in roosters, *Artery*, 10:237-249, 1982

34. Garbarsch, C., Matthiessen, M.E., Helin, P., Lorenzen, I.; Spontaneous aortic arteriosclerosis in rabbits of the Danish Country strain, *Atherosclerosis*, 12:291-300, 1970

35. Mersmann, H.J.; Lipid metabolism in Swine, in *Swine in Cardiovascular Research*, Vol. I, ed. by H.C. Stanton and J.J. Mersmann, CRC Press, Boca Raton, 1986

36. Lee, K.T., Kim, D.N., Thomas, W.A.; Atherosclerosis in Swine, Chp. 2 in *Swine in Cardiovascular Research*, Vol. II, ed. by H.C. Stanton and H.J. Mersmann, CRC Press, Boca Raton, 1986

37. Fuster, V., Bowie, E.J.W., Brown, A.L.; Spontaneous arterial lesions in normal pigs and pigs with von Willebrand's disease, in *Atherosclerosis: Metabolic, Morphologic and Clinical Aspects*, ed. by G.W. Manning and M.D. Haust, Plenum Press, New York, pp 315-317, 1977

38. Griggs, T.R.,m Reddick, R.L., Seltzer, D., et al.; Susceptibility to atherosclerosis in aortas and coronary arteries of swine with von Willebrand's disease, *Am J Pathol*, 102:137-145, 1981

39. McGill, H.C. Jr., McMahan, C.A., Kruski, A.W., et al.; Relationship in lipoprotein cholesterol concentrations to experimental atherosclerosis in baboons, *Arteriosclerosis*, 1:3-12, 1981

40. Blaton, V., Peeters, H.; The nonhuman primates as models for studying human atherosclerosis: Studies on the chimpanzee, the baboon and the rhesus macacus, in *Atherosclerosis Drug Discovery*, ed. by C.E. Day, Plenum Press, New York, pp. 33-64, 1976

41. Vesselinovitch, D., Getz, G.S., Hughes, R.H., et al.; Atherosclerosis in the rhesus monkey fed three food fats, *Atherosclerosis*,20:303-321, 1974

42. Vesselinovitch, D., Wissler, R.W., Schaffner, T.J. et al.; The effect of various diets on atherogenesis in rhesus monkeys, *Atherosclerosis*, 35:198-207, 1980

43. Masuda, J., Ross, R.; Atherogenesis during low level hypercholesterolemia in the nonhuman primate. II. Fatty streak conversion to fibrous plaque., *Arteriosclerosis*, 10:178-187, 1990

13. Animal models of hypertension

Introduction

Based upon the number of articles published each year the various animal models of hypertension are probably the most popular disease model used in cardiovascular research. The sheer volume of research accomplished demonstrates the potential usefulness of such a research tool. For example a Medline search of articles published between Jan., 1990 and Sept., 1993 found 26 articles dealing with renovascular hypertension in dogs, 206 in rats, 1 in cats, 15 in rabbits and 2 in swine.

As early as 1889 Tigerstedt and Bergman demonstrated that extracts from the kidney could produce a pressor effect. They named the active substance renin.[1] When Goldblatt and his associates, in 1934, produced chronic hypertension in dogs by a two-stage constriction of the renal arteries[2] the search for the humoral mechanism of this alteration was initiated. Within a few years Page and Helmer[3] working in the USA and Braun-Menendez and collaborators[4] working independently in Argentina, described the renin-angiotensin system.

Aside from the iatrogenic, surgically created, model of renovascular hypertension different forms of genetic hypertension have been created in rats. These, so-called, spontaneously hypertensive rats (SHR) are still the single most utilized animal model in cardiovascular research today, on the basis of the total numbers of animals used. There were 2315 different articles published using the SHR model between Jan., 1990 and Sept., 1993.[5]

Renovascular hypertension

Several different variations of the original Goldblatt renovascular hypertensive model have been developed. The original model in dogs was a 2-kidney, 1-clip model, which indicates that both kidneys were left intact but the renal arterial flow to one of the kidneys was markedly reduced by partial ligation.[2] In dogs the 2-kidney, 1-clip model has been well characterized. Following unilateral renal arterial constriction there is a decrease in extensibility of both arteries and veins during the first 24 hours. Within 32 days vascular stiffness is increased even more, along with a decrease in vascular smooth muscle contractility.[6]

Greenberg et al. modified the classical 2-kidney, 1-clip preparation by using a hydraulic occluder on a renal artery along with an electromagnetic flowmeter transducer. The flow was reduced to 5-15% of the pre-constriction flow as measured by the flowmeter. They found it was necessary to adjust the hydraulic occluder 3-4 times over the first 4 hours to maintain the flow reduced to that level, otherwise the renal blood flow increased again. This model produces a very stable hypertension.[7]

The early stages of the 2-kidney, 1-clip dog model are characterized by an increase in arterial pressure, an increase in aortic flow, a decrease in total peripheral resistance and enhanced responses to Angiotensin II and serotonin. As aortic flow increases the responses to norepinephrine increase and the dilator responses to acetylcholine and nitroglycerine decrease. Aortic flow then decreases to baseline levels and the increase in aortic pressure is maintained by an increase in total peripheral resistance.[8]

The 2-kidney, 1-clip model is also used in rats. The left renal artery is usually partially occluded with a silver clip (0.2 mm i.d.) while the right kidney is not disturbed. It usually takes about 4 weeks to develop mean pressures greater than 150 mmHg.[9] It is possible to reverse the hypertension in this model by removal of the affected kidney or by oral treatment with Captopril, an angiotensin converting enzyme inhibitor (50 mg/kg/day initially then 80 mg/kg/day as needed.[6,10,11]

The 1-kidney, 1-clip rat model has slightly different characteristics. The initial increases in blood pressure is accompanied by an increase in plasma renin activity. Within a few days the plasma renin activity returns to normal, sodium retention occurs and plasma and extracellular fluid volumes increase. The expansion of the plasma volume is not, however, necessarily dependent upon sodium retention, since it can occur in salt-deprived rats. The chronic phase of hypertension is presumably dependent upon increased blood volume in this model.[12]

It is also possible to produce severe hypertension in rats by occluding the aorta between the origins of the renal arteries. Approximately 8 days later the rats develop severe hypertension. It has been shown that the hypertension is not due to a mechanical increase in resistance caused by the coarctation but rather to an increase in renin release.[13] This model is also reversed by the administration by Captopril.[11,14]

The most common renovascular hypertension producing model in rabbits has been dubbed the 1-kidney, 1-wrap model. The surgical procedure involves removal of 1 kidney, usually the right kidney because the left is more accessible for wrapping, and then wrapping the remaining kidney with sterile cellophane or plastic wrap (Saran Wrap[(R)]).[7,15] It is possible to reverse the hypertension in this model by removing the cellophane and stripping the extensive fibrous thickening of the true renal capsule, which apparently allows the compressed kidney to expand.[16]

Perinephritis hypertension is also produced by wrapping both kidneys with cellophane or plastic wrap (Saran Wrap [(R)]). Unilateral wrapping of the remaining kidney following removal of a kidney results in enormous increases in total peripheral resistance, a decrease in heart rate and stroke volume and usually a greater than 35% decrease in cardiac output. With bilateral wrapping the hypertension produced is more moderate but is also maintained by an increase in total peripheral resistance.[17]

Renovascular hypertension has been demonstrated in 1-kidney and 2-kidney models, with and without wrapping, in other species, including non-human primates[18,19] and sheep, pigs and cats.[20] At least two different surgically produced models have been described in monkeys; surgical constriction of the midthoracic aorta, which produced a 40 mmHg gradient across the coarctation[18] and a modified 2-stage Goldblatt procedure.[19] All of the models described can be created in either a 1-stage or 2-stage procedure. In the 1-stage all surgery is completed during a single procedure. The 2-stage models usually involve the unilateral nephrectomy first and then, after a suitable time for recovery of the animal, a second operation to cause renal artery constriction or wrapping of the kidney.

Pathogenesis of the hypertension seems to differ with species. The renin-angiotensin system plays a primary role in the 2-kidney model in the rat. Other, as yet poorly defined, mechanisms have a primary role in 1-kidney hypertension in the rat and in both 1- and 2-kidney hypertension in the rabbit and dog.[1] Subcutaneous injection of renopressin into normal rabbits has been shown to produce a delayed, slow increase in blood pressure and then moderate, persistent hypertension after a few days. This substance has been shown to be produced in the kidney cortex of the 1-kidney, 1-clip rabbit model.[21]

Spontaneously hypertensive rats (SHR)

All strains of spontaneously hypertensive rats are derived from inbred strains of Wistar rats. They show an exaggerated cardiovascular responsiveness to environmental alerting stimuli, i.e. noise, vibration and light. If the external stimuli are decreased it is possible to delay the development of hypertension.[22] This seems to suggest an important sympathetic and/or central nervous system component in the pathogenesis of the hypertension in this model.

Pregnancy causes a decrease in blood pressure in the spontaneously hypertensive rat. Renal sodium ion handling is, apparently, not impaired in the SHR and angiotensin II does not seem to play an important role in maintaining blood pressure during gestation in this model.[23]

The early increase in cardiac output in the SHR seems to be related to an increase in central intravascular volume, possibly due to fluid retention. The later, further increase in blood pressure and total peripheral resistance seems to be caused by an independent, secondary, increase in vascular resistance.[24] Renal denervation has been shown to delay the onset and attenuate the severity of hypertension in both the Okamoto-Aoki and New Zealand strains of SHR (GH-Smirk).[25] Renal changes, characterized by a reduction in the glomerular filtration rate (GFR), probably provide a mechanism for the permanent establishment of hypertension in the Milan SHR model.[26] Sodium was retained to a greater extent by the Milan SHR during the early phases of development, from weaning to 4 weeks post-weaning. The sodium retention appears to be the result of a significant decrease in urinary sodium excretion.[27] This all suggests a causative role for the kidney in this model.

Other models available are the "stroke prone" and "stroke resistant" substrains of SHR, the arteriolipoidosis prone SHR and the obese SHR strain.[43] The Smirk's genetic hypotensive strain originated from the New Zealand breeding efforts.[43]

Studies in the SHR have shown that the percentage of energy derived from protein in the diet may markedly affect development of hypertension and survival of the animals. The more severely affected strains of this model, the stroke prone SHR, when fed a low-protein, excess salt, diet shows a marked decrease in stroke incidence. Methionine seems to be the most influential amino acid in this response in the stroke prone strain. When supplied in high levels there is a reduction in blood pressure in this model. Lysine and proline also have this effect but are less potent than methionine.[26] The angiotensin converting enzyme inhibitor Captopril also effectively reduces blood pressure in the SHR.[11] Bilateral nephrectomy, however, abolishes the antihypertensive activity of Captopril in this model.[14]

Dahl salt-sensitive rats

The Dahl, genetic, salt-sensitive rat was developed and characterized by selective inbreeding. Dahl and his associates produced two strains of rats with opposite genetic propensities for developing hypertension following feeding of a high salt (NaCl) diet. The two strains also showed opposite innate predispositions for developing experimental hypertension from deoxycorticosterone acetate (DOCA) and salt treatment, unilateral renal artery compression without salt, cortisone treatment or adrenal regeneration (cortisone treatment of adrenalectomized rats). All of this suggests that the basic pathogenic mechanism for all of these rat models may be the same.[28,29,30]

The Dahl strain of salt sensitive rats only develops hypertension when exposed to a high-salt diet. The hypertension is then maintained even if the salt is withdrawn. In most strains of SHR increased salt intake will exacerbate hypertension while salt restriction will not affect the normal course of hypertension development. In some cases salt loading may reverse experimentally induced malignant hypertension.[26,31] When two Dahl rats, one from a salt-sensitive and the other from a salt-resistant strain, are united in a parabiosis experiment (exchange of extracellular fluids) the salt-resistant animal rapidly develops chronic hypertension, provided a high-salt diet is fed to both rats.[29] The Dahl salt-sensitive rat is more sensitive than the salt-resistant rat to induction of hypertension by deoxycorticosterone (DOC) plus 7.3% NaCl, adrenal regeneration plus 1% NaCl or cortisone treatment of adrenalectomized rats (adrenal regeneration) drinking 0.85% saline. The salt-sensitive strain is also more prone to hypertension in experiments without excess salt but with renal artery constriction, the injection of cadmium or psychological stress.[28] Dahl salt-sensitive rats maintained on high-salt intake demonstrate a selective enhancement of vasoconstrictor responsiveness to sympathetic nerve stimulation. The fall in vascular resistance which results from sympathetic denervation is also enhanced in these animals. This seems to indicate that the induction of hypertension in Dahl salt-sensitive strains of rats might depend upon genetic transmission of hypersensitivity to both salt and stressful stimuli.[32]

Salt and DOCA-salt models

It is possible to create hypertension, at least in rats and primates, by feeding a high salt diet alone.[33,34] Another model has been used which involves the subcutaneous implantation of DOCA (200 mg/kg) impregnated in Silastic[(R)] strips (1 part DOCA to 2 parts Silastic). The rats used in these studies were unilaterally nephrectomized and given 1% NaCl and 0.2% KCl in the drinking water.[25,35]

Neurogenic hypertension and the central component

It is well known that atrial and cardiopulmonary receptors play a role in blood volume regulation, renal hemodynamics and renin release. All of these factors influence the development of hypertension. Continuous stimulation of the stellate ganglion or continuous stretching of the aorta in dogs has resulted in hypertension being maintained for as long as seven days.[36] Chronic electrical stimulation of the renal artery nerve or the splanchnic nerve, in conscious dogs, produces an increase in renal vascular resistance and results in hypertension. The hypertension is maintained as long as the stimulus is continued.[25] These results indicate some sort of spinal or CNS reflex loop. In dogs, rabbits and rats fed a low sodium diet renal denervation impairs the ability of the kidney to conserve sodium.[25] The delay in the development of hypertension produced by renal denervation in the Okamoto SHR and the DOCA-salt treated rat is due, in part, to an increase in sodium excretion. In the 1-kidney, 1-clip and 2-kidney, 1-clip Goldblatt rat model and in coarctation hypertension in the dog, the depressor effect of renal denervation is unrelated to changes in urinary sodium ion excretion or to plasma renin activity. The decrease in blood pressure in the later three models appears to be secondary to a decrease in peripheral sympathetic nervous activity.[35] It is well documented that efferent renal sympathetic nerves can effect control of the renal vasculature and influence renin release. They have been shown to regulate sodium and water excretion via arteriolar vasoconstriction.[25]

An interesting phenomena has been described concerning the central nervous system activity resulting from the arterial infusion of Angiotensin II. There is a greater pressor response from a carotid infusion than from infusion into the abdominal aorta. These studies seem to indicate that there are direct effects of Angiotensin II which induce neurally mediated vasoconstriction of the hindquarters, the renal and the mesenteric vascular beds.[37]

Following creation of bilateral lesions in the nucleus tractus solitari in dogs, renal sodium ion retention occurred during the first twenty-four hours after the lesions were made. This sodium ion retention was accompanied by hypertension.[25]

Kiline et al., using male Wistar rats, transected the aortic depressor nerve and dissected it and the cervical sympathetic nerves free from the vagus trunk. They were both then transected with a section of each removed. The carotid arteries were then stripped of all connective tissue. This resulted in a, so-called, "neurogenic" model of hypertension.[38] This type of selective aortic baroreceptor de-afferentation produces a persistent hypertension with increased neurogenic renal vasoconstrictor activity. No pressure diuresis or natriuresis is observed during the first week after these procedures are carried out.[25]

Bromocriptine, a Dopamine agonist which passes the blood-brain barrier, has been shown to reduce the hypertension in SHR. The effect, mediated through a central dopaminergic mechanism, seems to have limited peripheral components.[39]

This work also offers evidence of a centrally mediated mechanism in the genesis of hypertension in the SHR. It is well documented that vasopressin is essential for the production of DOC-salt hypertension in rats. Circulating levels of vasopressin are increased in SHR. Vasopressin secretion is greater in Dahl salt-sensitive rats on a high sodium diet than in similarly treated Dahl salt-resistant rats. Vasopressin appears to function as a pressor agent in some, but not all, rats with 2-kidneys, 1-clip hypertension and vasopressin is increased in nephrectomized-salt fed hypertensive rats.[5]

There has been considerable recent interest in the role of the endothelium in maintaining normal arterial pressures. Hypertension has been induced by the infusion of the endothelium-derived vasoconstrictor Endothelin 1[40] and by acute use of nitric oxide synthase inhibitors.[41,42]

Obesity-induced hypertension

A canine model of obesity-induced hypertension has been recently introduced. Adult dogs are fed a high-fat, high-calorie diet for 5-6 weeks. There is usually a 40-50% increase in body weight, compared to control groups of dogs which maintain the same weight while fed standard dog chow over the same period of time. The obese dogs typically demonstrate significant increases in aortic pressures and heart rates. Baroreceptor responses to nitroglycerine (hypotension) and phenylephrine (hypertension) are significantly enhanced in obese vs control dogs.[44] The natriuretic response to an acute sodium load is blunted in the obese hypertensive dog model.[45] Hyperinsulinemia has been hypothesized to be a factor in obesity-induced hypertension in dogs but insulin resistance and hyperinsulinemia alone cannot explain all the physiopathological mechanisms which are initiated in this apparently very complex model.[46,47,48]

References

1.   Davis, J.O.; The pathogenesis of chronic renovascular hypertension, *Circ. Res.*, 40:439-444, 1977
2.   Goldblatt, H.J., Lynch, J., Hanzel, R.F., Summerville, W.W.; Studies on experimental hypertension, *J. Exp. Med.*, 59:347-356, 1934
3.   Page, I.H., Helmer, O.M.; A crystalline pressor substance, angiotonin, resulting from the reaction between renin and renin activator, *Proc. Soc. Clin. Invest.*, 12:17, 1939
4.   Braun-Menendez, E., Fasciolo, J.C., Leloir, L.F., Munoz, J.M.; La substancia hipertensinora de la sangre del rinon es quemiado, *Ref. Soc. Argent. Biol. (Abs)*, 15:420, 1939
5.   Share, L., Crofton, J.T.; Contribution of vasopressin to hypertension, *Hypertension*, (5 Pt 2):III 85- III 92, 1982
6.   Greenberg, S.; Contractile properties of canine arteries and veins *in vitro* during the development of 2-kidney, one-clip Goldblatt hypertension, *Am. J. Physiol.*, 241:H525-H538, 1981
7.   Greenberg, S., McGowan, C., Gaida, M.; Vascular reactivity during the development of two-kidney, one-clip Goldblatt hypertension in conscious dogs, *Can. J. Physiol. Pharmacol.*, 60:1482-1492, 1982
8.   Greensberg, S., McGowan, C., Gaida, M.; Effect of an increased cardiac output on vascular responses to vasoactive agents in two-kidney, one-clip Goldblatt hypertension, *Clin. Exp. Hypertens.*, 4:1287-1302, 1982
9.   Russell, G.I., Bing, R.F., Swales, J.D., Thurston, H.; Hemodynamic changes induced by reversal of early and late renovascular hypertension, *Am. J. Physiol.*, 245(5 Pt 1):H734-H740, 1983

10. Ayobe, M.H., Tarazi, R.C.; reversal of changes in myocardial β-receptors and inotropic responsiveness with regression of cardiac hypertrophy in renal hypertensive rats (RHR), *Circ. Res.*, 54:125-134, 1984

11. Lai, F.M., Tanikella, T., Harzlinger, H., Goldstein, B., Chan, P.S., Cervoni, P.; Studies on the mechanism of the enhancement of the antihypertensive activity of captopril by a diuretic in spontaneously hypertensive rats, *Clin. Exp. Hypertens.*, 4:1001-1018, 1982

12. Share, L., Crofton, J.T., Lee-Kwon, W.J., Shade, R.E.; One-clip, one-kidney hypertension in rats with hereditary hypothalamic diabetes insipidus, *Clin. Exp. Hyperten.*, 4:1261-1270, 1982

13. Carretero, D.A., Kuk, P., Piwonska, S., Houle, J.A., Marin-Grez, M.; Role of the renin-angiotensin system in the pathogenesis of severe hypertension in rats, *Circ. Res.*, 29:645-663, 1971

14. Loffan, R.J., Goldberg, M.E., High, J.P., Schaeffer, T.R., Waugh, M.H., Rubin, B.; Antihypertensive activity in rats of SQ 14,225, an orally active inhibitor of angiotensin I-converting enzyme, *J. Pharmacol. Exp. Ther.*, 204:281-288, 1978

15. Fletcher, P.J., Korner, P.I., Angus, J.A., Oliver, J.R.; Changes in cardiac output and total peripheral resistance during the development of renal hypertension in the rabbit. Lack of conformity with the autoregulation theory, *Circ. Res.*, 39:633-639, 1976

16. Fletcher, P.J.; Baroreceptor heart rate reflex in rabbits after reversal of renal hypertension, *Am. J. Physiol.*, 246(2 Pt 2):H261-H266, 1984

17. Golt, G.R., Saxena, P.R.; Systemic and regional hemodynamic characteristics of bilateral cellophane perinephritis hypertension in conscious rabbits, *Clin. Exp. Hyperten.*, 5:885-901, 1983

18. Hollander, W., Madoff, J., Paddock, J., Kirkpatrick, B.; Aggravation of atherosclerosis by hypertension in a subhuman primate model with coarctation of the aorta, *Circ. Res. (Suppl II)*, 38:II-63- II-72, 1976

19. Dick, R., Johnson, P.J., Glick, G.; Deleterious effects of hypertension on the development of aortic and coronary atherosclerosis in stumptail macaques *(Macaca speciosa)* on an atherogenic diet, *Circ. Res.*, 35:472-482, 1974

20. Gross, D.R., unpublished observations

21. Sheggs, L.T., Kahn, J.R., Levine, M., Dorer, F.E., Lentz, K.E.; Chronic one-kidney hypertension in rabbits, *Circ. Res.*, 40:143-149, 1977

22. Galeno, T.M., Brody, M.J.; Hemodynamic responses to amygdaloid stimulation in spontaneously hypertensive rats, *Am. J. Physiol.*, 245:R281-R286, 1983

23. Lindheimer, M.D., Katz, A.I., Koeppen, B.M., Ordonez, N.G., Oparil, S.; Kidney function and sodium handling in the pregnant spontaneously hypertensive rat, *Hypertension*, 5:498-506, 1983

24. Evenwel, R.T., Kasbergen, C.M., Struyker-Boudier, H.H.; Central and regional hemodynamics and plasma volume distribution during the development of spontaneous hypertension in rats, *Clin. Exp. Hyperten.*, 5:1511-1536, 1983

25. Katholi, R.E.; Renal nerves in the pathogenesis of hypertension in experimental animals and humans, *Am. J. Physiol.*, 245:F1-F14, 1983

26. Sirtori, C.R., Lovati, M.R., Gianfranceschi, G., Farina, R., Franceschini, G.; Experimental studies on nutrition, hypertension, and cardiovascular diseases, *Prog. Biochem. Pharmacol.*, 19:192-207, 1983

27. Bianchi, G., Baer, P.G., Fox, U., Duzzi, L., Pagetti, D., Giovanetti, A.M.; Changes in renin, water balance, and sodium balance during development of high blood pressure in genetically hypertensive rats, *Circ. Res.*, 36/37 (Suppl.I):153-161, 1975

28. Dahl, L.K., Knudsen, K.D., Iwai, J.; Genetic influence of the kidney in hypertension-prone rats, *Circ. Res.*, 27(Suppl.II):II-277-II-281, 1970

29. Dahl, L.K., Kundsen, K.D., Heine, M. Leitl, G.; Effects of chronic excess salt ingestion. Genetic influence on the development of salt hypertension in parabiotic rats: evidence for a humoral factor, *J. Exp. Med.*, 126:687-693, 1967

30. Rapp, J.P.; Dahl salt-susceptible and salt-resistant rats, *Hypertension*, 4:73-76, 1982

31. Mohring, J., Petri, M., Szokol, M., Haack, D., Mohring, B.; Effects of saline drinking on malignant course of renal hypertension in rats, *Am. J. Physiol.*, 230:849-857, 1976

32. Bunag, R.D., Butterfield, J., Sasaki, S.; Hypothalamic pressor responses and salt-induced hypertension in Dahl rats, *Hypertension*, 5:460-467, 1983

33. Cherchovich, G.M., Capek, K., Jefremona, Z., Pohlova, I., Jelinek, J.; High salt intake and blood pressure in lower primates *(Papio hamadryas)*, *J. Appl. Physiol.*, 40:601-604, 1976

34.   Meneely, G.R., Tucker, R.G., Dorby, W.J., Auerback, S.H.; Chronic sodium chloride toxicity in the albino rat. II. Occurrence of hypertension and of a syndrome of oedema and renal failure, *J. Exp. Med.*, 98:71-80, 1955

35.   Winternitz, S.R., Oparil, S.; Importance of the renal nerves in the pathogenesis of experimental hypertension, *Hypertension*, 4(5 Pt 2):108-114, 1982

36.   Tarazi, R.C., Fouad, F.M., Ferrario, C.M.; Can the heart initiate some forms of hypertension?, *Fed. Proc.*, 42:2691-2697, 1983

37.   Lappe, R.W., Brody, M.J.; Mechanisms of the central pressor action of angiotensin II in conscious rats, *Am. J. Physiol.*, 246:R56-R62, 1984

38.   Kline, R.L. Patel, K.P., Ciriello, J., Mercer, P.F.; Effect of renal denervation on arterial pressure in rats with aortic nerve transection, *Hypertension*, 5:468-475, 1983

39.   Nagohama, S., Chen, Y.-F., Oparil, S.; Mechanism of the depressor effect of bromocriptine in the spontaneously hypertensive rat, *J. Pharmacol. Exp. Ther.*, 228:370-375, 1984

40.   Stacy, D.L., Scott, J.W., Granger, J.P.; Control of renal function during intrarenal infusion of endothelin, *Am. J. Physiol.*, 258:F1232-F1236, 1990

41.   Manning, R.D. Jr., Hu, L., Mizelle, H.L., Granger, J.P.; Role of nitric oxide in long-term angiotensin II-induced renal vasoconstriction, *Hypertension*, 21:949-955, 1993

42.   Toda, N., Kitamura, Y., Okamura, T.; Neural mechanism of hypertension by nitric oxide synthase inhibitor in dogs, *Hypertension*, 21:3-8, 1993

43.   Kiprov, D.; Experimental models of hypertension, *Cor Vasa*, 22:116-128, 1980

44.   Wehberg, K.E., West, D.B., Kieswetter, C., Granger, J.P.; Baroreflex sensitivity in the canine model of obesity-induced hypertension, *Am. J. Physiol.*, 259:R981-R985, 1990

45.   West, D.B., Wehberg, K.E., Kieswetter, K., Granger, J.P.; Blunted natriuretic response to an acute sodium load in obese hypertensive dogs, *Hypertension*, 19:I-96-I-100, 1992

46.   Brands, M.W., Hall, J.E.; Insulin resistance, hyperinsulinemia, and obesity-associated hypertension, *J. Am. Soc. Nephrol.*, 3:1064-1077, 1992

47.   Hall, J.E., Brands, M.W., Hildebrandt, D.A., Mizelle, H.L.; Obesity-associated hypertension. Hyperinsulinemia and renal mechanisms, *Hypertension*, 19(Suppl.I):I-45-I55, 1992

48.   Hall, J.E., Brands, M.W., Mizelle, H.L., Gaillard, C.A., Hildebrandt, D.A.; Chronic intrarenal hyperinsulinemia does not cause hypertension, *Am. J. Physiol.*, 260:F663-F669, 1991

Index

Developments in Cardiovascular Medicine

1. Ch.T. Lancée (ed.): *Echocardiology.* 1979   ISBN 90-247-2209-8
2. J. Baan, A.C. Arntzenius and E.L. Yellin (eds.): *Cardiac Dynamics.* 1980
                                                                ISBN 90-247-2212-8
3. H.J.Th. Thalen and C.C. Meere (eds.): *Fundamentals of Cardiac Pacing.* 1979
                                                                ISBN 90-247-2245-4
4. H.E. Kulbertus and H.J.J. Wellens (eds.): *Sudden Death.* 1980   ISBN 90-247-2290-X
5. L.S. Dreifus and A.N. Brest (eds.): *Clinical Applications of Cardiovascular Drugs.*
   1980   ISBN 90-247-2295-0
6. M.P. Spencer and J.M. Reid: *Cerebrovascular Evaluation with Doppler Ultrasound.*
   With contributions by E.C. Brockenbrough, R.S. Reneman, G.I. Thomas and D.L.
   Davis. 1981   ISBN 90-247-2384-1
7. D.P. Zipes, J.C. Bailey and V. Elharrar (eds.): *The Slow Inward Current and Cardiac
   Arrhythmias.* 1980   ISBN 90-247-2380-9
8. H. Kesteloot and J.V. Joossens (eds.): *Epidemiology of Arterial Blood Pressure.* 1980
                                                                ISBN 90-247-2386-8
9. F.J.Th. Wackers (ed.): *Thallium-201 and Technetium-99m-Pyrophosphate. Myocardial Imaging in the Coronary Care Unit.* 1980   ISBN 90-247-2396-5
10. A. Maseri, C. Marchesi, S. Chierchia and M.G. Trivella (eds.): *Coronary Care Units.*
    Proceedings of a European Seminar (1978). 1981   ISBN 90-247-2456-2
11. J. Morganroth, E.N. Moore, L.S. Dreifus and E.L. Michelson (eds.): *The Evaluation of
    New Antiarrhythmic Drugs.* Proceedings of the First Symposium on New Drugs and
    Devices, held in Philadelphia, Pa., U.S.A. (1980). 1981   ISBN 90-247-2474-0
12. P. Alboni: *Intraventricular Conduction Disturbances.* 1981   ISBN 90-247-2483-X
13. H. Rijsterborgh (ed.): *Echocardiology.* 1981   ISBN 90-247-2491-0
14. G.S. Wagner (ed.): *Myocardial Infarction.* Measurement and Intervention. 1982
                                                                ISBN 90-247-2513-5
15. R.S. Meltzer and J. Roelandt (eds.): *Contrast Echocardiography.* 1982
                                                                ISBN 90-247-2531-3
16. A. Amery, R. Fagard, P. Lijnen and J. Staessen (eds.): *Hypertensive Cardiovascular
    Disease.* Pathophysiology and Treatment. 1982   IBSN 90-247-2534-8
17. L.N. Bouman and H.J. Jongsma (eds.): *Cardiac Rate and Rhythm.* Physiological,
    Morphological and Developmental Aspects. 1982   ISBN 90-247-2626-3
18. J. Morganroth and E.N. Moore (eds.): *The Evaluation of Beta Blocker and Calcium
    Antagonist Drugs.* Proceedings of the 2nd Symposium on New Drugs and Devices,
    held in Philadelphia, Pa., U.S.A. (1981). 1982   ISBN 90-247-2642-5
19. M.B. Rosenbaum and M.V. Elizari (eds.): *Frontiers of Cardiac Electrophysiology.*
    1983   ISBN 90-247-2663-8
20. J. Roelandt and P.G. Hugenholtz (eds.): *Long-term Ambulatory Electrocardiography.*
    1982   ISBN 90-247-2664-6
21. A.A.J. Adgey (ed.): *Acute Phase of Ischemic Heart Disease and Myocardial Infarc-
    tion.* 1982   ISBN 90-247-2675-1
22. P. Hanrath, W. Bleifeld and J. Souquet (eds.): *Cardiovascular Diagnosis by Ultra-
    sound.* Transesophageal, Computerized, Contrast, Doppler Echocardiography. 1982
                                                                ISBN 90-247-2692-1
23. J. Roelandt (ed.): *The Practice of M-Mode and Two-dimensional Echocardiography.*
    1983   ISBN 90-247-2745-6
24. J. Meyer, P. Schweizer and R. Erbel (eds.): *Advances in Noninvasive Cardiology.*
    Ultrasound, Computed Tomography, Radioisotopes, Digital Angiography. 1983
                                                                ISBN 0-89838-576-8
25. J. Morganroth and E.N. Moore (eds.): *Sudden Cardiac Death and Congestive Heart
    Failure.* Diagnosis and Treatment. Proceedings of the 3rd Symposium on New Drugs
    and Devices, held in Philadelphia, Pa., U.S.A. (1982). 1983   ISBN 0-89838-580-6
26. H.M. Perry Jr. (ed.): *Lifelong Management of Hypertension.* 1983
                                                                ISBN 0-89838-582-2
27. E.A. Jaffe (ed.): *Biology of Endothelial Cells.* 1984   ISBN 0-89838-587-3

Developments in Cardiovascular Medicine

Developments in Cardiovascular Medicine

96. I. Cikes (ed.): *Echocardiography in Cardiac Interventions.* 1989
    ISBN 0-7923-0088-2
97. E. Rapaport (ed.): *Early Interventions in Acute Myocardial Infarction.* 1989
    ISBN 0-7923-0175-7
98. M.E. Safar and F. Fouad-Tarazi (eds.): *The Heart in Hypertension.* A Tribute to Robert C. Tarazi (1925-1986). 1989   ISBN 0-7923-0197-8
99. S. Meerbaum and R. Meltzer (eds.): *Myocardial Contrast Two-dimensional Echocardiography.* 1989   ISBN 0-7923-0205-2
100. J. Morganroth and E.N. Moore (eds.): *Risk/Benefit Analysis for the Use and Approval of Thrombolytic, Antiarrhythmic, and Hypolipidemic Agents.* Proceedings of the 9th Annual Symposium on New Drugs and Devices (1988). 1989   ISBN 0-7923-0294-X
101. P.W. Serruys, R. Simon and K.J. Beatt (eds.): *PTCA - An Investigational Tool and a Non-operative Treatment of Acute Ischemia.* 1990   ISBN 0-7923-0346-6
102. I.S. Anand, P.I. Wahi and N.S. Dhalla (eds.): *Pathophysiology and Pharmacology of Heart Disease.* 1989   ISBN 0-7923-0367-9
103. G.S. Abela (ed.): *Lasers in Cardiovascular Medicine and Surgery.* Fundamentals and Technique. 1990   ISBN 0-7923-0440-3
104. H.M. Piper (ed.): *Pathophysiology of Severe Ischemic Myocardial Injury.* 1990
    ISBN 0-7923-0459-4
105. S.M. Teague (ed.): *Stress Doppler Echocardiography.* 1990   ISBN 0-7923-0499-3
106. P.R. Saxena, D.I. Wallis, W. Wouters and P. Bevan (eds.): *Cardiovascular Pharmacology of 5-Hydroxytryptamine.* Prospective Therapeutic Applications. 1990
    ISBN 0-7923-0502-7
107. A.P. Shepherd and P.Å. Öberg (eds.): *Laser-Doppler Blood Flowmetry.* 1990
    ISBN 0-7923-0508-6
108. J. Soler-Soler, G. Permanyer-Miralda and J. Sagristà-Sauleda (eds.): *Pericardial Disease.* New Insights and Old Dilemmas. 1990   ISBN 0-7923-0510-8
109. J.P.M. Hamer: *Practical Echocardiography in the Adult.* With Doppler and Color-Doppler Flow Imaging. 1990   ISBN 0-7923-0670-8
110. A. Bayés de Luna, P. Brugada, J. Cosin Aguilar and F. Navarro Lopez (eds.): *Sudden Cardiac Death.* 1991   ISBN 0-7923-0716-X
111. E. Andries and R. Stroobandt (eds.): *Hemodynamics in Daily Practice.* 1991
    ISBN 0-7923-0725-9
112. J. Morganroth and E.N. Moore (eds.): *Use and Approval of Antihypertensive Agents and Surrogate Endpoints for the Approval of Drugs affecting Antiarrhythmic Heart Failure and Hypolipidemia.* Proceedings of the 10th Annual Symposium on New Drugs and Devices (1989). 1990   ISBN 0-7923-0756-9
113. S. Iliceto, P. Rizzon and J.R.T.C. Roelandt (eds.): *Ultrasound in Coronary Artery Disease.* Present Role and Future Perspectives. 1990   ISBN 0-7923-0784-4
114. J.V. Chapman and G.R. Sutherland (eds.): *The Noninvasive Evaluation of Hemodynamics in Congenital Heart Disease.* Doppler Ultrasound Applications in the Adult and Pediatric Patient with Congenital Heart Disease. 1990
    ISBN 0-7923-0836-0
115. G.T. Meester and F. Pinciroli (eds.): *Databases for Cardiology.* 1991
    ISBN 0-7923-0886-7
116. B. Korecky and N.S. Dhalla (eds.): *Subcellular Basis of Contractile Failure.* 1990
    ISBN 0-7923-0890-5
117. J.H.C. Reiber and P.W. Serruys (eds.): *Quantitative Coronary Arteriography.* 1991
    ISBN 0-7923-0913-8
118. E. van der Wall and A. de Roos (eds.): *Magnetic Resonance Imaging in Coronary Artery Disease.* 1991   ISBN 0-7923-0940-5
119. V. Hombach, M. Kochs and A.J. Camm (eds.): *Interventional Techniques in Cardiovascular Medicine.* 1991   ISBN 0-7923-0956-1
120. R. Vos: *Drugs Looking for Diseases.* Innovative Drug Research and the Development of the Beta Blockers and the Calcium Antagonists. 1991   ISBN 0-7923-0968-5

Developments in Cardiovascular Medicine

Developments in Cardiovascular Medicine

Previous volumes are still available

KLUWER ACADEMIC PUBLISHERS – DORDRECHT / BOSTON / LONDON